Rhinology: Evolution of Science and Surgery

Guest Editors

RODNEY J. SCHLOSSER, MD
RICHARD J. HARVEY, MD

OTOLARYNGOLOGIC CLINICS OF NORTH AMERICA

www.oto.theclinics.com

June 2010 • Volume 43 • Number 3

SAUNDERS an imprint of ELSEVIER, Inc.

W.B. SAUNDERS COMPANY

A Division of Elsevier Inc.

1600 John F. Kennedy Boulevard • Suite 1800 • Philadelphia, Pennsylvania 19103-2899

http://www.theclinics.com

OTOLARYNGOLOGIC CLINICS OF NORTH AMERICA Volume 43, Number 3
June 2010 ISSN 0030-6665, ISBN-13: 978-1-4377-2406-6

Editor: Joanne Husovski

Otolaryngologic Clinics of North America (ISSN 0030-6665) is published bimonthly by Elsevier, Inc., 360 Park Avenue South, New York, NY 10010-1710. Months of issue are February, April, June, August, October, and December. Business and Editorial Offices: 1600 John F. Kennedy Blvd., Suite 1800, Philadelphia, PA 19103-2899. Customer Service Office: 6277 Sea Harbor Drive, Orlando, FL 32887-4800. Periodicals postage paid at New York, NY and additional mailing offices. Subscription prices is $290.00 per year (US individuals), $527.00 per year (US institutions), $142.00 per year (US student/resident), $382.00 per year (Canadian individuals), $662.00 per year (Canadian institutions), $429.00 per year (international individuals), $662.00 per year (international institutions), $219.00 per year (international & Canadian student/resident). Foreign air speed delivery is included in all *Clinics*' subscription prices. All prices are subject to change without notice. **POSTMASTER:** Send address changes to *Otolaryngologic Clinics of North America*, Elsevier Health Sciences Division, Subscription Customer Service, 3251 Riverport Lane, Maryland Heights, MO 63043. **Telephone: 1-800-654-2452 (U.S. and Canada); 314-447-8871 (outside U.S. and Canada). Fax: 314-447-8029. E-mail: journalscustomerservice-usa@elsevier.com (for print support); journalsonlinesupport-usa@elsevier.com (for online support).**

Reprints. For copies of 100 or more of articles in this publication, please contact the Commercial Reprints Department, Elsevier Inc., 360 Park Avenue South, New York, NY 10010-1710. Tel.: 212-633-3812; Fax: 212-462-1935; E-mail: reprints@elsevier.com.

Otolaryngologic Clinics of North America is also published in Spanish by McGraw-Hill Interamericana Editores S.A., P.O. Box 5-237, 06500 Mexico D.F., Mexico.

Otolaryngologic Clinics of North America is covered in *MEDLINE/PubMed (Index Medicus), Current Contents/Clinical Medicine, Excerpta Medica, BIOSIS, Science Citation Index,* and *ISI/BIOMED.*

Printed and bound by CPI Group (UK) Ltd, Croydon, CR0 4YY

Transferred to Digital Print 2011

Contributors

GUEST EDITORS

RODNEY J. SCHLOSSER, MD
Professor and Director of Rhinology and Sinus Surgery, Department of Otolaryngology–Head and Neck Surgery, Medical University of South Carolina, Charleston, South Carolina

RICHARD J. HARVEY, MD
Clinical Associate Professor, Rhinology and Skull Base Surgery, Department of Otolaryngology/Skull Base Surgery, St Vincent's Hospital, Darlinghurst, Sydney, New South Wales, Australia

AUTHORS

BENJAMIN S. BLEIER, MD
Clinical Instructor, Division of Rhinology, Department of Otolaryngology–Head and Neck Surgery, Medical University of South Carolina, Charleston, South Carolina

ALEXANDER G. CHIU, MD
Associate Professor, Division of Rhinology, Department of Otorhinolaryngology–Head and Neck Surgery, University of Pennsylvania, Philadelphia, Pennsylvania

NOAM A. COHEN, MD, PhD
Assistant Professor, Division of Rhinology, Department of Otorhinolaryngology–Head and Neck Surgery, Hospital of the University of Pennsylvania, Philadelphia, Pennsylvania

MICHAEL A. DEMARCANTONIO, MD
Department of Otolaryngology–Head and Neck Surgery, Eastern Virginia Medical School, Norfolk, Virginia

RICHARD DOUGLAS, FRACS
Rhinologist, Department of Otorhinolaryngology–Head and Neck Surgery, North Shore Hospital, North Shore City; Auckland Hospital, Auckland, New Zealand

RICHARD M. GALLAGHER, MD
Rhinology and Skull Base, Department of Otolaryngology/Skull Base Surgery, St Vincent's Hospital, Darlinghurst, Sydney, New South Wales, Australia

DAVID A. GUDIS, MD
Department of Otorhinolaryngology–Head and Neck Surgery, University of Pennsylvania, Philadelphia, Pennsylvania

JOSEPH K. HAN, MD, FACS
Associate Professor; Director of Rhinology and Endoscopic Sinus and Skull Base Surgery; Director of Allergy Division, Department of Otolaryngology–Head and Neck Surgery, Eastern Virginia Medical School, Norfolk, Virginia

RICHARD J. HARVEY, MD
Clinical Associate Professor, Rhinology and Skull Base Surgery, Department
of Otolaryngology/Skull Base Surgery, St Vincent's Hospital, Darlinghurst, Sydney,
New South Wales, Australia

ELIZABETH K. HODDESON, MD
Department of Otolaryngology–Head and Neck Surgery, Emory University,
Atlanta, Georgia

JEAN SILVAIN LACROIX, MD, PhD
Professor of Rhinology-Olfactology, Rhinology-Olfaction Unit, Department
of Otorhinolaryngology–Head and Neck Surgery, Geneva University Hospital,
Geneva, Switzerland

JOHN M. LEE, MD, FRCSC
Lecturer, Department of Otolaryngology–Head and Neck Surgery, University of Toronto,
St Michael's Hospital, Toronto, Ontario, Canada

BRADLEY F. MARPLE, MD
Department of Otolaryngology–Head and Neck Surgery, University of Texas
Southwestern Medical Center, Dallas, Texas

JOÃO FLÁVIO NOGUEIRA, MD
ENT Institute of Fortaleza, Fortaleza, Brazil

ENG H. OOI, MBBS, PhD, FRACS
Rhinology Fellow, Department of Otolaryngology–Head and Neck Surgery, University
of Toronto, Mount Sinai Hospital, Toronto, Ontario, Canada

RICHARD R. ORLANDI, MD
Division of Otolaryngology–Head and Neck Surgery, University of Utah,
Salt Lake City, Utah

JAMES N. PALMER, MD
Department of Otorhinolaryngology–Head and Neck Surgery, Hospital of the University
of Pennsylvania, Philadelphia, Pennsylvania

ELEANOR PRATT, BS, BA
Department of Otolaryngology and Skull Base Surgery, St Vincent's Hospital,
Darlinghurst, Sydney; School of Biotechnology and Biomolecular Sciences,
University of New South Wales, Kensington, New South Wales, Australia

ALKIS J. PSALTIS, MBBS(Hons), PhD
Department of Otolaryngology Head and Neck Surgery, Flinders University; Department
of Otolaryngology Head and Neck Surgery, University of Adelaide, The Queen Elizabeth
Hospital, Woodville South, South Australia, Australia

VIJAY RAMAKRISHNAN, MD
Department of Otorhinolaryngology–Head and Neck Surgery, Hospital of the University of
Pennsylvania, Philadelphia, Pennsylvania

RAYMOND SACKS, MD
Associate Professor; Director of Rhinology and Skull Base Surgery, Department
of Otolaryngology–Head and Neck Surgery, Concord General Hospital, Concord,
Sydney, New South Wales, Australia

RODNEY J. SCHLOSSER, MD
Professor and Director of Rhinology and Sinus Surgery, Department
of Otolaryngology–Head and Neck Surgery, Medical University of South Carolina,
Charleston, South Carolina

TIMOTHY L. SMITH, MD, MPH
Division of Rhinology and Sinus Surgery, Department of Otolaryngology–Head and Neck
Surgery, Oregon Sinus Center, Oregon Health and Science University, Portland, Oregon

ZACHARY M. SOLER, MD
Division of Rhinology and Sinus Surgery, Department of Otolaryngology–Head and Neck
Surgery, Oregon Sinus Center, Oregon Health and Science University, Portland, Oregon

ALDO STAMM, MD, PhD
Director, São Paulo ENT Center – Hospital Professor Edmundo Vasconcelos,
São Paulo, Brazil

JAMES A. STANKIEWICZ, MD
Professor and Chairman, Department of Otolaryngology–Head and Neck Surgery, Loyola
University Medical Center, Maywood, Illinois

NICHOLAS W. STOW, FRACS
Rhinology Fellow, Department of Otorhinolaryngology–Head and Neck Surgery,
North Shore Hospital; Auckland Hospital, Auckland, New Zealand

JEFFREY D. SUH, MD
Department of Otorhinolaryngology–Head and Neck Surgery, Hospital of the University of
Pennsylvania, Philadelphia, Pennsylvania

PONGSAKORN TANTILIPIKORN, MD, FRCOT
Assistant Professor, Division of Rhinology and Allergy, Department of Otolaryngology,
Faculty of Medicine, Siriraj Hospital, Mahidol University, Thailand

EDUARDO VELLUTINI, MD
DFV Neuro, São Paulo, Brazil

FRANK W. VIRGIN, MD
PGY-4, Division of Otolaryngology–Head and Neck Surgery, Department of Surgery,
University of Alabama at Birmingham, Birmingham, Alabama

KEVIN C. WELCH, MD
Assistant Professor, Department of Otolaryngology–Head and Neck Surgery, Loyola
University Medical Center, Maywood, Illinois

SARAH K. WISE, MD
Department of Otolaryngology–Head and Neck Surgery, Emory University, Atlanta,
Georgia

IAN J. WITTERICK, MD, MSc, FRCSC
Professor, Department of Otolaryngology–Head and Neck Surgery, University of Toronto,
Mount Sinai Hospital, Toronto, Ontario, Canada

BRADFORD A. WOODWORTH, MD
Assistant Professor and James Johnston Hicks Endowed Chair of Otolaryngology, Division of Otolaryngology–Head and Neck Surgery, Department of Surgery, University of Alabama at Birmingham; Associate Scientist, Gregory Fleming James Cystic Fibrosis Research Center, University of Alabama at Birmingham, Birmingham, Alabama

PETER-JOHN WORMALD, MD, FRACS, FACS (SA)
Department of Otolaryngology–Head and Neck Surgery, Flinders University; Department of Otolaryngology–Head and Neck Surgery, University of Adelaide, The Queen Elizabeth Hospital, Woodville South, South Australia, Australia

ADVISORS TO OTOLARYNGOLOGIC CLINICS 2010:

SAMUEL BECKER, MD
Becker Nose and Sinus Center; Voorhees, New Jersey

DAVID HAYNES, MD
Vanderbilt University; Nashville, Tennessee

BRIAN KAPLAN, MD
Ear, Nose, and Throat Associates; Baltimore, Maryland

JOHN KROUSE, MD, PhD
Temple University Medicine; Philadelphia, Pennsylvania

ANIL KUMAR LALWANI, MD
New York University Langone Medical Center; New York, New York

ARLEN MEYERS, MD, MBA
University of Colorado; Denver, Colorado

MATTHEW RYAN, MD
University of Texas Southwestern Medical Center, Dallas, Texas

RALPH TUFANO, MD
Johns Hopkins Medicine; Baltimore, Maryland

Contents

Cilia are complex and powerful cellular structures that serve a multitude of functions across many types of organisms. In humans, one of the most critical roles of cilia is defense of the airway. The respiratory epithelium is lined with cilia that normally carry out an integrated and coordinated mechanism called mucociliary clearance. Mucociliary clearance, the process by which cilia transport the viscous mucus blanket of the upper airway to the gastrointestinal tract, is the primary means by which the upper airway clears itself of pathogens, allergens, debris, and toxins. The complex structure and regulatory mechanisms that dictate the form and function of normal cilia are not entirely understood, but it is clear that ciliary dysfunction results in impaired respiratory defense. Ciliary dysfunction may be primary, the result of genetic mutations resulting in abnormal cilia structure, or secondary, the result of environmental, infectious or inflammatory stimuli that disrupt normal motility or coordination.

Innate immunity is an exciting area of research in rhinology because emerging evidence suggests that abnormal local immune responses, rather than pathogen-specific adaptive immunity, may play a more important role in the pathogenesis of chronic rhinosinusitis (CRS). This article reviews important recent research regarding the innate immune system and CRS, with particular focus on the role of pattern recognition receptors, antimicrobial peptides and biofilms, epithelial ciliary function, cystic fibrosis, and cigarette smoking, and on areas for future research and therapy.

Superantigens (SAgs) are derived from diverse sources, including bacteria, viruses, and human hepatic tissue. SAgs initially cause lymphocyte activation but then result in clonal deletion and anergy, leading to immune tolerance. They can also act as superallergens by stimulating a broad spectrum of mast cells and basophils in patients with allergic conditions. The newly described staphylococcal SAg-like proteins subvert innate immune function by several mechanisms, which are distinct from SAgs' effects on lymphocytes and other acquired immune processes. There is mounting evidence to suggest that SAgs play a role in the pathophysiology of inflammatory airway disease. The pathophysiologic role of SAg-like proteins awaits clarification.

Traditional descriptions of type I hypersensitivity and its manifestations center on systemic immunoglobulin E (IgE)-mediated reactions to inciting antigens. Hence, many current diagnostic and therapeutic measures are based on systemic skin testing for allergy, systemic pharmacotherapy, and immunotherapy. Recent developments in rhinology and pulmonology, particularly in defining the phenomenon of local IgE production in various airway inflammatory conditions, have an impact on both medical and surgical diagnosis and management of these conditions. This review includes a discussion of allergy as a systemic disease, current systemic diagnostic and management strategies for allergy, and local IgE presence and synthesis in the upper and lower airways.

Bacterial biofilms are 3-dimensional aggregates of bacteria that have been shown to play a major role in many chronic infections. Evidence is growing that bacterial biofilms may play a role in certain cases of recalcitrant chronic sinusitis that do not respond to traditional medical and surgical therapies. Novel therapies may have clinical applications to prevent and destabilize biofilms. Future research will determine if topical antimicrobials, surfactants, and other adjuvant therapies can be used to treat biofilm-associated chronic rhinosinusitis.

Fungus has been cited as an etiologic factor (the etiologic factor?) in chronic rhinosinusitis (CRS), and a vigorous debate has ensued. Initial reports of in vitro observations promoted fungus as a potential origin of CRS, yet subsequent clinical trials of topical and systemic antifungal treatments have failed to demonstrate meaningful efficacy. More recent laboratory work has cast significant doubt on the universality of the fungal hypothesis by failing to replicate one of its basic science underpinnings. Combined with clinical data about antifungal therapy's ineffectiveness, these findings appear to tip the scales against fungus as the universal etiology of CRS.

Intranasal drug delivery is a rapidly growing field that offers the potential for enhanced treatment of local and systemic disease. Novel preclinical screening tools such as in vitro assays and 3-dimensional imaging are currently being used to improve drug design and delivery. In addition, new evidence has emerged underlining the importance of surgical marsupialization of the sinuses to allow for improved topical delivery. Although multiple barriers to administration and absorption exist, implantable therapeutics using new classes of drug-eluting polymers allow for prolonged, site-specific drug delivery and hold great promise in overcoming these obstacles.

Systemic Therapies in Managing Sinonasal Inflammation   551

Michael A. DeMarcantonio and Joseph K. Han

Chronic rhinosinusitis (CRS) is a condition characterized by persistent inflammation due to intrinsic mucosal hypersensitivity or persistent infection. Proper medical treatment with antibiotic, leukotriene modifiers, oral corticosteroids, or even aspirin desensitization for the sinus inflammation can prevent the need for surgical intervention. The key to delineating the specific medical application is to determine the cause of the sinus mucosa dysfunction and its specific inflammatory pathway. Such targeted antiinflammatory medical therapy will lead to improved efficacy in the management of CRS. Even if surgical intervention is required, postoperative medical treatment is essential to minimizing the intrinsic mucosal inflammation and therefore preventing revision endoscopic procedures.

Application of Minimally Invasive Endoscopic Sinus Surgery Techniques   565

Kevin C. Welch and James A. Stankiewicz

New instrumentation and techniques for endoscopic sinus surgery (ESS) are presently available that offer the potential of successfully treating recalcitrant chronic rhinosinusitis is a manner that minimizes operative times, sinus-mucosal trauma, and operative costs. This content describes current ESS techniques and quality-of-life outcomes, techniques for transnasal and transantral balloon catheter dilatation, and their outcomes. The authors address the changing medical climate that may open new avenues for surgeons to treat patients.

Role of Maximal Endoscopic Sinus Surgery Techniques in Chronic Rhinosinusitis   579

John M. Lee and Alexander G. Chiu

There remains a continued debate regarding the extent of endoscopic sinus surgery (ESS) required for patients with chronic rhinosinusitis (CRS). By examining anatomic, etiologic, and postoperative factors that may lead to recalcitrant CRS, this article aims to highlight some of the reasons for performing maximal techniques in ESS. This concept is further expanded in various surgical maneuvers including wide maxillary antrostomy, extended frontal sinus procedures, and intraoperative computed tomography–guided ESS.

Surgical Salvage for the Non-Functioning Sinus   591

Rodney J. Schlosser

The non-functioning or dysfunctional sinus is completely isolated from the remainder of the nasal cavity with no hope of normal ventilation despite the most aggressive medical therapy. Most often these sinuses are the result of mucosal stripping/removal during prior radical surgeries. The reason for these radical operations include treatment of neoplasm, but most often is for revision of inflammatory disease when prior procedures have not been successful at restoring ventilation and maintaining patent ostia. When faced with a dysfunctional sinus, rhinologists typically have two choices: repeat the radical obliterative procedure or attempt to restore function and ventilation by reestablishing a drainage pathway into the nasal cavity. This latter option seems to represent the best long-term chance for surgical success in these difficult cases, with repeat ablative procedures as a last resort.

Most patients with chronic rhinosinusitis seek medical treatment when the burden of symptoms negatively impacts their quality of life. The degree to which quality of life improves after sinus surgery is a critical indicator of surgical success. This article reviews quality of life outcomes after functional endoscopic sinus surgery, including relevant clinical factors, weaknesses in the current literature, and future research directions.

The evolution of endoscopic sinus surgery has led to a paradigm shift in the management of sinonasal and anterior skull base tumors in the past decade. Endoscopic resection is considered by many institutions to be the gold standard approach even for extensive pathology. Endoscopic tumor surgery should not imply less surgery but rather an alternative to external operations providing the same access and enabling equivalent or superior visualization for resection of tumors. It also avoids much of the potentially significant morbidity associated with external operations. Successful endoscopic tumor resection requires experience, an understanding of tumor behavior, and the development of a unique skill set. Tumor removal is often performed inside-out. Regions such as the anterolateral maxilla and frontal sinus require special access. Orientation of the surgeon is different to that of simple inflammatory disease. A structured approach to vascular control is important to ensure a workable surgical field. The final cavity and reconstruction need to be fashioned to ensure that reasonable sinonasal physiology and function are retained, including the lacrimal apparatus. The endoscopic cavity created after extensive surgery requires different care compared with the mucosal-preserving techniques of inflammatory disease. This article describes these key methodological differences that enable extended endoscopic surgery of the sinonasal tract and anterior skull base.

Endoscopic techniques have influenced almost all of the surgical specialties. From open procedures to minimally invasive approaches, the endoscope and its ability to reach areas within the human body has gained popularity among specialists, creating a revolution in some fields. Two of the fields in which endoscopes provided a true revolution are otolaryngology and neuro-surgery. The authors discuss some important factors for the evolution of endoscopic skull base surgery and expanded endonasal approaches, highlighting historical landmarks but also addressing the current concepts, complications, and the future of this promising field for clinical research and surgical techniques and technology.

THE CLINICS ARE NOW AVAILABLE ONLINE!

Access your subscription at:
www.theclinics.com

Preface

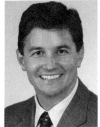 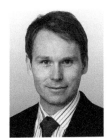

Rodney J. Schlosser, MD   Richard J. Harvey, MD
Guest Editors

Since the 1980s, the subspecialty of rhinology has arguably evolved faster than any other discipline within otolaryngology. Just 25 years ago, medical therapy for rhinosinusitis focused almost exclusively on antibiotics. Failure resulted in the removal of diseased mucosa via nonphysiologic sinus surgery performed through a variety of external incisions with headlights and noncutting hand instruments. The advent of the endoscope and video and digital image recording fueled the concept of functional sinus surgery, with an emphasis on mucociliary clearance and mucosal preservation. International collaborations and dissemination of scientific observation among researchers have resulted in a greater appreciation for the multiple factors that play a role in the heterogeneous disorder of rhinosinusitis that affects many of our patients. Our pathophysiologic understanding of chronic sinonasal conditions has progressed from simple models of obstruction and infection to a more comprehensive understanding of mucosal health, inflammation, and a concept of a unified airway. It is these innovations in surgical and scientific knowledge that have spawned greater clinical insight and allowed the development of rhinology into a recognized and respected subspecialty.

As technological advancements and novel surgical instruments were developed for use in inflammatory disorders, rhinologists began to perform complex procedures endoscopically, now encompassing the entire ventral skull base and paranasal sinuses. The evolution has yielded greater collaboration with other specialties, notably ophthalmologists and neurosurgeons. Subsequent multidisciplinary teams have defined the nascent field of neurorhinology, which is still in its infancy and will undoubtedly continue to evolve.

This issue brings together eight surgical and eight medical subjects from innovative researchers in the field. These authors represent a generation of dedicated rhinologists who build upon the contribution to the field by pioneers in rhinology. They have provided their expertise and insight into the application of recent advances in current clinical practice and for future research. The goal of this issue is to highlight key areas within rhinology that have rapidly developed during the past two decades.

Otolaryngol Clin N Am 43 (2010) xiii–xiv
doi:10.1016/j.otc.2010.02.019

As always, we also wish to acknowledge our spouses and families whose support has been an integral part of our careers.

Rodney J. Schlosser, MD
Department of Otolaryngology-Head and Neck Surgery
Medical University of South Carolina
135 Rutledge Avenue, Suite 1130
Charleston, SC 29425, USA

Richard J. Harvey, MD
Department of Otolaryngology/Skull Base Surgery
St Vincent's Hospital
354 Victoria Street, Darlinghurst
Sydney, NSW 2010, Australia

E-mail addresses:
schlossr@musc.edu (R.J. Schlosser)
rharvey@sydneyentclinic.com (R.J. Harvey)

Cilia Dysfunction

David A. Gudis, MD[a], Noam A. Cohen, MD, PhD[a,b],*

KEYWORDS

- Mucus • Mucociliary clearance • Ciliary beat frequency
- Chronic rhinosinusitis • Primary ciliary dyskinesia

Cilia are a ubiquitous organelle found on diverse cell types including sperm cells of vertebrates and some invertebrates, unicellular protozoa, and several vertebrate epithelial cell types. In mammals, for example, motile cilia found on cells lining the brain ventricles circulate cerebrospinal fluid; cilia in the respiratory tract sweep debris from the upper airway and the lungs; and oviduct cilia move the fertilized egg to the uterus. In addition, epithelial cilia present early in development are involved in left-right axis determination. Some epithelial cells, such as retinal photoreceptor cells and certain renal epithelial cells, possess immotile cilia that are now known to play important sensory roles in cell function. Individuals with motility-impaired cilia or defects in ciliary assembly may have any number of serious disorders, including respiratory disorders, hydrocephaly, retinal degeneration, polycystic kidney disease, liver disease, and infertility.

SINONASAL EPITHELIUM

The unique structure of the sinonasal epithelium facilitates normal cilia function and mucociliary clearance, thereby protecting the airway from debris, pathogens, and inhaled toxins. The anterior margin of the nasal vestibule is protected by a stratified squamous epithelium whose protective barrier includes sebaceous glands, sweat glands, and vibrissae. Near the nasal valves there is a histologic transition to pseudostratified columnar ciliated epithelium. Most of the nasal cavity epithelium consists of pseudostratified columnar ciliated cells, whereas the paranasal sinus epithelium is predominantly simple columnar ciliated cells.[1] In addition to the cilia projecting from their apical surface, the epithelial cells are lined with hundreds of immotile microvilli, hairlike projections of actin filaments, 1 to 2 μm in length, that lie beneath the cell membrane. By increasing the total mucosal surface area, the microvilli aid in sinonasal mucus production, sensation, secretion, and warming and humidifying inspired air.[2,3]

[a] Department of Otorhinolaryngology-Head and Neck Surgery, University of Pennsylvania, Ravdin Building, 5th Floor, 3400 Spruce Street, Philadelphia, PA 19104, USA
[b] Division of Rhinology, Department of Otorhinolaryngology-Head and Neck Surgery, Hospital of the University of Pennsylvania, Ravdin Building, 5th Floor, 3400 Spruce Street, Philadelphia, PA 19104, USA
* Corresponding author.
E-mail address: cohenn@uphs.upenn.edu

Otolaryngol Clin N Am 43 (2010) 461–472
doi:10.1016/j.otc.2010.02.007
0030-6665/10/$ – see front matter. Published by Elsevier Inc.

Ciliated columnar epithelial cells comprise approximately 80% of sinonasal mucosa, goblet cells that produce mucus approximately 20%, and progenitor basal cells less than 5%.

MUCUS

Mucus production and structure are integrally associated with normal cilia function. Just as abnormal mucus production can impair normal cilia function, abnormal cilia function can result in stagnant mucus containing abundant pathogens and debris and result in chronic inflammation. The mucus layer functions to trap inspired pathogens, particulate matter, and cellular debris, and through the process of mucociliary clearance this layer is continuously cleared and reproduced. The superficial layer of mucus is a viscous gel phase that rides along the tips of fully extended cilia. The deep layer is the sol phase that surrounds and bathes the shafts of cilia. The sol phase is a solution of water and electrolytes (Na1, K1, Ca^{2+}, Cl^-) of lower viscosity than the gel phase. Mucus is a complex immunologically active substance made of carbohydrates, enzymes, proteins, immunoglobulins, and other active molecules.

The composition of mucus is essential to normal mucociliary clearance, and disorders of mucus production can be debilitating by causing severe secondary ciliary dysfunction. Cystic fibrosis, an autosomal recessive disease resulting from a mutation in a single gene, involves several organ systems and is characterized by defective electrolyte transport resulting in abnormal mucus production.[4] The genetic defect is found in the cystic fibrosis transmembrane conductance regulator gene product, a cyclic adenosine monophosphate–mediated membrane glycoprotein that forms a chloride channel and regulates the open probability of the sodium channel, ENaC.[5] The defective sodium chloride transport yields abnormally viscous mucus. The goblet cells in such patients are subsequently engorged and distended. These patients have severely impaired mucociliary clearance and frequently develop severe recurrent sinopulmonary infections.[6]

CILIA STRUCTURE AND FUNCTION

Sinonasal cilia beat in a coordinated manner to clear the paranasal sinus cavities and upper airway of the mucus blanket containing pathogens and debris. Normal cilia are cylindrical projections from the apical surface of epithelial cells, anchored by intracellular basal bodies. Each epithelial cell is lined with approximately 50 to 200 cilia, measuring 5 to 7 μm in length and 0.2 to 0.3 μm in diameter.[7,8] The cilium is composed of interconnected microtubules bundled into axonemes, and its overlying membrane is continuous with the cell's plasma membrane. The microtubules are made of protofilaments, which in turn are composed of α- and β-tubulin dimers.

The axonemes of motile cilia contain 2 central singlet microtubules surrounded by 9 doublet microtubules. Each doublet consists of 1 α-tubule, a complete circle of 13 protofilaments, and 1 β-tubule, an incomplete circle of 10 protofilaments. This structure is consistent among the motile cilia of the respiratory epithelium, oviduct, and cerebral ventricular ependymal cells. The 2 central microtubules are attached by paired bridges whereas the peripheral doublets attach to the central pair via radial spoke heads. Each outer doublet interacts with the adjacent outer doublets via inner dynein arms (IDAs), outer dynein arms (ODAs), and nexin, each having a distinct role in the dynamic motion of cilia bending.[9] Activation of the dynein arms generates a sliding motion of 1 microtubule doublet against the adjacent doublet. It is thought that phosphorylation of the ODAs regulates cilia beat frequency while phosphorylation of the IDAs regulates the waveform pattern of beating.[10,11] Although the function of the radial spoke heads is not entirely understood, it seems they are involved in regionally limiting the sliding between the microtubules during the ciliary stroke, thus converting the sliding motion generated by the dynein arms into a bending motion of the axoneme.[12]

Each cilium has a forward power stroke followed by a recovery stroke. During the power stroke the cilium is fully extended, and the distal tip reaches the viscous outer gel phase of the mucus layer, transmitting directional force to the overlying mucus layer. During the recovery stroke, the cilium bends 90° and sweeps back to its starting point within the thinner periciliary sol phase. The mechanism of ciliary motion depends on a series of adenosine triphosphate (ATP)-dependent molecular motors that cause the outer doublets of the axoneme to slide relative to each other, producing a vectorial force. The coordination of cilia beating is thought to be secondary either to an intracellular calcium wave, via gap junctions between epithelial cells, that drives microtubule interactions,[13] or to a hydrodynamic wave that forces a timed coordination of nearby cilia.[14] Although the mechanism of coordination that results in this metachronous wave is not entirely understood, it is clear that disease states alter the normal function of cilia, thereby disrupting the critical process of mucociliary clearance.

DYNAMIC REGULATION

Ciliary activity accelerates in response to various mechanical,[15] chemical,[16,17] hormonal,[18-20] pH,[21] and thermal stimuli.[22,23] Extracellular nucleotides (adenosine and uridine) are especially potent regulators of epithelial functions stimulating mucociliary clearance through mucus secretion, increasing ciliary beat frequency (CBF), and gating ion channels involved in the maintenance of epithelial surface liquid volume.[24] Nucleotides released by the epithelium in response to mechanical and osmotic stimuli work in a paracrine fashion through metabotropic and ionotropic receptors to potentiate mucociliary clearance by recruiting adjacent cells to increase CBF.[24] Furthermore, adrenergic,[20,25,26] cholinergic,[27,28] and peptidergic[29,30] stimulations have also been demonstrated to stimulate ciliary motility. These environmental and host stimuli are transmitted via surface receptors and channels to trigger activation of second messenger cascades that regulate phosphorylation status of ciliary proteins, thereby modulating the kinetics of microtubules' sliding relative to each other. Inositol triphosphate (IP_3) mediated calcium transients have been correlated with increased CBF.[31-33] In addition, protein kinase A (PKA),[28,34] protein kinase G,[35,36] and a nitric oxide (NO)–dependent mechanism of CBF stimulation have been proposed,[17,37,38] while activation of protein kinase C (PKC) appears to decrease CBF.[30,39] To maintain rapid control of ciliary activity, kinase anchoring proteins, kinases, and phosphatases have been demonstrated to be tightly associated with the axoneme.[40-42] Experiments using fluorescence resonance energy transfer in primary ciliated cell culture demonstrated direct evidence that activation of PKA coincides with an increase in CBF, and that the return to baseline frequency lags PKA inactivation, indicating that dephosphorylation by phosphatases is required to terminate CBF stimulation.[43]

As mentioned earlier, environmental stimuli also modulate CBF. Small changes in extracellular and intracellular pH can have a profound impact on CBF. An increase in intracellular pH produces an increase in CBF, whereas a decrease in pH produces a decrease in CBF.[21] However, it is not known whether this effect is due to modulation of kinase activity, even though an acidic pH has been demonstrated to inhibit PKA function,[44] or due to direct regulation of the outer dynein arm of the axoneme.[45] Cilia beat has additionally been shown to be influenced by changes in temperature. Multiple investigations have demonstrated a direct correlation between temperature and CBF.[22,23,46] Furthermore, the temperature response appears to be mediated through kinase activity as activation of PKC shifts the temperature curve to the left.[22] Lastly, CBF is also regulated by mechanical factors. Direct mechanical stimulation of the cilia promotes an increase in CBF that coincides with an increase in intracellular Ca^{2+}.[15] In addition, shear stress applied to the apical surface of mouse tracheal explants stimulates CBF. The characteristics of this observation include a time-dependent component as well as a directional component with stimulation resulting from caudal applied shear stress. Furthermore, the response depends on purinergic receptor activation as well as intracellular Ca^{2+} and ATP.[47] Thus, these experiments suggest that CBF in the trachea coincides with the respiratory cycle, that is, CBF increases with inspiration and returns to baseline during exhalation, thereby preventing microaspirations.

MUCOCILIARY CLEARANCE

In the paranasal sinuses the coordinated function of cilia propels the mucus layer from the sinuses to the nasal cavity and then to the nasopharynx, where it is subsequently ingested into the gastrointestinal tract. In the maxillary sinus, mucus flows toward the natural sinus ostium in the superior medial wall of the sinus and then drains into the ethmoidal infundibulum. The anterior ethmoid cells drain into the middle meatus, and the posterior ethmoid cells into the superior meatus. The sphenoid sinus drains into the sphenoethmoidal recess. The frontal sinus drains into the infundibulum. The mucociliary flow from the anterior sinuses converges at the osteomeatal complex before traveling posterior to the nasopharynx. Once the mucus layer is in the nasopharynx, further mucociliary action and swallowing assist its ingestion. Microscopic cilia dysfunction at any step of this intricate transport system can result in significant and clinically evident sinonasal pathology.[48]

CILIA DYSFUNCTION
Genetic

Normal and effective mucociliary clearance is a critical component of sinonasal immunity and defense that is dependent on proper cilia function. In addition, unlike the lower airways where a compensation for decreased cilia function can be accomplished by a cough, the paranasal sinuses are solely dependent on ciliary function to propel mucus. There are several pathologic states, both genetic and acquired, in which cilia dysfunction results in impaired mucociliary clearance. These conditions are often a result of uncoordinated and dyssynchronous ciliary function or reduced motility of cilia, rather than complete cilia immotility. The hallmarks of cilia dysfunction in the otorhinolaryngologic evaluation are recurrent otitis media, sinus inflammation, and sinopulmonary infections caused by the accumulation of debris and infectious pathogens.

Primary ciliary dyskinesia (PCD) is an inherited disorder of abnormal cilia function that results in dysfunctional ciliary motility and impaired mucociliary clearance, with reported incidence ranging from 1 in 15,000 to 1 in 60,000 live births.[49] Patients with PCD typically present with chronic recurrent infections of the upper and lower airways, sinusitis, and otitis media. PCD and other syndromes of cilia dysfunction often manifest in several organ systems because cilia serve various systemic functions independent of mucociliary clearance. Approximately half of patients with PCD have situs inversus because normal embryonic nodal cilia are integral in the left-right orientation of visceral development.[50] Kartagener syndrome, described in 1933 before the discovery of the true structure and function of cilia, is the clinical triad of chronic sinusitis, bronchiectasis, and situs inversus.[51] In addition, as sperm motility and fallopian tube transport of ova are dependent on normal cilia motility, PCD patients may also suffer from infertility.

On clinical evaluation, PCD patients may present with symptoms and signs of chronic sinusitis, including nasal congestion, sinus pain and tenderness, mucopurulent nasal discharge, and anosmia. These patients often have a history of acute and chronic otitis media, with or without associated hearing loss and tympanic membrane inflammation, perforation, or scarring. PCD patients may have a chronic productive cough with associated bronchospasm, bronchiectasis, and a history of recurrent pneumonia, with associated wheezing, rales, or rhonchi. Physical examination may also reveal dextrocardia secondary to situs inversus. Because of the unusual constellation of clinical features crossing various organ systems, the diagnosis is often delayed even though the first signs may present in infancy. The differential diagnosis includes neonatal respiratory distress, asthma and allergic rhinitis or sinusitis, cystic fibrosis, or primary immunodeficiencies. A diagnosis of PCD can be confirmed by electron microscopy, genetics testing, immunofluorescent analysis, nasal NO measurement, and high-speed videomicroscopy.[52]

PCD is a genetically heterogeneous disorder. It is most commonly autosomal recessive, but other inheritance patterns have been identified. In more than 80% of PCD patients, the primary ciliary defect is in the outer dynein arm, the inner dynein arm, or both. When the outer dynein arm is defective, most but not all cilia are immotile, even if the inner arm is functional. When the inner dynein arm is defective, the cilia beat with an abnormal pattern and reduced amplitude of stroke. Some PCD patients have an abnormality of the central radial spoke complex connecting the 2 central singlet microtubules to the surrounding 9 doublet microtubules. Such cilia have a stiff repetitive beating motion but without sufficient bending to propel the overlying mucus layer.[53] The genetic mutations responsible for PCD have not been completely identified. The *DNAI1*, *DNAI2*, and *DNAH5* genes, for example, are all associated with outer dynein arm defects and have been implicated in the clinical manifestations of PCD, but many outer dynein arm defects have been described in the absence of identified mutations of these genes.[54]

Acquired

Whereas intrinsic factors can alter cilia function with catastrophic sequelae, extrinsic factors such as pollutants and microbial invaders can directly and indirectly, through induction of inflammatory mediators, affect normal cilia function. This is evident in patients with chronic rhinosinusitis (CRS) who experience relentless cycles of infection and inflammation, with clear clinical sequelae of mucociliary dysfunction (**Fig. 1**).

Microbial factors

Because normal mucociliary clearance is an extremely effective way to combat the continual influx of inspired pathogens and debris, many infectious organisms have developed mechanisms to interfere with and combat this process. Common bacterial pathogens such as *Haemophilus influenzae*, *Streptococcus pneumoniae*, *Staphylococcus aureus*, and *Pseudomonas aeruginosa* produce specific toxins to impair ciliary motion and coordination.[55] Viruses responsible for common upper respiratory tract infections disrupt the microtubule function of ciliated columnar cells and change the viscosity of surrounding mucus.[56] Impairing the local defense system facilitates the infectious pathogens' upper airway colonization.

P aeruginosa is a common respiratory pathogen that causes particularly severe infections in patients with a baseline mucociliary dysfunction, such as cystic fibrosis.

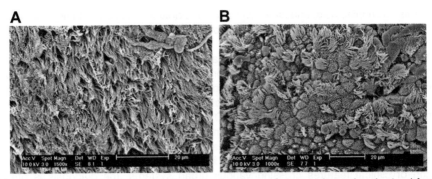

Fig. 1. Ciliary loss in CRS. Scanning electron microscopy of sinonasal samples obtained from a patient with no sinonasal disease (*A*) and CRS (*B*). Note the healthy-appearing cilia covering the entire epithelium (*A*) compared with the massive ciliary loss with just the short stubs of the microvilli evident in the CRS sample (*B*).

With abnormally thick mucus as described earlier, such patients are even more susceptible to the consequences of ciliary dysfunction. Pyocyanin, the pigment produced by *P aeruginosa* that gives it its characteristic blue-green color, is in fact a potent factor that aids in the bacteria's colonization and infection of respiratory epithelium. Several pathogenic mechanisms of pyocyanin, such as free radical generation, have been described. Pyocyanin has also been shown to cause a progressive and concentration-dependent slowing of human nasal CBF in vitro.[57] It has also been demonstrated that pyocyanin can reduce the velocity of mucus migration on rodent tracheal mucosa,[58] suggesting possible mechanisms for sinonasal mucociliary dysfunction in patients with chronic *P aeruginosa* infections.

H influenzae, another common respiratory pathogen, has been demonstrated to produce ciliotoxic substances that facilitate the bacteria's colonization of respiratory epithelium. *H influenzae* produces lipooligosaccharide and protein D, which have been shown to cause stasis and destruction of cilia and ciliated cells, although the specific mechanisms of these toxins remain unclear.[59] *S pneumoniae* produces several toxins including the cytolytic agent pneumolysin and the radical oxidant hydrogen peroxide. These toxins have been demonstrated, alone and in combination, to cause a dose-dependent slowing of CBF, in addition to damage of epithelium, on human ciliated epithelium in vitro harvested from inferior nasal turbinate brushings of healthy subjects.[60] In addition, the enterotoxin A produced by *S aureus* in high concentrations may also decrease CBF of ciliated sinus epithelium by unclear mechanisms.[61]

Inflammatory mediators

The inflammatory responses found in CRS can broadly be divided into T helper type 1 (T_H1) and T helper type 2 (T_H2) cascades according to the different cytokines they produce, with a predominance of T_H1 mediators found in CRS without nasal polyposis and T_H2 mediators found in CRS with nasal polyposis.[62] Although no general consensus regarding inflammatory cytokines has been compiled, several molecules are consistently upregulated in diseased mucosa by using various techniques including enzyme-linked immunosorbent assay (ELISA), reverse transcriptase coupled to quantitative polymerase chain reaction (RT-PCR), immunohistochemistry, and multiplex technology. The T_H1 cytokines consistently elevated in CRS include tumor necrosis factor (TNF)-α, interferon-γ, and interleukin (IL-8),[63,64] whereas IL-5, eotaxin, and RANTES represent consistently elevated T$_H$2 cytokines.[65–68] Furthermore, several of these factors are reduced following treatment with glucocorticoids,[63,68] a critical component of CRS medical management. Although chemokines and cytokines are primarily responsible for inducing migration, differentiation, activation, and degranulation of subpopulations of leukocytes, several studies have reported cytokine modulation of respiratory cilia function: IL-8 has been shown to inhibit isoproterenol-stimulated CBF in bovine bronchial epithelial cells,[69] and recently TNF-α has been shown to inhibit viscosity induced ciliary activity in primary human airway cultures.[70] These findings are further supported by recent work demonstrating a subset of patients with CRS having a reversible blunted ciliary response to environmental stimuli.[71,72] Furthermore, IL-13 has been shown to decrease basal CBF in human respiratory epithelial cells in a dose-dependent and time-dependent manner,[73] while IL-6 has demonstrated similar effects at high concentrations on human fallopian tube ciliary activity.[74] Conversely, TNF-α and IL-1β increase basal CBF in bovine bronchial epithelial cells.[18] Therefore, modulation of cilia physiology by CRS-specific inflammatory cytokines is a likely mechanism for decreased mucociliary clearance in the disease state.

Tobacco smoke

The effects of tobacco smoke on the mucociliary function of epithelia have been of interest for more than four decades.[75] Although studies reporting the effects of cigarette smoke on CBF have yielded conflicting results,[76–79] histologic studies of cilia from the airways of smokers consistently demonstrate decreased cilia number.[80,81] In addition, cigarette smoke increases mucus production by airway epithelial cells,[82–84] thus necessitating the epithelium, with sparse and most likely dysfunctional cilia, to increase the propulsive force to maintain homeostasis. Furthermore, to compound the insult to mucociliary clearance, tobacco-mediated blunting of stimulated CBF has been demonstrated in lower airway epithelium[79] as well as in sinonasal epithelial cultures.[85] Although no clear mechanism has been demonstrated to explain the decreased number of cilia in smokers,[80] recent reports have illustrated an inhibition of ciliogenesis by tobacco smoke exposure.[86]

SUMMARY

CRS, affecting more than 35 million Americans of all ages,[87] represents several distinct entities that are clinically indistinguishable. Although the mortality of the disease is low the morbidity is high, with patients with CRS demonstrating worse quality-of-life scores (for physical pain and social functioning) than those suffering from chronic obstructive pulmonary disease, congestive heart failure, or angina.[88] Multiple causes contribute to the development of CRS, but the common pathophysiologic sequela is ineffective sinonasal mucociliary clearance, resulting in stasis of sinonasal secretions. Although primary ciliopathies represent a minority of patients with CRS, secondary ciliopathies are most likely encountered in every patient with CRS. In addition to altered cilia structure resulting in persistent infection, many respiratory pathogens directly attack cilia function. Furthermore, inflammatory cytokines can also negatively modulate cilia function, resulting in blunted dynamic regulation and decreased basal cilia function, thereby resulting in decreased mucociliary clearance.

Implications for Research

Further comprehension of the biochemical processes regulating cilia function and disruption of these processes by microbes and inflammatory mediators should yield putative targets for design of pharmacologic agents capable of blocking the detrimental ciliary effects. Furthermore, understanding the molecular cascade regulating ciliogenesis would ultimately result in the ability to manipulate the epithelium for accelerated ciliary recovery and restoration of mucociliary clearance.

Implications for Clinical Practice

Restoring native mucociliary clearance in patients with primary cilia dysfunction is impossible. Thus, aggressive measures such as surgery directed at gravity drainage of the paranasal sinuses should be used. In patients with secondary ciliary dysfunction, attention should initially be directed at removing the offending agents and then focusing on aiding mucociliary clearance, through debridements and lavage, to maintain a relatively clean environment to help reciliation.

REFERENCES

1. Wagenmann M, Naclerio RM. Anatomic and physiologic considerations in sinusitis. J Allergy Clin Immunol 1992;90:419–23.
2. Eliezer N, Sade J, Silberberg A, et al. The role of mucus in transport by cilia. Am Rev Respir Dis 1970;102:48–52.
3. Naclerio RM, Durham SR, Mygind N. Rhinitis: mechanisms and management. New York: Dekker; 1999.
4. Accurso FJ. Update in cystic fibrosis 2005. Am J Respir Crit Care Med 2006;173: 944–7.
5. Wine JJ. The genesis of cystic fibrosis lung disease. J Clin Invest 1999;103: 309–12.
6. Van de Water TR, Staecker H. Otolaryngology: basic science and clinical review. New York: Thieme; 2005.
7. Houtmeyers E, Gosselink R, Gayan-Ramirez G, et al. Regulation of mucociliary clearance in health and disease. Eur Respir J 1999;13:1177–88.
8. Satir P, Sleigh MA. The physiology of cilia and mucociliary interactions. Annu Rev Physiol 1990;52:137–55.
9. Hard R, Blaustein K, Scarcello L. Reactivation of outer-arm-depleted lung axonemes: evidence for functional differences between inner and outer dynein arms in situ. Cell Motil Cytoskeleton 1992;21:199–209.
10. Brokaw CJ, Kamiya R. Bending patterns of *Chlamydomonas flagella*: IV. Mutants with defects in inner and outer dynein arms indicate differences in dynein arm function. Cell Motil Cytoskeleton 1987;8:68–75.
11. Brokaw CJ. Control of flagellar bending: a new agenda based on dynein diversity. Cell Motil Cytoskeleton 1994;28:199–204.
12. Satir P, Christensen ST. Overview of structure and function of mammalian cilia. Annu Rev Physiol 2007;69:377–400.
13. Yeh TH, Su MC, Hsu CJ, et al. Epithelial cells of nasal mucosa express functional gap junctions of connexin 43. Acta Otolaryngol 2003;123:314–20.
14. Gheber L, Priel Z. Synchronization between beating cilia. Biophys J 1989;55: 183–91.
15. Sanderson MJ, Dirksen ER. Mechanosensitivity of cultured ciliated cells from the mammalian respiratory tract: implications for the regulation of mucociliary transport. Proc Natl Acad Sci U S A 1986;83:7302–6.
16. Wong LB, Miller IF, Yeates DB. Stimulation of tracheal ciliary beat frequency by capsaicin. J Appl Phys 1990;68:2574–80.

17. Jain B, Rubinstein I, Robbins RA, et al. Modulation of airway epithelial cell ciliary beat frequency by nitric oxide. Biochem Biophys Res Commun 1993;191:83–8.
18. Jain B, Rubinstein I, Robbins RA, et al. TNF-alpha and IL-1 beta upregulate nitric oxide-dependent ciliary motility in bovine airway epithelium. Am J Physiol 1995; 268:L911–7.
19. Korngreen A, Ma W, Priel Z, et al. Extracellular ATP directly gates a cation-selective channel in rabbit airway ciliated epithelial cells. J Physiol 1998;508(Pt 3):703–20.
20. Sanderson MJ, Dirksen ER. Mechanosensitive and beta-adrenergic control of the ciliary beat frequency of mammalian respiratory tract cells in culture. Am Rev Respir Dis 1989;139:432–40.
21. Sutto Z, Conner GE, Salathe M. Regulation of human airway ciliary beat frequency by intracellular pH. J Physiol 2004;560:519–32.
22. Mwimbi XK, Muimo R, Green MW, et al. Making human nasal cilia beat in the cold: a real time assay for cell signalling. Cell Signal 2003;15:395–402.
23. Schipor I, Palmer JN, Cohen AS, et al. Quantification of ciliary beat frequency in sinonasal epithelial cells using differential interference contrast microscopy and high-speed digital video imaging. Am J Rhinol 2006;20:124–7.
24. Picher M, Boucher RC. Human airway ecto-adenylate kinase. A mechanism to propagate ATP signaling on airway surfaces. J Biol Chem 2003;278:11256–64.
25. Wyatt TA, Sisson JH. Chronic ethanol downregulates PKA activation and ciliary beating in bovine bronchial epithelial cells. Am J Physiol Lung Cell Mol Physiol 2001;281:L575–81.
26. Yang B, Schlosser RJ, McCaffrey TV. Dual signal transduction mechanisms modulate ciliary beat frequency in upper airway epithelium. Am J Physiol 1996; 270:L745–51.
27. Salathe M, Lipson EJ, Ivonnet PI, et al. Muscarinic signaling in ciliated tracheal epithelial cells: dual effects on Ca^{2+} and ciliary beating. Am J Physiol 1997; 272:L301–10.
28. Zagoory O, Braiman A, Priel Z. The mechanism of ciliary stimulation by acetylcholine: roles of calcium, PKA, and PKG. J Gen Physiol 2002;119:329–39.
29. Wong LB, Miller IF, Yeates DB. Pathways of substance P stimulation of canine tracheal ciliary beat frequency. J Appl Phys 1991;70:267–73.
30. Wong LB, Park CL, Yeates DB. Neuropeptide Y inhibits ciliary beat frequency in human ciliated cells via nPKC, independently of PKA. Am J Physiol 1998;275:C440–8.
31. Salathe M, Bookman RJ. Coupling of $[Ca^{2+}]i$ and ciliary beating in cultured tracheal epithelial cells. J Cell Sci 1995;108(Pt 2):431–40.
32. Korngreen A, Priel Z. Simultaneous measurement of ciliary beating and intracellular calcium. Biophys J 1994;67:377–80.
33. Lansley AB, Sanderson MJ. Regulation of airway ciliary activity by Ca^{2+}: simultaneous measurement of beat frequency and intracellular Ca^{2+}. Biophys J 1999;77: 629–38.
34. Braiman A, Zagoory O, Priel Z. PKA induces Ca^{2+} release and enhances ciliary beat frequency in a Ca^{2+}-dependent and -independent manner. Am J Physiol 1998;275:C790–7.
35. Zhang L, Sanderson MJ. The role of cGMP in the regulation of rabbit airway ciliary beat frequency. J Physiol 2003;551:765–76.
36. Wyatt TA, Spurzem JR, May K, et al. Regulation of ciliary beat frequency by both PKA and PKG in bovine airway epithelial cells. Am J Physiol 1998;275:L827–35.
37. Yang B, Schlosser RJ, McCaffrey TV. Signal transduction pathways in modulation of ciliary beat frequency by methacholine. Ann Otol Rhinol Laryngol 1997;106: 230–6.

38. Uzlaner N, Priel Z. Interplay between the NO pathway and elevated $[Ca^{2+}]i$ enhances ciliary activity in rabbit trachea. J Physiol 1999;516(Pt 1):179–90.

39. Mwimbi XK, Muimo R, Green M, et al. Protein kinase C regulates the flow rate-dependent decline in human nasal ciliary beat frequency in vitro. J Aerosol Med 2000;13:273–9.

40. Porter ME, Sale WS. The 9+2 axoneme anchors multiple inner arm dyneins and a network of kinases and phosphatases that control motility. J Cell Biol 2000;151: F37–42.

41. Kamiya R. Functional diversity of axonemal dyneins as studied in *Chlamydomonas* mutants. Int Rev Cytol 2002;219:115–55.

42. Smith EF. Regulation of flagellar dynein by the axonemal central apparatus. Cell Motil Cytoskeleton 2002;52:33–42.

43. Schmid A, Bai G, Schmid N, et al. Real-time analysis of cAMP-mediated regulation of ciliary motility in single primary human airway epithelial cells. J Cell Sci 2006;119:4176–86.

44. Reddy MM, Kopito RR, Quinton PM. Cytosolic pH regulates GCl through control of phosphorylation states of CFTR. Am J Physiol 1998;275:C1040–7.

45. Keskes L, Giroux-Widemann V, Serres C, et al. The reactivation of demembranated human spermatozoa lacking outer dynein arms is independent of pH. Mol Reprod Dev 1998;49:416–25.

46. Green A, Smallman LA, Logan AC, et al. The effect of temperature on nasal ciliary beat frequency. Clin Otolaryngol 1995;20:178–80.

47. Winters SL, Davis CW, Boucher RC. Mechanosensitivity of mouse tracheal ciliary beat frequency: roles for Ca^{2+}, purinergic signaling, tonicity, and viscosity. Am J Physiol Lung Cell Mol Physiol 2007;292:L614–24.

48. Donald PJ, Gluckman JL, Rice DH. The sinuses. New York: Raven Press; 1995.

49. Afzelius BA. The immotile-cilia syndrome: a microtubule-associated defect. CRC Crit Rev Biochem 1985;19:63–87.

50. Noone PG, Leigh MW, Sannuti A, et al. Primary ciliary dyskinesia: diagnostic and phenotypic features. Am J Respir Crit Care Med 2004;169:459–67.

51. Kartagener M. Zur pathogene der bronkiectasein:bronkiectasein bei situs viscerum inversus. Beitr Klin Tuberk 1933;82:489.

52. Leigh MW, Pittman JE, Carson JL, et al. Clinical and genetic aspects of primary ciliary dyskinesia/Kartagener syndrome. Genet Med 2009;11:473–87.

53. Chilvers MA, Rutman A, O'Callaghan C. Ciliary beat pattern is associated with specific ultrastructural defects in primary ciliary dyskinesia. J Allergy Clin Immunol 2003;112:518–24.

54. Escudier E, Duquesnoy P, Papon JF, et al. Ciliary defects and genetics of primary ciliary dyskinesia. Paediatr Respir Rev 2009;10:51–4.

55. Ferguson JL, McCaffrey TV, Kern EB, et al. The effects of sinus bacteria on human ciliated nasal epithelium in vitro. Otolaryngol Head Neck Surg 1988;98: 299–304.

56. Jones N. The nose and paranasal sinuses physiology and anatomy. Adv Drug Deliv Rev 2001;51:5–19.

57. Kanthakumar K, Taylor G, Tsang KW, et al. Mechanisms of action of Pseudomonas aeruginosa pyocyanin on human ciliary beat in vitro. Infect Immun 1993;61:2848–53.

58. Munro NC, Barker A, Rutman A, et al. Effect of pyocyanin and 1-hydroxyphenazine on in vivo tracheal mucus velocity. J Appl Phys 1989;67:316–23.

59. St Geme JW 3rd. The pathogenesis of nontypable *Haemophilus influenzae* otitis media. Vaccine 2000;19(Suppl 1):S41–50.

60. Feldman C, Anderson R, Cockeran R, et al. The effects of pneumolysin and hydrogen peroxide, alone and in combination, on human ciliated epithelium in vitro. Respir Med 2002;96:580–5.
61. Min YG, Oh SJ, Won TB, et al. Effects of staphylococcal enterotoxin on ciliary activity and histology of the sinus mucosa. Acta Otolaryngol 2006;126:941–7.
62. Hamilos DL. Chronic sinusitis. J Allergy Clin Immunol 2000;106:213–27.
63. Lennard CM, Mann EA, Sun LL, et al. Interleukin-1 beta, interleukin-5, interleukin-6, interleukin-8, and tumor necrosis factor-alpha in chronic sinusitis: response to systemic corticosteroids. Am J Rhinol 2000;14:367–73.
64. Kuehnemund M, Ismail C, Brieger J, et al. Untreated chronic rhinosinusitis: a comparison of symptoms and mediator profiles. Laryngoscope 2004;114:561–5.
65. Bachert C, Wagenmann M, Rudack C, et al. The role of cytokines in infectious sinusitis and nasal polyposis. Allergy 1998;53:2–13.
66. Bachert C, Wagenmann M, Hauser U, et al. IL-5 synthesis is upregulated in human nasal polyp tissue. J Allergy Clin Immunol 1997;99:837–42.
67. Bachert C, Van Cauwenberge PB. Inflammatory mechanisms in chronic sinusitis. Acta Otorhinolaryngol Belg 1997;51:209–17.
68. Woodworth BA, Joseph K, Kaplan AP, et al. Alterations in eotaxin, monocyte chemoattractant protein-4, interleukin-5, and interleukin-13 after systemic steroid treatment for nasal polyps. Otolaryngol Head Neck Surg 2004;131:585–9.
69. Allen-Gipson DS, Romberger DJ, Forget MA, et al. IL-8 inhibits isoproterenol-stimulated ciliary beat frequency in bovine bronchial epithelial cells. J Aerosol Med 2004;17:107–15.
70. Gonzalez C, Sanchez MT, Perez-Sepulveda A, et al. Effect of TNF alpha and viscosity in airway epithelial cells. In: The Proceedings of the American Academy of Otolaryngology-Head and Neck Surgery. Washington, DC: Elsevier; 2007. p. 200.
71. Chen B, Shaari J, Claire SE, et al. Altered sinonasal ciliary dynamics in chronic rhinosinusitis. Am J Rhinol 2006;20:325–9.
72. Chen B, Antunes MB, Claire SE, et al. Reversal of chronic rhinosinusitis-associated sinonasal ciliary dysfunction. Am J Rhinol 2007;21:346–53.
73. Laoukili J, Perret E, Willems T, et al. IL-13 alters mucociliary differentiation and ciliary beating of human respiratory epithelial cells. J Clin Invest 2001;108:1817–24.
74. Papathanasiou A, Djahanbakhch O, Saridogan E, et al. The effect of interleukin-6 on ciliary beat frequency in the human fallopian tube. Fertil Steril 2008;90:391–4.
75. Falk HL, Tremer HM, Kotin P. Effect of cigarette smoke and its constituents on ciliated mucus-secreting epithelium. J Natl Cancer Inst 1959;23:999–1012.
76. Hybbinette JC. A pharmacological evaluation of the short-term effect of cigarette smoke on mucociliary activity. Acta Otolaryngol 1982;94:351–9.
77. Pettersson B, Curvall M, Enzell C. The inhibitory effect of tobacco smoke compound on ciliary activity. Eur J Respir Dis Suppl 1985;139:89–92.
78. Wyatt TA, Gentry-Nielsen MJ, Pavlik JA, et al. Desensitization of PKA-stimulated ciliary beat frequency in an ethanol-fed rat model of cigarette smoke exposure. Alcohol Clin Exp Res 2004;28:998–1004.
79. Elliott MK, Sisson JH, West WW, et al. Differential in vivo effects of whole cigarette smoke exposure versus cigarette smoke extract on mouse ciliated tracheal epithelium. Exp Lung Res 2006;32:99–118.
80. Wanner A, Salathe M, O'Riordan TG. Mucociliary clearance in the airways. Am J Respir Crit Care Med 1996;154:1868–902.
81. Isik AC, Yardimci S, Guven C, et al. Morphologic alteration induced by short-term smoke exposure in rats. ORL J Otorhinolaryngol Relat Spec 2007;69:13–7.

82. Gensch E, Gallup M, Sucher A, et al. Tobacco smoke control of mucin production in lung cells requires oxygen radicals AP-1 and JNK. J Biol Chem 2004;279: 39085–93.

83. Takeyama K, Jung B, Shim JJ, et al. Activation of epidermal growth factor receptors is responsible for mucin synthesis induced by cigarette smoke. Am J Physiol Lung Cell Mol Physiol 2001;280:L165–72.

84. Kreindler JL, Jackson AD, Kemp PA, et al. Inhibition of chloride secretion in human bronchial epithelial cells by cigarette smoke extract. Am J Physiol Lung Cell Mol Physiol 2005;288:L894–902.

85. Cohen NA, Zhang S, Sharp DB, et al. Cigarette smoke condensate inhibits transepithelial chloride transport and ciliary beat frequency. Laryngoscope 2009; 119(11):2269–74.

86. Tamashiro E, Xiong G, Anselmo-Lima WT, et al. Cigarette smoke exposure impairs respiratory epithelial ciliogenesis. Am J Rhinol Allergy 2009;23:117–22.

87. Murphy MP, Fishman P, Short SO, et al. Health care utilization and cost among adults with chronic rhinosinusitis enrolled in a health maintenance organization. Otolaryngol Head Neck Surg 2002;127:367–76.

88. Gliklich RE, Metson R. The health impact of chronic sinusitis in patients seeking otolaryngologic care. Otolaryngol Head Neck Surg 1995;113:104–9.

Innate Immunity

Eng H. Ooi, MBBS, PhD, FRACS[a], Alkis J. Psaltis, MBBS(Hons), PhD[b,c],
Ian J. Witterick, MD, MSc, FRCSC[a],
Peter-John Wormald, MD, FRACS[b,c],*

KEYWORDS

• Innate immunity • Rhinosinusitis • Biofilms • Cigarette smoke
• Toll-like receptors • Cystic fibrosis

The sinonasal tract is continuously exposed to environmental particulates and pathogens, which are normally cleared by efficient host defenses.[1] The innate immune system forms the first line of defense against these aerosolized pathogens and, although typically constitutive, has also been found to be inducible. One significant component of the innate immune system is the cellular structure of the sinonasal mucosal lining itself. This lining consists of the ciliated respiratory epithelium, goblet cells, subepithelial cells (dendritic cells, macrophages, leucocytes, plasma cells), and glands, which all contribute to pathogen clearance in several ways.[2]

The epithelial cells provide a physical barrier to pathogen invasion and secrete mucus to trap the particulates and facilitate their removal toward the pharynx through coordinated mucociliary action. The mucosal cells possess receptors that recognize certain conserved structures present on microorganisms, resulting in not only the prompt induction of innate immune responses but also activation and amplification of the T- and B-cell responses of the acquired immune system. These mucosal cells also secrete antimicrobial peptides, immunoglobulins, opsonins, cytokines, chemokines, and complement to help remove potential pathogens.[1] The actions of the innate immune system and the cross-talk between it and the slower but longer-lasting adaptive immune system enable pathogen clearance, restoration of mucosal homeostasis, and prevention of ongoing inflammation (**Fig. 1**). Impairment of the innate immune

Disclosure: Funding for this work: Dr Ooi is supported by the RACS Margorie Hooper travelling scholarship and the SAPMEA Mark Jolly travelling scholarship.
Disclosure of potential conflict of interests: Dr Wormald receives royalties for instruments designed from Medtronic ENT and is a consultant for Neilmed.
a Department of Otolaryngology Head and Neck Surgery, University of Toronto, Mount Sinai Hospital, 600 University Avenue, Room 413, Toronto, ON M5G 1X5, Canada
b Department of Otolaryngology Head and Neck Surgery, Flinders University, The Queen Elizabeth Hospital, 28 Woodville Road, Woodville South, South Australia 5011, Australia
c Department of Otolaryngology Head and Neck Surgery, University of Adelaide, The Queen Elizabeth Hospital, 28 Woodville Road, Woodville South, South Australia 5011, Australia
* Corresponding author. Department of Otolaryngology Head and Neck Surgery, Flinders University, The Queen Elizabeth Hospital, 28 Woodville Road, Woodville South, South Australia 5011, Australia.
E-mail address: Peterj.wormald@adelaide.edu.au

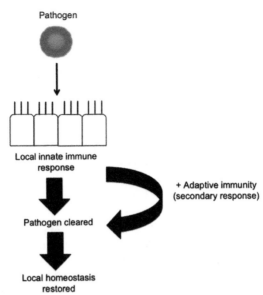

Fig. 1. Schematic diagram of normal local innate immunity responding to pathogens and secondary activation of adaptive immunity if required. Local homeostasis is restored with clearance of the pathogen and subsequent braking of both innate and adaptive immune activation.

system and failure to restore homeostasis is believed to result in chronic inflammation.[3]

Research on innate immunity in the field of rhinology has predominantly focused on chronic rhinosinusitis (CRS) as a group of disorders characterized by chronic inflammation of the mucosa of the paranasal sinuses.[4] CRS is common, affecting nearly 16% of the United State population, consuming a large proportion of health expenditure (estimated $6 billion per year), and having adverse effects on quality of life scores.[5-7]

A consensus statement proposed classifying CRS in the presence (CRSwNP) or absence of nasal polyps (CRSsNP) based on differences in their clinical features and histologic and cytokine profile. Further subclassification depends on presence of eosinophilic inflammation, fungal hyphae in the sinus mucus, and aspirin intolerance.[8] Patients with CRSwNP tend to have predominantly nasal obstruction, facial pressure, decreased sense of smell, and eosinophilic inflammation with a Th2 cytokine profile. CRSsNP is more commonly associated with colored rhinorrhea, facial pain, and more neutrophilic inflammation with a Th1 cytokine profile. Whether these entities are truly different in terms of pathophysiology or are variable manifestations of the same disease spectrum remains unclear.

Previously, CRS was believed to be a disorder of the adaptive immune system, but recent research suggests that changes in the adaptive immunity are secondary to disorders in the innate immune system. Understanding of immunity has evolved to appreciate that adaptive immune responses are secondary to changes in innate immunity. Research into the cause and pathogenesis of CRS remains unclear despite the identification of numerous infectious and noninfectious agents. Recent studies have implicated the presence of biofilms,[9] superantigens,[10] and fungus[11] in the cause of CRS because of their identification in tissue biopsies or cultures. However, their detection in healthy individuals and absence in a proportion of patients with CRS makes it unlikely that they are responsible for all forms of CRS.[12,13]

Recently, the immune barrier hypothesis was proposed, suggesting that bacteria and fungi are more likely to be disease modifiers than primary causative agents in predisposed individuals.[14] However, further research on innate immunity is needed to examine this hypothesis.

PATTERN RECOGNITION RECEPTORS

The innate immune system recognizes specific molecular structures known as *pathogen-associated molecular patterns* (PAMPs), which are conserved and considered essential for the survival of pathogens.[1] The responses of the innate immune system against these PAMPs signal the adaptive immune system to develop memory and subsequent longer-lasting immune responses.

Toll proteins were originally discovered in the fruit fly *Drosophila* and led to the identification of a family of transmembrane pattern recognition receptors known as *Toll-like receptors* (TLRs) in humans.[15] TLRs are transmembrane glycoproteins with an extracellular *N*-terminal leucine-rich domain and an intracellular *C*-terminal domain, known as the *Toll/interleukin (IL)-1 receptor* (TIR) domain because it shows homology with the IL-1 receptor. TLRs are differentially expressed between cells, with some expressed on the cell surface and others expressed intracellularly within endosomes and the endoplasmic reticulum (**Table 1**). The recognition of various PAMPs by the TLRs induces a cascade of downstream signaling to induce inflammatory cytokine signaling that can be the Th1, Th2, or type I interferon (IFN)-γ cytokine profile. TLR signaling pathways are complex but can be essentially categorized as myeloid differentiation primary response (MyD88)–dependent or TIR-containing adaptor-inducing IFN-γ–dependent pathways.[15] The MyD88-dependent pathway is used by all TLRs except for TLR3.

Table 1
Summary of Toll-like receptors

	TLR Location	PAMPs Recognized
TLR1	Cell surface	Triacyl lipopeptides (bacteria and mycobacteria)
TLR2	Cell surface	Hemagglutinin protein (viruses), peptidoglycan and LTA (gram-positive bacteria), lipoarabinomannan (mycobacteria)
TLR3	Endosome	ssRNA, dsRNA viruses
TLR4	Cell surface	LPS (gram-negative bacteria), glycoinositolphospholipids (*Trypanosoma*), mannan (*Candida*), fusion protein (respiratory syncytial virus)
TLR5	Cell surface	Flagellin, an important protein in bacteria motility, adhesion, and invasion
TLR6	Cell surface	LTA (gram-positive bacteria), zymosan (*Saccharomyces*)
TLR7	Endosome	ssRNA viruses
TLR8	Endosome	ssRNA viruses
TLR9	Endosome	dsDNA viruses, unmethylated CpG motifs
TLR11	Cell surface	Profilins from toxoplasmosis gondii, uropathogenic *Escherichia coli*

Abbreviations: dsDNA, double stranded deoxyribonucleic acid; LPS, lipopolysaccharide; LTA, lipoteichoic acid; PAMP, pathogen-associated molecular patterns; ssRNA, single stranded ribonucleic acid; TLR, Toll-like receptor.

Data from Kumar H, Kawai T, Akira S. Pathogen recognition in the innate immune response. Biochem J 2009;420(1):1–16.

Research in the area of TLRs and rhinology has shown mRNA expression of TLRs in cultured nasal epithelial cells[16,17] and sinonasal biopsies from patients with CRS.[18] Immunostaining of sinonasal biopsy specimens has shown that TLR-2 is localized to the stroma deep to the epithelial surface, whereas TLR-4 is predominantly in the submucosal seromucinous glands.[19] Patients with both allergic and nonallergic rhinitis show reduced mRNA expression of TLR-2 in turbinate tissue biopsies compared with controls.[20] TLR-2 and -4 mRNA expression was reduced in patients with nasal polyp with fungal and bacterial colonization, suggesting a possible relationship between fungus and TLR expression in nasal polyps. Stimulation of TLR-2 and -4 increased the in vitro phagocytic ability of neutrophils and eosinophils against *Aspergillus conidia*, suggesting that manipulation of TLRs may aid in the clearance of fungi.[21]

The genome of DNA viruses contains unmethylated CpG DNA that are DNA motifs recognized by TLR-9. Host CpG DNA, however, is highly methylated and therefore host DNA does not stimulate TLR activation. This mechanism is useful to promote tolerance of normal cells. Use of CpG-oligonucleotides in a nasal mucosal explant model in vitro showed some possibility in reducing the expression of the cytokine IL-5.[22]

Other innate immune pattern recognition receptors have been discovered recently. These include retinoic acid–inducible–like receptors (RLRs) and nucleotide binding and oligomerization domain (NOD)–like receptors (NLRs).[15] Although little is known about the molecules in the field of rhinology, other areas of scientific research have provided some insight into their possible function. RLRs are intracellular receptors important for detecting RNA derived from RNA and DNA viruses. NLRs are another family of intracellular receptors consisting of 23 proteins in humans. These proteins consist of a central NOD and a *C*-terminal domain with leucine-rich repeats.[15]

In summary many questions remain regarding the role of TLRs, RLRs, and NLRs and their role in CRS. These include defining their expression in different subgroups of CRS, and how they respond to various bacteria, fungi, biofilms, and in association with other innate immune peptides. Research is being conducted in these areas.

CYSTIC FIBROSIS AND CHRONIC RHINOSINUSITIS

Cystic fibrosis is an autosomal recessive disorder caused by mutations of the *cystic fibrosis transmembrane regulator* (*CFTR*) gene, with the most common being the ΔF508 mutation.[23] Cystic fibrosis is a recognized genetic predisposition condition associated with CRS because of its mucociliary dysfunction and chronic bacterial or fungal colonization.[4,23,24] Nasal polyps are present in approximately 40% of patients with cystic fibrosis, but the polyps exhibit predominantly neutrophilic, rather than eosinophilic, inflammation. Recently, Pinto and colleagues[25] identified eight individuals with CRS within an isolated small group of people who practice a communal lifestyle and share common environmental exposures. Linkage analysis and DNA genome screening were used on these eight individuals, who were also related to each other. A strong linkage signal among these individuals was identified at 7q31.1 to 7q32.1, which is near the *CFTR* gene.

Previous studies have shown that carriers with a cystic fibrosis mutation have a higher prevalence of CRS compared with the general population.[26] Similarly, pediatric patients with CRS who did not meet the criteria for a diagnosis of cystic fibrosis were screened for and found to have a higher prevalence of cystic fibrosis variant mutations than would be expected in a general population.[27] Other innate immune defects have been identified in cystic fibrosis. Epithelial cells use CFTR to internalize *Pseudomonas aeruginosa* and thereby remove it from the airway surface.[28] Experts believe that in patients with cystic fibrosis, epithelial cells are unable to remove *P aeruginosa* because of mutations in the *CFTR* gene. These patients also show reduced activity of antimicrobial peptides in lung surface fluid, which is believed to be caused partly by the high salt conditions in cystic fibrosis.[29] Further studies are required to investigate the possibility that carriers of variant mutations in the *CFTR* gene who do not have clinical cystic fibrosis are predisposed to the development of recalcitrant CRS.

MUCOCILIARY FUNCTION AND INNATE IMMUNITY

The mucociliary clearing action of epithelium in the sinonasal tract is a key innate immune function and the primary defense mechanism against inhaled particles.[30] This function occurs through the production of mucus, which traps inhaled particles, followed by the active process of ciliary beating, transporting the trapped mucus and particles toward the pharynx where they are swallowed. The sinonasal mucosa is lined by ciliated respiratory epithelium with goblet cells that produce mucus.

Messerklinger[31] is credited with showing the distinct pattern of flow of mucociliary clearance and mucus in each sinus. The sinuses are dependent on healthy mucociliary clearing to transport mucus, bacteria, fungus, and other material from the sinus. Stripping of the mucosa has been shown to result in abnormal mucosal regeneration, thus removing this essential innate immune function.[32] This finding has been the basis for the mucosa preservation approach of endoscopic sinus surgery.[33] CRS is associated with decreased mucociliary clearing, with demonstration of reduced saccharin transit time.[34,35] Impaired mucociliary clearing leads to stasis of the mucus and secretions, theoretically leading to ongoing colonization and potentially inflammation. However, more than 3 months after endoscopic sinus surgery, the mucociliary clearing showed significant improvement with regeneration of cilia, suggesting that impaired mucociliary clearing was secondary to the chronic inflammation rather than was the primary defect.[35,36]

The anatomy, physiology, and biochemistry of mucociliary clearing have been reviewed previously.[30] Briefly, mucociliary clearing is dependent on the properties of mucus and coordinated beating action of the cilia, and uncertainty still exists as to whether a decrease in mucociliary clearing in patients with CRS is caused by the mucus, ciliary dysfunction, or both. Cilia beat spontaneously at a basal ciliary beat frequency (CBF), a function that is dependent on intracellular ATP and increases in response to various stimuli. Ciliary beating increases in response to fever, stress, exercise, adrenergic, cholinergic, and purinergic stimuli.[30]

A study by Chen and colleagues[37] showed a significant difference in basal and stimulated CBF of sinonasal mucosal explants between patients who had CRSwNP and controls. In another study, the same investigators compared controls and patients with CRSsNP using cholinergic and adrenergic stimulation to determine if the stimulating effect seen with ATP was unique to purinergic stimuli.[38] The most significant effect with impairment of stimulated CBF was seen in the CRSsNP group. Tissue dissociation was performed to isolate the epithelial cells and maintained ex vivo in submersion. Daily observation of basal and stimulated CBF found that 72% of these cultures resumed ciliary action within 36 hours, suggesting that the blunting of ciliary effects was caused by chronic inflammation and that epithelial cells isolated from this chronic inflammatory environment have a chance of regaining normal ciliary function.

Future work investigating immunomodulatory agents that can stimulate CBF or improve ciliogenesis (eg, topical retinoic acid[39]) will improve understanding and treatment of CRS.

CIGARETTE SMOKING, INNATE IMMUNITY, AND CHRONIC RHINOSINUSITIS

Smoking is a well-recognized adverse factor in CRS associated with worse outcomes after endoscopic sinus surgery.[40] A retrospective chart review and complex multiple linear logistic statistical analysis found that patients who ever smoked had a 43-fold risk for developing nasal polyps.[41] Smokers and nonsmokers undergoing septoplasty surgery were recently compared.[42] The group that did not smoke had significantly shorter mucociliary clearing times. Cigarette smoke is known to cause airway epithelial hyperplasia, submucosal gland hypertrophy, goblet cell hyperplasia, epithelial permeability, and squamous cell metaplasia.[43] The effects of cigarette smoke may be caused by mainstream, side stream, or exhaled smoke; gaseous, particulate, or aqueous phase components; or individual chemical compounds.[43] The chemical compounds in cigarette smoke include nicotine, tar, ammonia, carbon monoxide, formaldehyde, acrolein, acetone, benzopyrenes, hydroxyquinone, nitrogen oxides, and cadmium.[44] Cigarette smoke extract at high concentrations causes cytotoxicity of primary human nasal epithelial cells.[45] Cigarette smoke condensates (particle phase) and extracts (volatile phase) significantly impaired ciliogenesis in an in vitro mouse nasal epithelium culture model. These findings may explain the poorer outcomes seen in patients who continue to smoke after surgery.

The effects of cigarette smoke on the innate immune system are not as well studied, but several recent papers suggest that cigarette smoke suppresses the innate immune function of sinonasal epithelial cells.[46,47] Cantin and colleagues[48] showed that cigarette smoke exposure using gaseous and aqueous extracts can suppress CFTR mRNA and protein expression in airway cell lines in vitro. Therefore, they surmised that cigarette smoke might induce a form of CFTR suppression. CFTR is important for internalization of *P aeruginosa*,[49] and cigarette smoke may affect CFTR function in patients who do not have cystic fibrosis, therefore impairing the innate immune system.

TLR-4 mRNA expression was found to be down-regulated in nasal brushings of smokers and in a dose-dependent fashion in vitro in an airway epithelial cell line.[50] The effects of acrolein, an aldehyde compound in cigarette smoke, on primary culture of human sinonasal epithelial cells were recently studied.[46] Real-time polymerase chain reaction and enzyme-linked immunosorbent assay (ELISA) showed that IL-8 and human ß-defensin 2 mRNA and protein expression decreased in a dose-dependent manner because of acrolein. Unfortunately, this study did not include a normal control group for comparison.

Smoking has a substantial effect on reducing surfactant protein (SP)-D levels in bronchoalveolar fluid (BALF), with former smokers having reduced levels compared with those who never smoked, suggesting that cigarette smoke may have a long-lasting effect on SP-D even after they have stopped smoking.[51] Further research is required to determine if a similar reduction in SP levels are seen in sinonasal mucosa of smokers.

In summary, these studies indicate that various components of cigarette smoke can affect the innate immune response in many ways.[44] Most studies on cigarette smoke and innate immunity study the effects from an acute exposure rather than chronic exposure standpoint. Studies on innate immunity in CRS usually do not stratify patients who smoke as a separate subgroup for study. However, the effects of cigarette smoking on innate immunity seem significant, and therefore a need exists to determine what these are.

ANTIMICROBIAL PEPTIDES, BIOFILMS, AND CHRONIC RHINOSINUSITIS

Numerous antimicrobial peptides are expressed in the sinonasal and lower airway epithelium.[3] These include lactoferrrin,[52] lysozyme,[53] cathelicidins,[54] defensins,[55]

SP-A and -D,[56,57] acid mammalian chitinase,[58] collectins,[18] serum amyloid A,[18] and secretory leukocyte proteinase inhibitor.[59] Lysozyme, lactoferrin, and secretory leukocyte proteinase inhibitor are the most abundant antimicrobial peptides in nasal secretions.[60] The antimicrobial peptides are secreted in response to microbes, thus inhibiting or directly lysing the microorganism through endogenous antibiotics. These peptides also have other immune functions and can attract and activate effector cells of the innate and adaptive immune system. For example, the human cathelicidin LL-37 is chemotactic for neutrophils, monocytes, and T cells.[61] Conversely, these peptides can also suppress or modulate the adaptive immune system. SP-D has been shown to inhibit lymphocyte proliferation,[62] cause a shift from a Th1 to Th2 cytokine response, and regulate dendritic cell responses.[63]

SP-A and -D are members of the collectin family of proteins involved in innate immunity.[1] Deficiency of SP-A and -D in patients with cystic fibrosis is believed to result in increased frequency of bacterial colonization, infections, and inflammation.[64] In the study by Postle and colleagues,[64] the levels of SP-D protein in BALF were significantly decreased in patients with cystic fibrosis (median, 0.1 μg/mL) compared with the acute infection (12.17 μg/mL) and control (641 μg/mL) groups.

SP-A and -D mRNA and protein have been identified in the sinonasal mucosa of healthy controls and patients with CRS.[56,57,65] Woodworth and colleagues[66] showed that SP-A and -D mRNA levels were up-regulated in the CRS and cystic fibrosis groups. Ooi and colleagues showed[56] that SP-D protein levels were undetectable using ELISA or immunohistochemistry in patients with allergic fungal rhinosinusitis (AFRS) and were decreased in those with CRS relative to the normal controls.

SP-A, -D, and tumor necrosis factor α protein levels were investigated in sinus mucosal biopsies from cystic fibrosis, AFRS, and controls using semiquantitative Western blot analysis.[67] The cystic fibrosis group had reduced SP-A, -D, and tumor necrosis factor α protein levels compared with controls but higher levels than the AFRS group.

BALF collected from patients with chronic obstructive pulmonary disease (COPD) and healthy control subjects was subjected to multivariate linear regression analysis.[51] This study showed reduced SP-D levels in the group with COPD but higher levels in those using inhaled corticosteroids. The investigators evaluated the effects of dexamethasone on type II alveolar epithelial cells from rat lungs and found that SP-D mRNA and protein, but not SP-A, increased after 4 days of culture with dexamethasone (10 ng/mL). Experts speculate that corticosteroids in CRS may boost SP-D levels and be a potent anti-inflammatory treatment.

In summary, several studies have shown reduced levels of secreted SP-A and -D in patients with cystic fibrosis. However, no studies have investigated secreted SP levels in CRS. One study showed reduced secreted SP-D levels in CRS in response to fungal extract challenge compared with normal controls, but that was a mucosal explant in vitro model.[56] Further research is required to investigate the levels of SPs produced and secreted in patients with CRS compared with normal controls, and to study the effects of corticosteroids on SP-A and -D levels in larger studies with sinus biopsies and human cell cultures.

Biofilms are organized communities of microbial cells encased in a self-produced exopolysaccharide matrix and irreversibly attached to an inert or living surface.[9] Most bacteria exist in this biofilm form, with only 1% residing in the free-floating or planktonic form, which is the form that clinicians commonly culture. Through intercellular signaling called *quorum sensing*, planktonic bacteria are believed to undergo genotypic and phenotypic alterations, converting them into the more robust and resistant biofilm form. This form has a much slower growth and metabolic rate, and in its dormant state can evade the host's immune system.

Biofilms have been implicated as a potential cause of CRS in a subset of patients, with these structures identified in sinus biopsies taken from patients undergoing sinus surgery.[13,68,69] The study by Psaltis and colleagues[68] also found that patients with biofilms seemed to have more clinical and endoscopic evidence of ongoing postoperative inflammation, and speculated that these structures may explain the recalcitrant nature of CRS. This study also showed that the presence of fungus was associated with an adverse outcome after endoscopic sinus surgery. Using the modified Calgary Biofilm Detection Assay, Prince and colleagues[70] showed that 28.6% (45/157 samples) of bacteria cultured in sinuses from bacterial swabs of patients with CRS undergoing endoscopic sinus surgery can form biofilms in vitro. The most common organism cultured was *Staphylococcus aureus*, followed by polymicrobial infections and *P aeruginosa*. More recently, pan-fungal and specific bacterial fluorescent in situ hybridization probes showed the presence of fungus within bacterial biofilms of patients with AFRS, CRS and eosinophilic mucin rhinosinsitis.[69]

Topical treatments are an evolving area of interest in the medical management of refractory CRS that has failed to respond to standard treatments.[71–78] Their use partly evolved from experience with topical tobramycin in treating chronic *Pseudomonas* infections in patients with cystic fibrosis, in whom a much higher dose of antibiotic can be delivered locally to achieve a higher minimal inhibitory concentration without causing adverse effects usually associated with systemic administration.[79]

Research on topical treatments has focused mainly on biofilms and fungus.[80,81] For example, regular treatment with topical mupirocin for 7 days has been shown to have the most significant effect on inhibiting biofilm formation in a sheep model of Staphylococcal biofilm sinusitis.[81]

One area of interest is the possibility of using endogenous antimicrobial peptides as topical treatments for CRS. The cathelicidin LL-37 has antibacterial and antifungal properties and is being explored as a novel approach to treating infections and inflammation.[82] Synthetic LL-37 has recently been shown in vitro to have antibiofilm properties when cultured with *P aeruginosa* at concentrations below what is required to kill the bacteria.[83] *P aeruginosa* cultured with 0.5 μg/mL LL-37, which is far below the concentration required to kill or inhibit bacterial growth (1/128 minimal inhibitory concentration), led to a 40% decrease in biofilm mass. An increasing dose-dependent effect was seen, with a maximum of 80% inhibition at 16 μg/mL LL-37 (1/4 minimal inhibitory concentration).

LL-37 was also shown to affect established *P aeruginosa* biofilms, with loss of the characteristic mature untreated biofilm architecture when 4 μg/mL LL-37 was added and incubated for 2 days after mature biofilm formation was observed. Confocal scanning laser microscopy was used to identify biofilms with the BacLight kit (Invitrogen, Carlsbad, CA, USA) to identify live and dead bacteria, and crystal violet staining and absorbance were used to assess growth of biofilm. LL-37 was further shown to affect biofilm formation through decreasing the attachment of bacterial cells, stimulating twitch motility, and down-regulating the genes responsible for the quorum-sensing system of biofilms (Las and Rhi).

Chennupati and colleagues[77] showed that synthetic LL-37 used in an animal model of biofilm *Pseudomonas* sinusitis successfully eradicated the biofilm and decreased bacterial counts. However, this occurred at the higher concentration of 2.5 mg/mL, whereas at the lowest concentration of 0.1 mg/mL, evidence of rods was still present on scanning electron microscopy, suggesting biofilm formation, although the highest concentration of LL-37 (2.5 mg/mL) caused increasing inflammation and ciliotoxicity. LL-37 can cause apoptosis in vitro of human airway epithelial cells.[84]

Overhage and colleagues[83] observed significant inhibition of biofilm growth with much lower concentrations of LL-37 compared with the study by Chennupati and colleagues[77] (4 μg/mL vs 2.5 mg/mL, respectively). Different biofilm detection methods may explain the findings, because Overhage and colleagues[83] used confocal scanning laser microscopy, which is reported to be more accurate in detecting biofilms than scanning electron microscopy.[85,86] Alternatively differences in LL-37 peptide synthesis may explain the differences in concentration findings. Mucus may not be easily distinguished from the biofilm exopolysaccharide matrix, and the rods seen may represent architectural distortion or artifact when using scanning electron microscopy.[86]

Lipopolysaccharide (LPS) and lipoteichoic acid (LTA) are major components of gram-negative and -positive bacteria, respectively. LPS and LTA increase epithelial cell thickness and squamous metaplasia, impairing mucociliary clearance. A novel LL-37–derived antimicrobial peptide P60.4-Ac inhibited the ability of LPS or LTA to cause these epithelial changes in an in vitro air–liquid interface culture of primary cells from the sinus mucosa.[87]

In summary, recent in vitro results support LL-37 as a potential therapeutic option against biofilms, but evidence in an animal model of biofilm sinusitis indicates that loss of cilia at high concentration would limit its use as topical therapy.[77,83]

Lactoferrin is another innate immune molecule known to inhibit P aeruginosa biofilm formation at concentrations again below those that kill or inhibit bacterial growth.[88] Lactoferrin chelates iron, thus stimulating twitching and causing the bacteria to migrate across the surface instead of coalescing to form biofilms. Lactoferrin also has direct bactericidal and fungicidal activity independent of its iron-binding capacity.[89] The mRNA and protein expression of lactoferrin are significantly reduced in patients with CRS and eosinophilic mucus CRS compared with normal controls, suggesting a defect in innate immunity perhaps predisposing to CRS development.[52]

Psaltis and colleagues[90] analyzed patients with CRS for the presence of biofilms and found that patients who tested positive for the presence of biofilm had a significantly reduced lactoferrin expression compared with those who tested negative. The association between lactoferrin down-regulation and presence of biofilms is intriguing and requires further exploration.

Lysozyme is found to be expressed strongly in neutrophils, serous cells of the submucosal glands, and goblet cells.[91,92] It is an enzyme directed against the peptidoglycan component of the bacterial cell wall, causing cell lysis.[93] It also has anti-fungal properties and acts synergistically with antimycotic agents.[94] More recently, lysozyme was shown to inhibit biofilm formation against Candida on denture acrylic surfaces.[95] Lysozyme precursor C was down-regulated in patients with CRS compared with normal controls using proteomic techniques to analyze aspirated nasal mucus.[96]

Currently, a paucity of research exists on lysozyme in rhinology, despite its being one of the most abundant antimicrobials in nasal fluid[60] and its recently shown antifungal and antibiofilm properties.[95] In summary, evidence is emerging on the use of these peptides for treating CRS, especially in preventing biofilm formation. The antimicrobial properties of naturally occurring compounds, such as honey, may be caused by antimicrobial peptides.[97] Further studies are required to explore the role of these antimicrobial peptides and whether they can be used, either topically or systemically, as disease-modifying therapy in CRS.

SUMMARY
Implications for Research

Increasing evidence shows innate immunity abnormalities in CRS. Whether these are associated abnormalities or a direct cause of CRS is currently unknown. Evidence

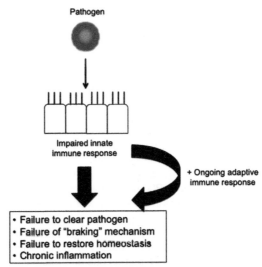

Fig. 2. Schematic of impaired innate immunity in chronic rhinosinusitis with proposed multiple abnormalities resulting in chronic inflammation.

indicates that failure of the local innate immune mucosal braking mechanism and persistent activation of adaptive immunity may lead to chronic inflammation (**Fig. 2**). If experts believe that innate immunity abnormalities result in an abnormal local response to the pathogen rather than are caused by the pathogen itself, this possibility has implications as a likely important differentiating factor between healthy individuals and those with CRS.[1] Future research will need to be directed toward improved diagnostic methods and treatment of specific innate immunity abnormalities (**Fig. 3**).

Implications for Clinical Practice

Clinicians should continue to discourage smoking in patients with CRS, because it appears to adversely affect innate immunity. Testing for *CFTR* mutations should be considered in younger patients with recalcitrant CRS. Biopsies taken at surgery reflect the preexisting CRS condition, but few studies have obtained biopsies after surgery to determine if mucosal innate immunity returns to normal after surgery. Failure of improvement in CRS after standard medical therapy and endoscopic sinus surgery may be from underlying innate immunity abnormalities. Management of CRS can be

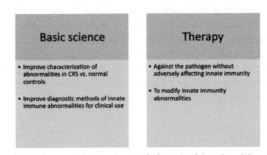

Fig. 3. Future research for innate immunity and chronic rhinosinusitis with implications for basic science and therapy.

improved in the future with better understanding of innate immunity and development of novel therapies to enhance innate immunity (see **Fig. 3**).

REFERENCES

1. Ooi EH, Wormald PJ, Tan LW. Innate immunity in the paranasal sinuses: a review of nasal host defenses. Am J Rhinol 2008;22(1):13–9.
2. Bals R, Hiemstra PS. Innate immunity in the lung: how epithelial cells fight against respiratory pathogens. Eur Respir J 2004;23(2):327–33.
3. Lane AP. The role of innate immunity in the pathogenesis of chronic rhinosinusitis. Curr Allergy Asthma Rep 2009;9(3):205–12.
4. Benninger MS, Ferguson BJ, Hadley JA, et al. Adult chronic rhinosinusitis: definitions, diagnosis, epidemiology, and pathophysiology. Otolaryngol Head Neck Surg 2003;129(Suppl 3):S1–32.
5. Anand VK. Epidemiology and economic impact of rhinosinusitis. Ann Otol Rhinol Laryngol Suppl 2004;193:3–5.
6. Metson RB, Gliklich RE. Clinical outcomes in patients with chronic sinusitis. Laryngoscope 2000;110(3 Pt 3):24–8.
7. Van Cauwenberge P, Watelet JB. Epidemiology of chronic rhinosinusitis. Thorax 2000;55(Suppl 2):S20–1.
8. Meltzer EO, Hamilos DL, Hadley JA, et al. Rhinosinusitis: establishing definitions for clinical research and patient care. J Allergy Clin Immunol 2004;114(6 Suppl): 155–212.
9. Cohen M, Kofonow J, Nayak JV, et al. Biofilms in chronic rhinosinusitis: a review. Am J Rhinol Allergy 2009;23(3):255–60.
10. Seiberling KA, Grammer L, Kern RC. Chronic rhinosinusitis and superantigens. Otolaryngol Clin North Am 2005;38(6):1215–36, ix.
11. Sasama J, Sherris DA, Shin SH, et al. New paradigm for the roles of fungi and eosinophils in chronic rhinosinusitis. Curr Opin Otolaryngol Head Neck Surg 2005;13(1):2–8.
12. Braun H, Buzina W, Freudenschuss K, et al. 'Eosinophilic fungal rhinosinusitis': a common disorder in Europe? Laryngoscope 2003;113(2):264–9.
13. Sanderson AR, Leid JG, Hunsaker D. Bacterial biofilms on the sinus mucosa of human subjects with chronic rhinosinusitis. Laryngoscope 2006;116(7):1121–6.
14. Kern RC, Conley DB, Walsh W, et al. Perspectives on the etiology of chronic rhinosinusitis: an immune barrier hypothesis. Am J Rhinol 2008;22(6):549–59.
15. Kumar H, Kawai T, Akira S. Pathogen recognition in the innate immune response. Biochem J 2009;420(1):1–16.
16. Lin CF, Tsai CH, Cheng CH, et al. Expression of Toll-like receptors in cultured nasal epithelial cells. Acta Otolaryngol 2007;127(4):395–402.
17. Dong Z, Yang Z, Wang C. Expression of TLR2 and TLR4 messenger RNA in the epithelial cells of the nasal airway. Am J Rhinol 2005;19(3):236–9.
18. Lane AP, Truong-Tran QA, Myers A, et al. Serum amyloid A, properdin, complement 3, and toll-like receptors are expressed locally in human sinonasal tissue. Am J Rhinol 2006;20(1):117–23.
19. Rampey AM, Lathers DM, Woodworth BA, et al. Immunolocalization of dendritic cells and pattern recognition receptors in chronic rhinosinusitis. Am J Rhinol 2007;21(1):117–21.
20. Vanhinsbergh LJ, Powe DG, Jones NS. Reduction of TLR2 gene expression in allergic and nonallergic rhinitis. Ann Allergy Asthma Immunol 2007;99(6): 509–16.

21. Pitzurra L, Bellocchio S, Nocentini A, et al. Antifungal immune reactivity in nasal polyposis. Infect Immun 2004;72(12):7275–81.
22. Tan L, Rogers TJ, Hatzirodos N, et al. Immunomodulatory effect of cytosine-phosphate-guanosine (CpG)-oligonucleotides in nonasthmatic chronic rhinosinusitis: an explant model. Am J Rhinol Allergy 2009;23(2):123–9.
23. Fokkens W, Lund V, Mullol J. European position paper on rhinosinusitis and nasal polyps 2007. Rhinol Suppl 2007;20:1–136.
24. Wise SK, Kingdom TT, McKean L, et al. Presence of fungus in sinus cultures of cystic fibrosis patients. Am J Rhinol 2005;19(1):47–51.
25. Pinto JM, Hayes MG, Schneider D, et al. A genomewide screen for chronic rhinosinusitis genes identifies a locus on chromosome 7q. Laryngoscope 2008; 118(11):2067–72.
26. Wang X, Kim J, McWilliams R, et al. Increased prevalence of chronic rhinosinusitis in carriers of a cystic fibrosis mutation. Arch Otolaryngol Head Neck Surg 2005;131(3):237–40.
27. Raman V, Clary R, Siegrist KL, et al. Increased prevalence of mutations in the cystic fibrosis transmembrane conductance regulator in children with chronic rhinosinusitis. Pediatrics 2002;109(1):E13.
28. Doring G, Gulbins E. Cystic fibrosis and innate immunity: how chloride channel mutations provoke lung disease. Cell Microbiol 2009;11(2):208–16.
29. Smith JJ, Travis SM, Greenberg EP, et al. Cystic fibrosis airway epithelia fail to kill bacteria because of abnormal airway surface fluid. Cell 1996;85(2): 229–36.
30. Cohen NA. Sinonasal mucociliary clearance in health and disease. Ann Otol Rhinol Laryngol Suppl 2006;196:20–6.
31. Messerklinger W. [On the drainage of the human paranasal sinuses under normal and pathological conditions 1]. Monatsschr Ohrenheilkd Laryngorhinol 1966; 100(1–2):56–68 [in German].
32. Schenck NL. Frontal sinus disease. III. Experimental and clinical factors in failure of the frontal osteoplastic operation. Laryngoscope 1975;85(1):76–92.
33. Kennedy DW. Functional endoscopic sinus surgery. Technique. Arch Otolaryngol 1985;111(10):643–9.
34. Sakakura Y, Majima Y, Saida S, et al. Reversibility of reduced mucociliary clearance in chronic sinusitis. Clin Otolaryngol 1985;10(2):79–83.
35. Elwany S, Hisham M, Gamaee R. The effect of endoscopic sinus surgery on mucociliary clearance in patients with chronic sinusitis. Eur Arch Otorhinolaryngol 1998;255(10):511–4.
36. Inanli S, Tutkun A, Batman C, et al. The effect of endoscopic sinus surgery on mucociliary activity and healing of maxillary sinus mucosa. Rhinology 2000;38(3): 120–3.
37. Chen B, Shaari J, Claire SE, et al. Altered sinonasal ciliary dynamics in chronic rhinosinusitis. Am J Rhinol 2006;20(3):325–9.
38. Chen B, Antunes MB, Claire SE, et al. Reversal of chronic rhinosinusitis-associated sinonasal ciliary dysfunction. Am J Rhinol 2007;21(3):346–53.
39. Maccabee MS, Trune DR, Hwang PH. Paranasal sinus mucosal regeneration: the effect of topical retinoic acid. Am J Rhinol 2003;17(3):133–7.
40. Briggs RD, Wright ST, Cordes S, et al. Smoking in chronic rhinosinusitis: a predictor of poor long-term outcome after endoscopic sinus surgery. Laryngoscope 2004;114(1):126–8.
41. Houser SM, Keen KJ. The role of allergy and smoking in chronic rhinosinusitis and polyposis. Laryngoscope 2008;118(9):1521–7.

42. Karaman M, Tek A. Deleterious effect of smoking and nasal septal deviation on mucociliary clearance and improvement after septoplasty. Am J Rhinol Allergy 2009;23(1):2–7.
43. Dye JA, Adler KB. Effects of cigarette smoke on epithelial cells of the respiratory tract. Thorax 1994;49(8):825–34.
44. Mehta H, Nazzal K, Sadikot RT. Cigarette smoking and innate immunity. Inflamm Res 2008;57(11):497–503.
45. Lan MY, Ho CY, Lee TC, et al. Cigarette smoke extract induces cytotoxicity on human nasal epithelial cells. Am J Rhinol 2007;21(2):218–23.
46. Lee WK, Ramanathan M Jr, Spannhake EW, et al. The cigarette smoke component acrolein inhibits expression of the innate immune components IL-8 and human beta-defensin 2 by sinonasal epithelial cells. Am J Rhinol 2007;21(6): 658–63.
47. Tamashiro E, Xiong G, Anselmo-Lima WT, et al. Cigarette smoke exposure impairs respiratory epithelial ciliogenesis. Am J Rhinol Allergy 2009;23(2): 117–22.
48. Cantin AM, Hanrahan JW, Bilodeau G, et al. Cystic fibrosis transmembrane conductance regulator function is suppressed in cigarette smokers. Am J Respir Crit Care Med 2006;173(10):1139–44.
49. Bajmoczi M, Gadjeva M, Alper SL, et al. Cystic fibrosis transmembrane conductance regulator and caveolin-1 regulate epithelial cell internalization of Pseudomonas aeruginosa. Am J Physiol Cell Physiol 2009;297(2):C263–77.
50. MacRedmond RE, Greene CM, Dorscheid DR, et al. Epithelial expression of TLR4 is modulated in COPD and by steroids, salmeterol and cigarette smoke. Respir Res 2007;8:84.
51. Sims MW, Tal-Singer RM, Kierstein S, et al. Chronic obstructive pulmonary disease and inhaled steroids alter surfactant protein D (SP-D) levels: a cross-sectional study. Respir Res 2008;9:13.
52. Psaltis AJ, Bruhn MA, Ooi EH, et al. Nasal mucosa expression of lactoferrin in patients with chronic rhinosinusitis. Laryngoscope 2007;117(11):2030–5.
53. Kalfa VC, Spector SL, Ganz T, et al. Lysozyme levels in the nasal secretions of patients with perennial allergic rhinitis and recurrent sinusitis. Ann Allergy Asthma Immunol 2004;93(3):288–92.
54. Ooi EH, Wormald PJ, Carney AS, et al. Human cathelicidin antimicrobial peptide is up-regulated in the eosinophilic mucus subgroup of chronic rhinosinusitis patients. Am J Rhinol 2007;21(4):395–401.
55. Lee SH, Kim JE, Lim HH, et al. Antimicrobial defensin peptides of the human nasal mucosa. Ann Otol Rhinol Laryngol 2002;111(2):135–41.
56. Ooi EH, Wormald PJ, Carney AS, et al. Surfactant protein D expression in chronic rhinosinusitis patients and immune responses in vitro to Aspergillus and Alternaria in a nasal explant model. Laryngoscope 2007;117(1):51–7.
57. Woodworth BA, Neal JG, Newton D, et al. Surfactant protein A and D in human sinus mucosa: a preliminary report. ORL J Otorhinolaryngol Relat Spec 2007; 69(1):57–60.
58. Ramanathan M Jr, Lee WK, Lane AP. Increased expression of acidic mammalian chitinase in chronic rhinosinusitis with nasal polyps. Am J Rhinol 2006;20(3):330–5.
59. Singh PK, Tack BF, McCray PB Jr, et al. Synergistic and additive killing by antimicrobial factors found in human airway surface liquid. Am J Physiol Lung Cell Mol Physiol 2000;279(5):L799–805.
60. Cole AM, Liao HI, Stuchlik O, et al. Cationic polypeptides are required for antibacterial activity of human airway fluid. J Immunol 2002;169(12):6985–91.

61. De Y, Chen Q, Schmidt AP, et al. LL-37, the neutrophil granule- and epithelial cell-derived cathelicidin, utilizes formyl peptide receptor-like 1 (FPRL1) as a receptor to chemoattract human peripheral blood neutrophils, monocytes, and T cells. J Exp Med 2000;192(7):1069–74.

62. Borron PJ, Mostaghel EA, Doyle C, et al. Pulmonary surfactant proteins A and D directly suppress CD3+/CD4+ cell function: evidence for two shared mechanisms. J Immunol 2002;169(10):5844–50.

63. Haczku A. Protective role of the lung collectins surfactant protein A and surfactant protein D in airway inflammation. J Allergy Clin Immunol 2008;122(5): 861–79 [quiz: 880–1].

64. Postle AD, Mander A, Reid KB, et al. Deficient hydrophilic lung surfactant proteins A and D with normal surfactant phospholipid molecular species in cystic fibrosis. Am J Respir Cell Mol Biol 1999;20(1):90–8.

65. Woodworth BA, Lathers D, Neal JG, et al. Immunolocalization of surfactant protein A and D in sinonasal mucosa. Am J Rhinol 2006;20(4):461–5.

66. Woodworth BA, Wood R, Baatz JE, et al. Sinonasal surfactant protein A1, A2, and D gene expression in cystic fibrosis: a preliminary report. Otolaryngol Head Neck Surg 2007;137(1):34–8.

67. Skinner ML, Schlosser RJ, Lathers D, et al. Innate and adaptive mediators in cystic fibrosis and allergic fungal rhinosinusitis. Am J Rhinol 2007;21(5):538–41.

68. Psaltis AJ, Weitzel EK, Ha KR, et al. The effect of bacterial biofilms on post-sinus surgical outcomes. Am J Rhinol 2008;22(1):1–6.

69. Healy DY, Leid JG, Sanderson AR, et al. Biofilms with fungi in chronic rhinosinusitis. Otolaryngol Head Neck Surg 2008;138(5):641–7.

70. Prince AA, Steiger JD, Khalid AN, et al. Prevalence of biofilm-forming bacteria in chronic rhinosinusitis. Am J Rhinol 2008;22(3):239–45.

71. Ha KR, Psaltis AJ, Butcher AR, et al. In vitro activity of mupirocin on clinical isolates of Staphylococcus aureus and its potential implications in chronic rhinosinusitis. Laryngoscope 2008;118(3):535–40.

72. Alandejani T, Marsan J, Ferris W, et al. Effectiveness of honey on Staphylococcus aureus and Pseudomonas aeruginosa biofilms. Otolaryngol Head Neck Surg 2009;141(1):114–8.

73. Lim M, Citardi MJ, Leong JL. Topical antimicrobials in the management of chronic rhinosinusitis: a systematic review. Am J Rhinol 2008;22(4):381–9.

74. Uren B, Psaltis A, Wormald PJ. Nasal lavage with mupirocin for the treatment of surgically recalcitrant chronic rhinosinusitis. Laryngoscope 2008;118(9):1677–80.

75. Elliott KA, Stringer SP. Evidence-based recommendations for antimicrobial nasal washes in chronic rhinosinusitis. Am J Rhinol 2006;20(1):1–6.

76. Chiu AG, Antunes MB, Palmer JN, et al. Evaluation of the in vivo efficacy of topical tobramycin against Pseudomonas sinonasal biofilms. J Antimicrob Chemother 2007;59(6):1130–4.

77. Chennupati SK, Chiu AG, Tamashiro E, et al. Effects of an LL-37-derived antimicrobial peptide in an animal model of biofilm Pseudomonas sinusitis. Am J Rhinol Allergy 2009;23(1):46–51.

78. Antunes MB, Feldman MD, Cohen NA, et al. Dose-dependent effects of topical tobramycin in an animal model of Pseudomonas sinusitis. Am J Rhinol 2007; 21(4):423–7.

79. Geller DE. Aerosol antibiotics in cystic fibrosis. Respir Care 2009;54(5):658–70.

80. Ebbens FA, Scadding GK, Badia L, et al. Amphotericin B nasal lavages: Not a solution for patients with chronic rhinosinusitis. J Allergy Clin Immunol 2006; 118(5):1149–56.

81. Le T, Psaltis A, Tan LW, et al. The efficacy of topical antibiofilm agents in a sheep model of rhinosinusitis. Am J Rhinol 2008;22(6):560–7.
82. Nijnik A, Hancock RE. The roles of cathelicidin LL-37 in immune defenses and novel clinical applications. Curr Opin Hematol 2009;16(1):41–7.
83. Overhage J, Campisano A, Bains M, et al. Human host defense peptide LL-37 prevents bacterial biofilm formation. Infect Immun 2008;76(9):4176–82.
84. Lau YE, Bowdish DM, Cosseau C, et al. Apoptosis of airway epithelial cells: human serum sensitive induction by the cathelicidin LL-37. Am J Respir Cell Mol Biol 2006;34(4):399–409.
85. Psaltis AJ, Ha KR, Beule AG, et al. Confocal scanning laser microscopy evidence of biofilms in patients with chronic rhinosinusitis. Laryngoscope 2007;117(7):1302–6.
86. Ha KR, Psaltis AJ, Tan L, et al. A sheep model for the study of biofilms in rhinosinusitis. Am J Rhinol 2007;21(3):339–45.
87. Vonk MJ, Hiemstra PS, Grote JJ. An antimicrobial peptide modulates epithelial responses to bacterial products. Laryngoscope 2008;118(5):816–20.
88. Singh PK, Parsek MR, Greenberg EP, et al. A component of innate immunity prevents bacterial biofilm development. Nature 2002;417(6888):552–5.
89. Farnaud S, Evans RW. Lactoferrin–a multifunctional protein with antimicrobial properties. Mol Immunol 2003;40(7):395–405.
90. Psaltis AJ, Wormald PJ, Ha KR, et al. Reduced levels of lactoferrin in biofilm-associated chronic rhinosinusitis. Laryngoscope 2008;118(5):895–901.
91. Raphael GD, Jeney EV, Baraniuk JN, et al. Pathophysiology of rhinitis. Lactoferrin and lysozyme in nasal secretions. J Clin Invest 1989;84(5):1528–35.
92. Fukami M, Stierna P, Veress B, et al. Lysozyme and lactoferrin in human maxillary sinus mucosa during chronic sinusitis. An immunohistochemical study. Eur Arch Otorhinolaryngol 1993;250(3):133–9.
93. Ellison RT 3rd, Giehl TJ. Killing of gram-negative bacteria by lactoferrin and lysozyme. J Clin Invest 1991;88(4):1080–91.
94. Anil S, Samaranayake LP. Impact of lysozyme and lactoferrin on oral Candida isolates exposed to polyene antimycotics and fluconazole. Oral Dis 2002;8(4):199–206.
95. Samaranayake YH, Cheung BP, Parahitiyawa N, et al. Synergistic activity of lysozyme and antifungal agents against Candida albicans biofilms on denture acrylic surfaces. Arch Oral Biol 2009;54(2):115–26.
96. Tewfik MA, Latterich M, DiFalco MR, et al. Proteomics of nasal mucus in chronic rhinosinusitis. Am J Rhinol 2007;21(6):680–5.
97. Lee H, Churey JJ, Worobo RW. Antimicrobial activity of bacterial isolates from different floral sources of honey. Int J Food Microbiol 2008;126(1–2):240–4.

Superantigens

Nicholas W. Stow, FRACS[a,b,*], Richard Douglas, FRACS[a,b],
Pongsakorn Tantilipikorn, MD, FRCOT[c],
Jean Silvain Lacroix, MD, PhD[d]

KEYWORDS

- Superantigen • Enterotoxin • Rhinosinusitis • Rhinitis
- Allergy • *Staphylococcus aureus*

The concept of superantigens (SAgs) was first described in 1989 in reference to the polyclonal activation of T lymphocytes by the staphylococcal enterotoxin B.[1] Since then, many other proteins with SAg properties have been reported. A new group of SAgs, which act as superallergens by stimulating mast cells and basophils with a wide range of immunoglobulin (Ig) E specificities, have been observed. In addition, a group of SAg-like proteins, which have multiple effects on the innate immune system, have been recently described.

It is now known that SAgs are derived from diverse sources, including gram-positive and gram-negative bacteria, viruses, and even human hepatic tissue. There is evidence that SAgs have actions not only on T lymphocytes but also more broadly within the immune system, affecting B lymphocytes, mast cells, basophils, and chemokine production. Of particular relevance to otorhinolaryngologists is the involvement of SAgs in the pathogenesis of inflammatory airway conditions, including allergic rhinitis, chronic rhinosinusitis with nasal polyposis (CRSwNP), and asthma.

This article aims to summarize the current knowledge of SAgs and their relevance to current clinical rhinologic practice and research.

IMMUNE RESPONSE TO CONVENTIONAL ANTIGENS

To explain the actions of SAgs, the immune response to conventional antigens is very briefly outlined. Antigen-presenting cells (APCs), such as monocyte-macrophage

Disclaimer: Financial support: none to declare.

[a] Department of Otorhinolaryngology–Head and Neck Surgery, North Shore Hospital, Private Bag 93-503 Takapuna, North Shore City 0740, Auckland, New Zealand

[b] Department of Otorhinolaryngology-Head and Neck Surgery, Auckland City Hospital, 2 Park Road, Grafton 1010, New Zealand

[c] Division of Rhinology and Allergy, Department of Otolaryngology, Faculty of Medicine, Siriraj Hospital, Mahidol University, 2 Prannok Street, Bangkok 10700, Thailand

[d] Rhinology-Olfaction Unit, Department of Otorhinolaryngology–Head and Neck Surgery, Geneva University Hospital, 4 Rue Gabrielle-Perret-Gentil, CH-1211, Geneva 14, Switzerland

* Corresponding author. Department of Otorhinolaryngology–Head and Neck Surgery, North Shore Hospital, Private Bag 93-503 Takapuna, North Shore City 0740, Auckland, New Zealand.

E-mail address: nickstow@hotmail.com

Otolaryngol Clin N Am 43 (2010) 489–502
doi:10.1016/j.otc.2010.02.008
0030-6665/10/$ – see front matter © 2010 Elsevier Inc. All rights reserved.

cells, dendritic cells, or B lymphocytes, encounter an antigen, internalize and process it, and then present it on their cell membranes held within the antigen-presenting groove of major histocompatibility complex (MHC) class II proteins. Subsequent activation of a CD4+ helper T lymphocyte occurs when its cell surface receptor (T lymphocyte cell receptor [TCR]) interacts with the presented antigen–MHC II complex on the APC (**Fig. 1**). This interaction, which requires CD4 as a coreceptor, is highly specific; only a few T-lymphocyte clones will possess the particular TCR capable of binding to a given antigen. The conventional antigen–MHC II interaction involves the variable regions of both the TCR's α and β chains (TCRV$_\alpha$ and TCRV$_\beta$). The result is a T-lymphocyte clonal response in which there is a selective activation and proliferation of less than 0.1% of the naive T-lymphocyte repertoire.[2] Subsequently, some clones are deleted but others persist as memory T lymphocytes, which facilitate a more rapid and vigorous secondary immune response after reexposure to the same antigen.

The humoral immune system also plays a role in the response to conventional antigens. Natural antibodies (usually IgM) act as a first line of defense by binding to antigens, which enter the circulation.[3] In a manner analogous to the TCR-antigen interaction, B lymphocytes have membrane-bound Immunoglobulins, which act as antigen receptors (B lymphocyte cell receptors [BCRs]). Antigen binds to a specific BCR, leading to a B-lymphocyte clonal response. B lymphocytes also present the processed antigen to T lymphocytes, and this interaction stimulates transformation of B lymphocytes into plasma cells and the synthesis of immunoglobulins specific for that antigen.

The innate immune system plays an important role in sinonasal mucosal defense and has several components (**Fig. 2**).

THE ACTIONS OF SAGS ON THE IMMUNE SYSTEM

The initial report of the effect of a staphylococcal SAg on T lymphocytes described a non–antigen specific activation.[1] Subsequent research has shown that the biologic effects of these proteins are much more diverse. Although many of the effects of SAgs are proinflammatory, it is now understood that during the early stages of bacterial colonization or infection SAgs may in fact facilitate the avoidance or suppression of local immune mechanisms.[4] In this way, SAgs may confer an evolutionary advantage on bacteria.

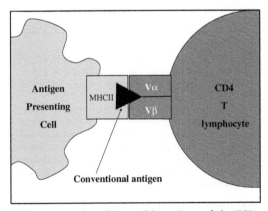

Fig. 1. Conventional antigens bind to the variable regions of the TCR's α and β chains and the MHC class II molecules on the surface of APCs.

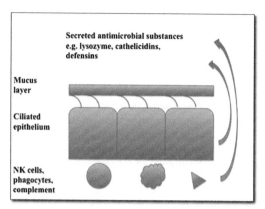

Fig. 2. The sinonasal mucosal innate immune system has several components: an intact epithelium with a mucociliary layer, phagocytic cells, natural killer cells, and the complement cascade.

The classical SAgs are *Staphylococcus aureus* exotoxins. These proteins have 3 targets in the adaptive immune system: the TCR, the BCR, and the MHC class II proteins on APCs.[5] In this manner, SAgs may be classified as T- or B-lymphocyte SAgs.

The Actions of SAgs on T Lymphocytes

SAgs are the most powerful of all known T-lymphocyte mitogens.[6] Unlike conventional antigens, T-lymphocyte SAgs do not undergo processing by APCs. Instead, they possess structural features that allow them to bind directly and sequentially to the MHC class II proteins on APCs and then to the TCR's β chain at a region that lies outside the conventional antigen–specific binding site (**Fig. 3**).[4] In this manner, the conventional antigen-specific T-lymphocyte activation is bypassed and a T-lymphocyte supraclonal response follows, involving more than 5% of the naive T-lymphocyte repertoire.[2] This widespread activation may induce massive cytokine release from CD4[+] lymphocytes (predominantly interleukin [IL] 2 and tumor necrosis factor α)

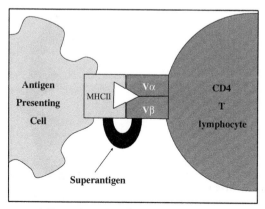

Fig. 3. SAgs bind sequentially to the MHC class II proteins on APCs and then to the TCR's β chain, outside the conventional antigen–specific binding site.

and CD8[+] lymphocytes (predominantly interferon gamma). In contrast to the response to conventional antigens, most of the activated T lymphocytes are subsequently deleted, sometimes to such an extent that their numbers decrease below original levels.[7] This clonal deletion benefits both the host, by moving toward resolution of the inflammation, and the microbe, by allowing it to subvert the immune response, because the clones that are not deleted become anergic rather than becoming memory cells.[7–9] In addition, SAgs activate CD4[+] regulatory T lymphocytes, which then act to suppress the immune response via secretion of IL-10 and transforming growth factor β.[7]

Different SAgs show different binding preferences for various MHC class II alleles and TCR profiles. However, the affinity of SAgs binding to MHC class II molecules is consistently more than 10 times greater than their affinity for binding to TCR.[4] There exist low-affinity and high-affinity binding interfaces between SAgs and different MHC class II alleles. Of the human MHCs, HLA-DR tends to have the greatest affinity for SAg binding, followed by HLA-DQ, and then HLA-DP.[10] With regard to TCR interactions, SAgs have been divided into 3 groups based on their specificity of binding to regions of TCRV$_\beta$ proteins.[9] Human T lymphocytes have about 50 possible TCRV$_\beta$ regions, and each SAg may stimulate up to 20% of these regions.[6]

Unlike conventional antigens, SAgs do not need CD4 as a coreceptor in the activation of T lymphocytes, and their structure does not change significantly after binding.[9]

The Actions of SAgs on B Lymphocytes

B lymphocytes have cell surface immunoglobulins, which interact with antigens without requiring presentation of the antigen by MHC class II proteins of APCs. B-lymphocyte SAgs bypass the conventional antigen–binding site of human immunoglobulin molecules. Conventional antigens bind to the hypervariable region of surface immunoglobulins (**Fig 4**), whereas SAgs bind to certain areas of the variable regions of the heavy or light chain of membrane-associated immunoglobulin (which is the B lymphocyte equivalent of the TCR, **Fig 5**). These areas have been conserved over the course of human evolution so that a large proportion of B lymphocytes possess them.[3] B-lymphocyte SAgs then activate BCRs by cross-linking them. The cross-linking is possible because the SAgs are composed of oligovalent or multivalent arrays of

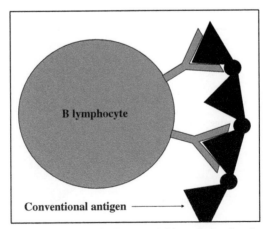

Fig. 4. Conventional antigens bind to the hypervariable regions of surface immunoglobulins on B lymphocytes.

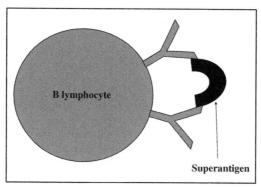

Fig. 5. SAgs bind to the variable regions of the heavy or light chains of surface immunoglobulins on B lymphocytes, outside the conventional antigen–specific binding site.

antigen-binding fragment (Fab)–binding domains. The result is a supraclonal B-lymphocyte proliferation, which is followed by cell death in some clones. In vivo studies have shown that administration of B-lymphocyte SAgs can deplete subsets of B cells, which have innatelike immune functions (such as secretion of natural antibodies).[3,11] In particular, B1 and marginal zone B lymphocytes, which have innate immune functions, are inherently more sensitive to BCR-mediated signaling than other subsets of B lymphocytes, and strong stimulation results in apoptosis of these cells. B-lymphocyte SAgs exploit this tendency and cause deletion of these B-lymphocyte clones.[3] There has been a speculation that this then leads to a weakened–host immune response to the bacteria.[3]

Different SAgs show different binding preferences for the areas within the variable region of the BCR. The prototypic B-lymphocyte SAg is staphylococcal protein A, which targets the Fab portion of the heavy chain of between 15% and 50% of polyclonal IgG, IgM, IgA, and IgE.[12] In contrast, *Peptostreptococcus magnus* protein L (PpL) targets immunoglobulin light chains. *S aureus* enterotoxins A (SEA) and D are also B-lymphocyte SAgs, and they enhance the survival of the B cells to which they bind in vitro.[5]

The Actions of SAgs on Chemokine Production

Chemokines are a superfamily of proteins produced by immune cells, which regulate innate and adaptive immune responses and are especially involved with leukocyte chemotaxis, including leukocyte adhesion to vascular endothelium, extravasation, and migration through tissue.[13] Chemokines interact with cell surface receptors and one group, the cluster chemokines, binds to many different receptors.[14]

There is evidence that staphylococcal SAgs are able to increase chemokine output in atopic dermatitis.[15] SAgs may directly increase production of chemokine (C-C motif) ligand 1 (CCL1) and CCL18 by dermal dendritic cells, after these cells have interacted with T lymphocytes.[15] CCL1, which binds to the receptor CCR8, may then promote survival of T lymphocytes and dendritic cells at the sites of inflammation. Also, SAgs may induce memory T lymphocytes to secrete cytokines, especially IL-31 that causes increased chemokine expression by keratinocytes.[14] IL-31 is significantly associated with pruritis, which leads to scratching, skin trauma, and subsequent amplification of the inflammatory cascade.[16]

DIVERSITY AMONG SOURCES OF SAGS

Although the classical SAgs are produced by gram-positive bacteria, it is now known that SAgs are also synthesized by gram-negative bacteria, viruses, and human hepatic tissue.

Gram-Positive Bacterial SAgs

Protein toxins secreted by some *Staphylococcus* and *Streptococcus* spp are proto-typic SAgs. They seem to have evolved from a single common ancestor and share a signature in their amino acid sequences (designated the PROSITE sequence).[6] According to crystallographic studies, their structures share a core 3-dimensional fold (the oligosaccharide- or oligonucleotide-binding fold or OB fold).[17] Despite this shared structure, their modes of binding to MHC class II proteins and TCRs differ, they possess different potencies for stimulating lymphocyte proliferation, and they target different subsections of the TCRV$_\beta$ region.[6] Often more than 1 SAg is present in a particular bacterial strain, and it may be advantageous for 1 bacterial strain to produce several SAgs to target different subsets of T-cell clones.[6]

The largest group of bacterial SAgs are proteins secreted by *S aureus*. There are currently 22 known *S aureus* secreted toxins (exotoxins): enterotoxins A to E, G to R, and U, toxic shock syndrome toxin 1 (TSST-1), exfoliatin toxins A and B, and Pan-ton-Valentine leukocidin.[18–20] Their genes (*se*) are generally located in mobile genetic elements, most commonly in pathogenicity islands and also in plasmids, transposons, or phages.[4,21] Because more than 1 *se* (gene) may be encoded within a mobile genetic element, some *se* genes are transferred as a group between bacteria, so that certain genes usually exist in a cluster. For example, *seg, sei, sem, sen, seo,* and *seu* form a cluster named *egc* (enterotoxin gene cluster).[20] Different strains of *S aureus* carry different *se*.

Another large group of bacterial SAgs are those produced by group A streptococci, most commonly *Streptococcus pyogenes*. Examples include streptococcal pyrogenic exotoxins (SPE) A, C, and G to M, streptococcal SAg, and streptococcal mitogenic exotoxins 1 and 2.[17] Group C *Streptococcus equi* pyrogenic toxins H, I, L, and M and group G *Streptococcus dysgalactiae* toxins SDM (*Streptococcus dysgalactiae*–derived mitogen) and SPE-G^{dys} have similar structures and identical functions like the SAgs from group A streptococci.[17] Streptococcal SAg genes are mostly located on prophages.[4] Some streptococcal SAgs are more similar to staphylococcal SAgs than other streptococcal ones, due to genetic transfers between species. Strepto-coccal SAgs show a greater variation in their abilities to stimulate lymphocytes than staphylococcal SAgs.[4]

Gram-Negative Bacterial SAgs

Mycoplasma arthritidis mitogen and *Yersinia pseudotuberculosis* mitogens A, B, and C are SAgs, which are structurally distinct from gram-positive bacterial SAgs and target different TCRV$_\beta$ profiles.[6] These proteins do not have the PROSITE signature of the prototypic SAgs.[4]

Viral SAgs

Mouse mammary tumor virus (MMTV) is a retrovirus that acts as an SAg. This protein is structurally distinct but functionally similar to the bacterial SAgs, causing supraclonal expansion of certain TCRV$_\beta$ subsets and B-lymphocyte proliferation.[6] MMTV is trans-mitted via the breast milk of mice and infects B lymphocytes in the gut. This SAg prob-ably acts to increase the number of B lymphocytes available for viral replication.[6]

Human endogenous retrovirus K18 is associated with Epstein-Barr virus and has SAg activity against certain $TCRV_\beta$ subsets, encouraging T-lymphocyte activation and subsequent B-lymphocyte proliferation.[6] Again, this may increase the number of lymphocytes available for viral replication.[6]

Endogenously Synthesized Human SAg

Protein Fv (so-named because it binds to the variable domain of immunoglobulin heavy chains) is usually synthesized by the liver in small quantities, secreted into bile, and then transported to the gut lumen. It may bind to at least 6 sites on each molecule of the variable region of the heavy chain of human immunoglobulin.[22,23] It usually binds to IgA and as for other SAgs, the site of attachment is outside the conventional antigen–binding site. In the gut, Fv binds to secreted IgA, enhancing its immune function by forming IgA polymers.[22]

The production of protein Fv increases in viral hepatitis.[24] In this setting, it may act as an endogenous SAg by binding to the variable region of the heavy chain of IgE, which is bound to the surface of basophils and mast cells. This interaction may induce prostaglandin D2 and leukotriene C4 release from lung and heart mast cells and IL-4 release from basophils.[25–27] This may be the mechanism by which it plays a role in the cardiac complications of hepatitis C virus. This is the first reported example of a virus causing increased production of an endogenous SAg, which then leads to allergic inflammatory changes.[22]

STAPHYLOCOCCAL SAG-LIKE PROTEINS

Genes for 14 staphylococcal SAg-like proteins (SSLs) have been found on staphylococcal pathogenicity islands, which are mobile genetic elements that encode virulence factors.[4,21] The gene for TSST-1 is in fact closer in sequence to SSL genes than to other classical SAg genes. In general, the tertiary structure of SSLs is similar to that of staphylococcal SAgs, including the presence of the PROSITE motif and OB fold. Unlike SAgs, however, SSLs neither bind MHC class II proteins nor stimulate T lymphocytes. Instead, different SSLs subvert innate immune functions by several mechanisms.[28]

For example, SSL7 binds to the Fc domain of IgA, inhibiting the usual interaction of IgA with its surface receptor (FcαRI) and possibly prolonging the survival of bacteria at mucosal surfaces. Another region of SSL7 binds to complement factor C5, inhibiting the usual hemolytic activity of C5.[28]

SSL5 inhibits the interaction of P-selectin and its glycoprotein ligand 1 (PSGL-1), a crucial step that allows neutrophils to adhere to vascular endothelium in preparation for extravasation into tissues.[29] The result of this inhibition by SSL5 is a reduction in neutrophil adhesion.[29] SSL11 also binds FcαRI and PSGL-1, which also reduces neutrophil adherence to endothelium.

THE ACTIVITY OF SAGS AS SUPERALLERGENS

Conventional allergens stimulate production of specific IgE, which then binds to receptors (FcϵRI) on tissue mast cells and blood basophils. Subsequent allergen exposure can cause cross-linking of the IgE-FcϵRI complexes and activation of the mast cells and basophils.[23] It has been recognized that various SAg may lead to the activation of mast cells and basophils by nonconventional mechanisms. This effect has been described as a superallergen action.[23]

The mechanism of superallergen action seems to involve the binding of SAgs to the IgE component of surface IgE-FcϵRI complexes of basophils and mast cells. For example, staphylococcal protein A binds to the heavy chain of IgE, stimulating histamine release from lung and skin mast cells and circulating basophils.[23] This is a mechanism by which *S aureus* may trigger inflammation in allergic conditions such as chronic atopic dermatitis, allergic rhinitis, and atopic asthma.[5,23,30] As discussed earlier, hepatitis viruses may cause increased synthesis of protein Fv from the liver, which then activates IgE bound to basophils and mast cells causing these cells to secrete cytokines that may contribute to allergic inflammatory changes.[25–27]

Another potential superallergen is PpL, which binds with high affinity to the variable domain of κ light chains of IgE on basophils. This induces the basophils to secrete IL-4 and IL-13, which lead to a T_H2 pattern of inflammation.[31] In a similar manner, the envelope glycoprotein 120 of human immunodeficiency virus 1 (HIV-1) binds to the variable domain of IgE heavy chains on basophils, causing a similar cytokine response.[32] This observation may partly explain the increased incidence of allergic rhinitis in patients with HIV.[33]

Other mechanisms by which *S aureus* SAgs may act as superallergens have been proposed. In a previously sensitized patient, T and B lymphocytes specific to the relevant allergen may be among the many clones stimulated to proliferate by T-lymphocyte SAgs.[5] This may lead to greater numbers of antigen-specific B lymphocytes differentiating into plasma cells and secreting IgE specific to conventional antigens, potentially worsening allergic inflammation. B-lymphocyte SAgs may have a similar effect.[5]

THE ROLE OF SAGS IN INFLAMMATORY AIRWAY DISEASES

There is an increasing body of evidence linking SAg to the pathogenesis of allergic rhinitis, NP, and asthma.

Allergic Rhinitis

There is evidence that *S aureus* SAgs promote inflammation in some perennial allergic rhinitic patients.[34] The prevalence of nasal *S aureus* carriage in patients with perennial allergic rhinitis is higher than in controls (44% vs 20%), and this carriage is associated with increased eosinophilic inflammatory markers and total IgE levels in the local nasal tissue.[35] The strains present in patients with allergic rhinitis are more likely to produce SAg exotoxins than those present in controls (22% vs 7%).[34] Allergic rhinitic patients with antibodies to SAg exotoxins are more likely to have higher levels of both total IgE and house dust mite–specific IgE.[36]

CRSwNP

Patients with CRSwNP may have higher rates of nasal *S aureus* colonization than in controls or patients with CRS without NP (64%, 33%, and 27%, respectively).[37] *S aureus* exotoxin SAgs have been directly detected in the nasal mucosa or mucus of 48% of patients with CRSwNP, which is significantly more than in controls or patients with CRS without NP.[38] Furthermore, levels of IgE directed against *S aureus* exotoxin SAgs are higher in patients with CRSwNP than in controls or patients with CRS without NP (28%, 15%, and 6%, respectively).[37] The presence of IgE directed against staphylococcal SAgs is associated with higher rates of eosinophilic inflammation.[37] Also, in patients with higher specific-IgE levels, levels of IgG are increased in NP tissue, with relatively increased IgG4 and decreased IgG2 levels. It has been suggested that, in these patients, IgG4 may promote IgE production.[39]

The higher levels of IgE to SAgs in these patients may reflect a compensatory local immune response to defects in immune defenses against *S aureus*. Evidence for such a local immune deficiency includes the observation that macrophages in polyp tissue may have a reduced capacity to phagocytose *S aureus*.[39] Also, a deficiency in the level of IgG2 directed against *S aureus* enterotoxin C1 has been reported in a subgroup of patients with severe atopic dermatitis and CRSwNP.[39,40] Hence, there is evidence that deficiencies in innate and adaptive immune responses to *S aureus* may contribute to subsequent colonization, SAg production, and exacerbation of inflammation.

Secondary lymphoid structures in NP tissue, including B and T lymphocytes in follicles and a diffuse plasma cell distribution, have been detected using immunohistochemical techniques.[41] Half of these patients had IgE to staphylococcal SAg in their NP tissue. It has been suggested that this SAg-specific IgE is being produced within these nasal mucosal lymphoid aggregates (rather than in regional secondary lymphoid tissues, as is more usual).

An analysis of T lymphocytes derived from NP tissue showed skewing toward TCRV$_\beta$ regions associated with SAg in 35% of cases of CRSwNP but not in antrochoanal polyps.[42] In a study by the same group, there was a dramatic skewing of TCRV$_\beta$ regions toward those associated with SAg in T lymphocytes derived from NP tissue compared with circulating T lymphocytes.[43] These TCRV$_\beta$ regions had undergone oligoclonal expansion in all cases. This provided further compelling evidence for a local nasal stimulus to the T-lymphocyte immune response to SAgs.[43]

Asthma

In patients with asthma, serum levels of IgE directed against *S aureus* exotoxin SAgs are higher than in controls (62% vs 13%).[44] Furthermore, the levels are even higher in clinically severe asthmatic patients and correlate with the degree of eosinophilic inflammation and total IgE levels.[44] Clinical severity of asthma does not correlate with the levels of IgE directed against common allergens.[39]

Application of *S aureus* SAg onto nasal and bronchial mucosa in mice induced changes consistent with asthma, including eosinophilia.[45] It seems plausible that nasal colonization may exacerbate asthma, supporting the concept of united airway disease.[39] Several studies performed in patients with asthma have provided evidence for the involvement of a B-lymphocyte SAg. Such a B-lymphocyte SAg may be responsible for the overrepresentation of the V$_H$5 family of IgE that has been reported. There is also evidence for this finding in allergic rhinitis and atopic dermatitis.[39,46] However, such B-lymphocyte SAgs with specificity for the V$_H$5 family of IgE remain to be identified.[5]

Insensitivity to Glucocorticoid Therapy

S aureus exotoxin SAgs may play a role in glucocorticoid insensitivity, which affects up to 25% of patients with asthma and also occurs in allergic rhinitis.[47] Glucocorticoids usually inhibit T-lymphocyte activation and proliferation. In glucocorticoid insensitivity, circulating T lymphocytes remain persistently activated despite therapy with glucocorticoids. A combination of high levels of IL-2 and IL-4 and the overexpression of the cytoplasmic glucocorticoid receptor (GCR) splice variant GCRβ in peripheral blood monocytes seems to be responsible for this insensitivity.[48–50] The result is a reduction of the usual inhibitory effect of glucocorticoids on the production of the inflammatory mediators that are stimulated by cytokines. This inhibition is usually performed by glucocorticoid binding to cytoplasmic GCRα, which then interacts with transcription factors in the nucleus and binds to DNA. SAgs may lead to glucocorticoid insensitivity by stimulating the production of GCRβ, which then inhibits GCRα translocation to the nucleus for DNA binding.[5,51,52]

IMPLICATIONS FOR CLINICAL PRACTICE

Increasing evidence supports a role for SAgs in the pathogenesis of inflammatory airway diseases in some patients. Therapeutic options directed at SAg effects may include eradication of the bacteria producing SAgs, neutralization of the SAgs once they are released, or inhibition of the SAgs' immune effects. In the future, it could be possible to prevent inflammation caused by SAgs by the administration of antistaphylococcal or antiexotoxin vaccines.[39]

Studies of potential anti-SAg treatments have been performed. Results with pooled intravenous immunoglobulin, peptide SAg antagonists, and SAg receptor mimics have not yet yielded promising results.[4] Attempts have also been made to inhibit the inflammatory effects of SAgs. The anti-IL-5 agent reslizumab has been shown to temporarily reduce nasal polyp size in about half of patients. The anti-IgE agent omalizumab used in monotherapy or in combination with immunotherapy has been proven to be effective in allergic rhinitis. However, neither of these interventions are specific in their actions against SAgs.[53,54]

A new therapeutic focus on antibiotics with intracellular activity may be appropriate. S aureus has been shown to survive within nasal epithelial cells, thus avoiding exposure to antibiotics and contributing to disease recurrence or chronicity.[55–57] Indeed, antibiotics commonly used in the treatment of chronic rhinosinusitis may lead to intracellular persistence of S aureus.[58] These intracellular bacteria may be a source of SAg secretion, leading to exacerbation of inflammation.

IMPLICATIONS FOR RESEARCH

Standard microbiological techniques, such as culture of middle meatal swabs, are less than ideal for detecting bacteria present in biofilms, mucus, intracellular reservoirs, or small colony variants. Bacteria in these sites may be potentially producing SAgs, and further research is needed to investigate the importance of SAgs from these sources in chronic sinonasal inflammatory conditions.[59–65]

The regulation of SAg-gene expression is not yet well understood, but it could potentially be important to the development of both disease and new therapies. The quorum-sensing accessory gene regulator system of S aureus is activated at high cell densities, which results in upregulation of most SAgs. SEA is constitutively expressed but not upregulated.[4] TSST-1 and S aureus enterotoxin B may act to suppress transcription of all SAg genes.[66] Streptococcal SAg may be upregulated in the presence of infection, under the influence of host factors that have yet to be defined.[4]

The role of host genetic profiles seems to be important in SAg-related diseases. As already described, different alleles of MHC class II proteins and TCRs have different binding affinities for SAgs, and further understanding of these relationships may prove fruitful.

SUMMARY

SAgs are fascinating proteins. Although they were initially thought to be powerful proinflammatory agents, now they appear to also play a role in the subversion of the immune response to bacteria. SAgs have been found in several skin and mucosal inflammatory conditions, but their precise role in the pathogenesis of these conditions remains to be elucidated.

- SAgs are derived from diverse sources, including gram-positive and gram-negative bacteria, viruses, and human hepatic tissue.
- SAgs have diverse effects upon the immune system, involving T lymphocytes, B lymphocytes, chemokine production, basophils, and mast cells.
- T-lymphocyte SAgs bypass conventional antigen processing by binding directly to the MHC class II proteins of APCs and the variable β chain of the TCR, which lies outside of the conventional antigen groove.
- Although T-lymphocyte SAgs initially activate T lymphocytes by causing a supraclonal response, this is followed by T-lymphocyte clonal deletion or the induction of anergy and activation of regulatory T lymphocytes, all of which may lead to an immune tolerance.
- Similarly, B-lymphocyte SAgs cause a supraclonal B-lymphocyte response by binding to BCRs outside the conventional antigen groove. This is followed by deletion of subsets of B lymphocytes, which have innate immune functions.
- SAgs may act as superallergens by binding to IgE on the surface of basophils and mast cells, thereby worsening inflammation in allergic conditions, such as chronic atopic dermatitis, allergic rhinitis, and atopic asthma.
- SSLs subvert innate immune functions by several mechanisms, but unlike SAgs they neither bind MHC class II proteins nor stimulate T lymphocytes.

REFERENCES

1. White J, Herman A, Pullen AM, et al. The V beta-specific superantigen staphylococcal enterotoxin B: stimulation of mature T cells and clonal deletion in neonatal mice. Cell 1989;56(1):27–35.
2. Silverman GJ, Goodyear CS. Confounding B-cell defences: lessons from a staphylococcal superantigen. Nat Rev Immunol 2006;6(6):465–75.
3. Goodyear CS, Silverman GJ. B cell superantigens: a microbe's answer to innate-like B cells and natural antibodies. Springer Semin Immunopathol 2005;26(4):463–84.
4. Fraser JD, Proft T. The bacterial superantigen and superantigen-like proteins. Immunol Rev 2008;225:226–43.
5. Gould HJ, Takhar P, Harries HE, et al. The allergic march from *Staphylococcus aureus* superantigens to immunoglobulin E. Chem Immunol Allergy 2007;93:106–36.
6. Proft T, Fraser JD. Bacterial superantigens. Clin Exp Immunol 2003;133(3):299–306.
7. Ivars F. Superantigen-induced regulatory T cells in vivo. Chem Immunol Allergy 2007;93:137–60.
8. Lynch DH, Ramsdell F, Alderson MR. Fas and FasL in the homeostatic regulation of immune responses. Immunol Today 1995;16(12):569–74.
9. Bueno C, Criado G, McCormick JK, et al. T cell signalling induced by bacterial superantigens. Chem Immunol Allergy 2007;93:161–80.
10. Herman A, Kappler JW, Marrack P, et al. Superantigens: mechanism of T-cell stimulation and role in immune responses. Annu Rev Immunol 1991;9:745–72.
11. Zouali M. B cell superantigens subvert innate functions of B cells. Chem Immunol Allergy 2007;93:92–105.
12. Inganas M. Comparison of mechanisms of interaction between protein A from *Staphylococcus aureus* and human monoclonal IgG, IgA and IgM in relation to the classical FC gamma and the alternative F(ab')2 epsilon protein A interactions. Scand J Immunol 1981;13(4):343–52.

13. Butcher EC, Picker LJ. Lymphocyte homing and homeostasis. Science 1996; 272(5258):60–6.
14. Homey B, Meller S, Savinko T, et al. Modulation of chemokines by staphylococcal superantigen in atopic dermatitis. Chem Immunol Allergy 2007;93:181–94.
15. Pivarcsi A, Gombert M, Dieu-Nosjean MC, et al. CC chemokine ligand 18, an atopic dermatitis-associated and dendritic cell-derived chemokine, is regulated by staphylococcal products and allergen exposure. J Immunol 2004;173(9): 5810–7.
16. Sonkoly E, Muller A, Lauerma AI, et al. IL-31: a new link between T cells and pruritus in atopic skin inflammation. J Allergy Clin Immunol 2006;117(2):411–7.
17. Proft T, Fraser JD. Streptococcal superantigens. Chem Immunol Allergy 2007;93: 1–23.
18. Alouf JE, Muller-Alouf H. Staphylococcal and streptococcal superantigens: molecular, biological and clinical aspects. Int J Med Microbiol 2003;292(7-8): 429–40.
19. Chiang YC, Liao WW, Fan CM, et al. PCR detection of staphylococcal enterotoxins (SEs) N, O, P, Q, R, U, and survey of SE types in Staphylococcus aureus isolates from food-poisoning cases in Taiwan. Int J Food Microbiol 2008;121(1):66–73.
20. Letertre C, Perelle S, Dilasser F, et al. Identification of a new putative enterotoxin SEU encoded by the egc cluster of Staphylococcus aureus. J Appl Microbiol 2003;95(1):38–43.
21. Novick RP, Subedi A. The SaPIs: mobile pathogenicity islands of Staphylococcus. Chem Immunol Allergy 2007;93:42–57.
22. Bouvet JP, Marone G. Protein Fv: an endogenous immunoglobulin superantigen and superallergen. Chem Immunol Allergy 2007;93:58–76.
23. Marone G, Rossi FW, Detoraki A, et al. Role of superallergens in allergic disorders. Chem Immunol Allergy 2007;93:195–213.
24. Bouvet JP, Pires R, Lunel-Fabiani F, et al. Protein F. A novel F(ab)-binding factor, present in normal liver, and largely released in the digestive tract during hepatitis. J Immunol 1990;145(4):1176–80.
25. Patella V, Bouvet JP, Marone G. Protein Fv produced during vital hepatitis is a novel activator of human basophils and mast cells. J Immunol 1993;151(10): 5685–98.
26. Genovese A, Borgia G, Bouvet JP, et al. Protein Fv produced during viral hepatitis is an endogenous immunoglobulin superantigen activating human heart mast cells. Int Arch Allergy Immunol 2003;132(4):336–45.
27. Patella V, Giuliano A, Bouvet JP, et al. Endogenous superallergen protein Fv induces IL-4 secretion from human Fc epsilon RI+ cells through interaction with the VH3 region of IgE. J Immunol 1998;161(10):5647–55.
28. Langley R, Wines B, Willoughby N, et al. The staphylococcal superantigen-like protein 7 binds IgA and complement C5 and inhibits IgA-Fc alpha RI binding and serum killing of bacteria. J Immunol 2005;174(5):2926–33.
29. Bestebroer J, Poppelier MJ, Ulfman LH, et al. Staphylococcal superantigen-like 5 binds PSGL-1 and inhibits P-selectin-mediated neutrophil rolling. Blood 2007; 109(7):2936–43.
30. Breuer K, Haussler S, Kapp A, et al. Staphylococcus aureus: colonizing features and influence of an antibacterial treatment in adults with atopic dermatitis. Br J Dermatol 2002;147(1):55–61.
31. Genovese A, Borgia G, Bjorck L, et al. Immunoglobulin superantigen protein L induces IL-4 and IL-13 secretion from human Fc epsilon RI+ cells through interaction with the kappa light chains of IgE. J Immunol 2003;170(4):1854–61.

32. Patella V, Florio G, Petraroli A, et al. HIV-1 gp120 induces IL-4 and IL-13 release from human Fc epsilon RI+ cells through interaction with the VH3 region of IgE. J Immunol 2000;164(2):589–95.
33. Porter JP, Patel AA, Dewey CM, et al. Prevalence of sinonasal symptoms in patients with HIV infection. Am J Rhinol 1999;13(3):203–8.
34. Shiomori T, Yoshida S, Miyamoto H, et al. Relationship of nasal carriage of *Staphylococcus aureus* to pathogenesis of perennial allergic rhinitis. J Allergy Clin Immunol 2000;105(3):449–54.
35. Riechelmann H, Essig A, Deutschle T, et al. Nasal carriage of *Staphylococcus aureus* in house dust mite allergic patients and healthy controls. Allergy 2005; 60(11):1418–23.
36. Rossi RE, Monasterolo G. Prevalence of serum IgE antibodies to the *Staphylococcus aureus* enterotoxins (SAE, SEB, SEC, SED, TSST-1) in patients with persistent allergic rhinitis. Int Arch Allergy Immunol 2004;133(3):261–6.
37. Van Zele T, Gevaert P, Watelet JB, et al. *Staphylococcus aureus* colonization and IgE antibody formation to enterotoxins is increased in nasal polyposis. J Allergy Clin Immunol 2004;114(4):981–3.
38. Seiberling KA, Conley DB, Tripathi A, et al. Superantigens and chronic rhinosinusitis: detection of staphylococcal exotoxins in nasal polyps. Laryngoscope 2005; 115(9):1580–5.
39. Bachert C, Gevaert P, Zhang N, et al. Role of staphylococcal superantigens in airway disease. Chem Immunol Allergy 2007;93:214–36.
40. Mrabet-Dahbi S, Breuer K, Klotz M, et al. Deficiency in immunoglobulin G2 antibodies against staphylococcal enterotoxin C1 defines a subgroup of patients with atopic dermatitis. Clin Exp Allergy 2005;35(3):274–81.
41. Gevaert P, Holtappels G, Johansson SG, et al. Organization of secondary lymphoid tissue and local IgE formation to *Staphylococcus aureus* enterotoxins in nasal polyp tissue. Allergy 2005;60(1):71–9.
42. Conley DB, Tripathi A, Seiberling KA, et al. Superantigens and chronic rhinosinusitis: skewing of T-cell receptor V beta-distributions in polyp-derived CD4+ and CD8+ T cells. Am J Rhinol 2006;20(5):534–9.
43. Conley DB, Tripathi A, Seiberling KA, et al. Superantigens and chronic rhinosinusitis II: analysis of T-cell receptor V beta domains in nasal polyps. Am J Rhinol 2006;20(4):451–5.
44. Bachert C, Gevaert P, Howarth P, et al. IgE to *Staphylococcus aureus* enterotoxins in serum is related to severity of asthma. J Allergy Clin Immunol 2003; 111(5):1131–2.
45. Hellings PW, Hens G, Meyts I, et al. Aggravation of bronchial eosinophilia in mice by nasal and bronchial exposure to *Staphylococcus aureus* enterotoxin B. Clin Exp Allergy 2006;36(8):1063–71.
46. Coker HA, Harries HE, Banfield GK, et al. Biased use of VH5 IgE-positive B cells in the nasal mucosa in allergic rhinitis. J Allergy Clin Immunol 2005;116(2): 445–52.
47. Chan MT, Leung DY, Szefler SJ, et al. Difficult-to-control asthma: clinical characteristics of steroid-insensitive asthma. J Allergy Clin Immunol 1998;101(5): 594–601.
48. Kam JC, Szefler SJ, Surs W, et al. Combination IL-2 and IL-4 reduces glucocorticoid receptor-binding affinity and T cell response to glucocorticoids. J Immunol 1993;151(7):3460–6.
49. Adcock IM, Lane SJ, Brown CR, et al. Differences in binding of glucocorticoid receptor to DNA in steroid-resistant asthma. J Immunol 1995;154(7):3500–5.

50. Sousa AR, Lane SJ, Cidlowski JA, et al. Glucocorticoid resistance in asthma is associated with elevated in vivo expression of the glucocorticoid receptor beta-isoform. J Allergy Clin Immunol 2000;105(5):943–50.

51. Fakhri S, Tulic M, Christodoulopoulos P, et al. Microbial superantigens induce glucocorticoid receptor beta and steroid resistance in a nasal explant model. Laryngoscope 2004;114(5):887–92.

52. Hauk PJ, Hamid QA, Chrousos GP, et al. Induction of corticosteroid insensitivity in human PBMCs by microbial superantigens. J Allergy Clin Immunol 2000;105(4): 782–7.

53. Gevaert P, Lang-Loidolt D, Lackner A, et al. Nasal IL-5 levels determine the response to anti-IL-5 treatment in patients with nasal polyps. J Allergy Clin Immunol 2006;118(5):1133–41.

54. Verbruggen K, Van Cauwenberge P, Bachert C. Anti-IgE for the treatment of allergic rhinitis–and eventually nasal polyps? Int Arch Allergy Immunol 2009; 148(2):87–98.

55. Clement S, Vaudaux P, Francois P, et al. Evidence of an intracellular reservoir in the nasal mucosa of patients with recurrent Staphylococcus aureus rhinosinusitis. J Infect Dis 2005;192(6):1023–8.

56. Garzoni C, Kelley WL. Staphylococcus aureus: new evidence for intracellular persistence. Trends Microbiol 2009;17(2):59–65.

57. Plouin-Gaudon I, Clement S, Huggler E, et al. Intracellular residency is frequently associated with recurrent Staphylococcus aureus rhinosinusitis. Rhinology 2006; 44(4):249–54.

58. Krut O, Sommer H, Kronke M. Antibiotic-induced persistence of cytotoxic Staphylococcus aureus in non-phagocytic cells. J Antimicrob Chemother 2004;53(2): 167–73.

59. Kern RC, Conley DB, Walsh W, et al. Perspectives on the etiology of chronic rhinosinusitis: an immune barrier hypothesis. Am J Rhinol 2008;22(6):549–59.

60. Zhang N, Gevaert P, van Zele T, et al. An update on the impact of Staphylococcus aureus enterotoxins in chronic sinusitis with nasal polyposis. Rhinology 2005; 43(3):162–8.

61. Seiberling KA, Grammer L, Kern RC. Chronic rhinosinusitis and superantigens. Otolaryngol Clin North Am 2005;38(6):1215–36, ix.

62. Proctor RA, van Langevelde P, Kristjansson M, et al. Persistent and relapsing infections associated with small-colony variants of Staphylococcus aureus. Clin Infect Dis 1995;20(1):95–102.

63. Hall-Stoodley L, Stoodley P. Biofilm formation and dispersal and the transmission of human pathogens. Trends Microbiol 2005;13(1):7–10.

64. Harvey RJ, Lund VJ. Biofilms and chronic rhinosinusitis: systematic review of evidence, current concepts and directions for research. Rhinology 2007;45(1): 3–13.

65. Hunsaker DH, Leid JG. The relationship of biofilms to chronic rhinosinusitis. Curr Opin Otolaryngol Head Neck Surg 2008;16(3):237–41.

66. Vojtov N, Ross HF, Novick RP. Global repression of exotoxin synthesis by staphylococcal superantigens. Proc Natl Acad Sci U S A 2002;99(15):10102–7.

Local and Systemic IgE in the Evaluation and Treatment of Allergy

Elizabeth K. Hoddeson, MD[a], Eleanor Pratt, BS, BA[b,c],
Richard J. Harvey, MD[b], Sarah K. Wise, MD[a],*

KEYWORDS

• Immunoglobulin E • IgE • Allergy • Nasal polyp
• Chronic rhinosinusitis • Allergic fungal rhinosinusitis
• Allergic rhinitis • Asthma

Allergy is a clinical manifestation of an exaggerated immune response following repeated exposures in a genetically predisposed "atopic" patient. In allergic patients, the body responds to usually harmless substances as though they were pathogens. Allergy may present as a variety of systemic conditions, most commonly hay fever, allergic rhinitis, asthma, and eczema. The symptoms of allergy are predictable when considered in context of chemical mediators released by mast cells during a type I immunoglobulin E (IgE)-mediated hypersensitivity reaction. Mast cells are concentrated in the submucosal layer of the respiratory tract, gastrointestinal tract, conjunctiva of the eye, and subcutaneous layer of the skin, which correlates directly to the target organs that manifest symptoms during an allergic reaction. Histamine and other mediators released from mast cells and basophils during allergic reactions contribute to vasodilation, glandular secretion, and increased vascular permeability.

It is estimated that 20% to 25% of the general population manifests clinical symptoms of allergy.[1] A nationwide survey in 2006 showed that 54.6% of people in the United States tested positive to at least one allergen.[2] The profound economic impact of allergy is increasing. Between 2000 and 2005, the cost of treating allergic rhinitis

Conflict of Interest statement: Preparation of this manuscript was not supported by an external funding source. Dr Harvey has served on an advisory board for Schering Plough and has received grant support from NeilMed. Dr Wise has received grant support from Arthrocare, Inc. Dr Hoddeson and Eleanor Pratt have no financial interests to declare.

[a] Department of Otolaryngology-Head and Neck Surgery, Emory University, 1365A Clifton Road NE, Suite A2300, Atlanta, GA 30322, USA
[b] Department of Otolaryngology and Skull Base Surgery, St Vincent's Hospital, 354 Victoria Street, Darlinghurst, Sydney, New South Wales 2010, Australia
[c] School of Biotechnology and Biomolecular Sciences, University of New South Wales, Kensington, New South Wales 2052, Australia
* Corresponding author.
E-mail address: sarah.wise@emoryhealthcare.org

Otolaryngol Clin N Am 43 (2010) 503–520
doi:10.1016/j.otc.2010.02.009
0030-6665/10/$ – see front matter © 2010 Elsevier Inc. All rights reserved.

oto.theclinics.com

almost doubled from \$6.1 to \$11.2 billion, with more than half of this money spent on prescription medications.[3,4] Costs related to lost productivity, missed work, and health care costs incurred by exacerbation of coexisting medical conditions by allergy are more difficult to quantify.[1]

IMMUNOLOGY

A discussion of allergy and its treatment would be incomplete without an understanding of the effector cells involved. An IgE-mediated allergic reaction consists of 2 phases: early humoral reaction and a late cellular reaction.[5] An almost immediate response to an allergen occurs with a preformed specific IgE molecule presenting an antigen to an attached mast cell. This antigen presentation results in degranulation and release of histamine from mast cells in the submucosal layer, with subsequent vasodilatation and increased vascular permeability. In addition to histamine, mast cells release a cascade of other proinflammatory mediators (prostaglandins, leukotrienes, platelet-activating factor, bradykinin, and cytokines) within minutes of the antigen-antibody reaction. The presence of cytokines and leukotrienes up-regulate or induce de novo expression of adhesion molecules, selectins, and integrins. This release of mediators inspires an influx of other inflammatory cells, primarily eosinophils, but also basophils and neutrophils into the reaction site within several hours following the humoral reaction. This cellular influx comprises the late or cellular reaction, and may enhance the allergic symptom expression for up to several days.[6]

In a milieu of cytokines and other mediators, B lymphocytes proceed to generate further antigen-specific IgE that will be displayed on the B cells in preparation for subsequent exposures.[7] The critical step in the commitment of B cells to synthesis of IgE is heavy chain class switching, which involves recombination within the immunoglobulin heavy chain gene cluster, thus changing the ε germ line gene into the rearranged gene. This gives rise to the ε mRNA for the ε heavy chain of IgE.[8] Several signals are necessary for heavy chain switching, whether in vivo *or* in vitro. When provoked by allergen exposure, mast cells and Th2-type lymphocytes release interleukin (IL)-4 and IL-13.[9] These signals target the ε gene for recombination by binding to CD40. CD40 ligand is constitutively expressed on mast cells and expressed after allergen activation on T cells. Cross-linking of CD40 on B-cell membrane induces the cell to undergo heavy chain switching.[8,9] Immunoglobulin subclasses vary in abundance. The 4 IgG subclasses make up 75% of the immunoglobulins found in serum, with a concentration in healthy individuals of about 10 mg/mL.[10] IgG responds to a wide range of antigens, including many bacterial proteins.[10] In contrast, the least-abundant Ig in serum is IgE, with a normal concentration of approximately 150 ng/mL.[11]

TRADITIONAL SYSTEMIC ALLERGY TESTING

Current diagnostic and treatment regimens for allergic patients revolve around systemic IgE. Diagnostic techniques are dependent on sufficiently detectable levels of systemic IgE, and treatment is administered for local and systemic symptom control with pharmaceutical agents or antigen-specific immunotherapy. Increased evidence for local IgE production and concomitant disease manifestations incurred by local inundation with IgE has abounded recently. Local IgE production and its effects have been hypothesized to explain the discrepancy between sensitization detected by systemic allergy testing and clinical expression of allergy. Despite research evidencing increased local tissue IgE levels, the development of routine testing for local IgE and treatment regimens centered on elevated local IgE have not been routinely used.

Systemic Skin Testing for Allergy

The gold standard for allergy testing is in vivo antigen-specific skin testing, which is essentially a semiquantitative measurement of the early-phase type I hypersensitivity reaction. Antigens are selected by the tester according to their likelihood to induce a reaction based on the patient's medical history. These are applied to the skin by an epicutaneous screening method or an intracutaneous diluted fashion. If a sensitized mast cell to that specific antigen exists, a humoral reaction will ensue with development of a wheal and flare that reaches its maximum at about 20 minutes after exposure. The diameter of the early-phase wheal is measured and the exuberance of the allergy inferred. A late-phase cellular reaction may ensue, but this is not interpreted as part of standard testing. Therefore, despite manifestations of allergy typically occurring at local intranasal, ocular, or bronchial sites, gold standard allergy testing methods have traditionally been undertaken via systemic skin-testing protocols.

The most commonly used epicutaneous test is the prick or puncture method initially described by Lewis and Grant in 1924 and later modified by Pepys in 1975.[7] A drop of purified antigen or control fluid is applied to the skin, and a needle or similar device is used to puncture the epidermis through the fluid without inciting bleeding. After allowing time for a humoral reaction to develop, based on presence or absence of antigen-specific IgE-sensitized mast cells in the skin, the resulting reaction is graded. More exuberant reactions develop in patients with higher levels of systemic antigen-specific IgE; however, negative prick tests do not preclude existence of allergen-specific IgE at lower levels that may still result in clinical allergy symptoms.

Intracutaneous or intradermal systemic allergy testing may complement prick testing, or be used alone to quantify systemic antigen-specific responses. Although the antigen concentration used in intradermal testing is far weaker than antigen concentration in prick testing, the volume of antigen to which the patient is exposed is much greater, increasing a risk of an anaphylactic reaction. The intradermal test was reported as an allergy skin testing method by Cooke in 1915.[7] The 2 most common methods for intradermal testing are single-dilution and intradermal dilution testing, previously known as skin-endpoint titration. Intradermal dilution testing is more clinically relevant given the ability to accurately quantitate a patient's sensitivity and infer the starting concentration for immunotherapy. Single-dilution testing provides only a positive or negative result, and all immunotherapy is begun at an extremely low dose to ensure safety, prolonging overall time of escalation dosing.

Systemic In Vitro Testing for Allergy

Systemic in vivo skin testing, despite remaining the gold standard, inherently presents several drawbacks. The degree of reactivity is suppressed by antihistamines, which must be avoided for at least 72 hours before testing. Patients often experience an increase in symptoms with withdrawal of antihistamine medications. Skin-testing methods have been refined to encompass exposure to very low doses or diluted antigen to maximize the safety profile; however, a small risk of anaphylactic reaction persists with in vivo testing. Rates of untoward reactions during skin testing, both large local reactions and systemic reactions, are reported at a rate of 0.02% to 1.40%.[12,13] Protocols to manage these life-threatening reactions are mandated for administering centers to maximize success for management of anaphylaxis.

An alternative to in vivo testing exists for patients who are advised against or unlikely to be able to tolerate skin testing. Radioallergosorbent testing, or RAST testing, involves a radioimmunoassay capable of detecting specific IgE antibodies in serum. A solid phase is manufactured in which allergens react with serum drawn from a patient. Antigen-specific IgE binds to the solid phase antigens. This solid phase antigen-antibody complex is then incubated with radiolabeled rabbit antibodies to human IgE. The amount of antibody present is calculated by measurement of the radioactive marker.[7] The modified RAST was introduced in 1979 by Fadal and Nalebuff[14] to increase the sensitivity of the test while maintaining its specificity. Adjustments were made not only to the technical aspects of the testing procedure but also to the scoring and interpretation mechanisms. The modified RAST is more useful to the clinician as correlations to intradermal dilutional testing can be made to facilitate initiation of immunotherapy.[15] Some advocate that total quantitative measurement of serum systemic IgE provides additional diagnostic value in addition to modified RAST. Even modified RAST, however, remains less sensitive than in vivo skin testing for allergy detection.[12,16]

TREATMENT OF ALLERGY

Management options for allergy consist of avoidance measures and several classes of pharmacotherapeutic agents, but the only "cure" for this disorder requires immunotherapy. A tailored regimen, largely designed by trial and error, can be designed for the patient with the goal of symptom control, from antihistamines, decongestants, mast cell stabilizers, corticosteroids, anticholinergics, and leukotriene modifiers. Unsatisfactory relief with these mechanisms prompts consideration of immunotherapy.

Avoidance

The best and most effective management of allergy is avoidance of allergens when possible. Patient education can be provided by verbal counseling as well as administration of printed materials with specific control regimens for various antigens, such as dust mites, molds, and animal dander. Antigens are not always avoidable, and even when immunotherapy is instituted, overwhelming exposure to antigens both during treatment and following therapy may continue to provoke symptoms. As such, pharmacotherapeutic management of symptoms is a cornerstone in treating the allergic patient.

Pharmacotherapy

Antihistamines help to control symptoms of sneezing and rhinorrhea, symptoms induced by vasodilation, increased vascular permeability, and increased glandular production that occurs with direct effects of histamine. First-generation antihistamines, or "sedating" antihistamines, compete with histamine for H1 receptor sites on target organs (**Table 1**). Second-generation, or "nonsedating," antihistamines do not cross the blood-brain barrier, and as such, have a better tolerated side-effect profile. Topical, intranasal antihistamines are now available and offer benefits of antihistamine and anti-inflammatory actions. Third-generation antihistamines seek to offer equal or superior potency with further-enhanced safety profile and longer duration of action.[7]

Decongestants are alpha-adrenergic agonists that oppose vasodilation and decrease symptoms of nasal congestion.[7] Systemic administration carries a risk profile characterized by the vasopressive actions, mainly exacerbation of hypertension. They readily cross the blood-brain barrier, and can cause central nervous system stimulation. When applied topically to the nose, systemic effects are minimized, but risk of rebound rhinitis and cycles of addiction can ensue.

Mast cell stabilizers have multiple actions, but retain their original description in name. They are used topically intranasally, and are most effective when administered

Table 1
Summary of pharmacotherapeutic agents used to treat allergic and related disease

Drug Class		Example	Mechanism of Action	Current Indication
Oral antihistamine	1st generation	Diphenhydramine	Blocks H1 receptor sites on target organs	Allergic rhinitis
	2nd	Loratadine		
	3rd	Desloratadine		
Topical antihistamine		Azelastine	Blocks H1 receptor site	Allergic rhinitis
Topical decongestant		Neosynephrine	Alpha-adrenergic agonist	Acute nasal congestion
Oral decongestant		Phenylephrine	Alpha-adrenergic agonist	Nasal congestion
Oral steroid		Prednisone	Decreases capillary permeability, stabilizes lysosomal membranes, blocks action of migratory inhibitory factor, inhibits phospholipase	Late-phase allergic reactions
Intranasal steroid		Mometasone	See above	Chronic allergic rhinitis
Leukotriene modifier		Monteleukast	Inhibits formation of leukotrienes	Asthma, nasal polyposis, allergic rhinitis
Chromones		Sodium cromoglycate	Mast cell stabilizer	Before allergen exposure
Topical anticholinergic		Ipratropium bromide	Blocks muscarinic receptors (M2 and M3)	Allergic rhinitis with prominent rhinorrhea, Asthma
Sympathomimetic		Epinephrine	α and β adrenergic receptor activation	Anaphylaxis
Inhaled short-acting selective beta2-adrenergic agonists		Albuterol	Directly activates $\beta2$-receptors	Bronchospasm
Inhaled long-acting selective $\beta2$ agonist		Salmeterol	Directly activates $\beta2$-receptors	Asthma, COPD
Methylxanthine		Theophylline	Nonselective phosphodiesterase inhibitor, ↑ apoptosis of inflammatory cells, ↑ histone deacetylase activity	Asthma
Anti-IgE antibodies		Omalizumab	Prevents IgE binding to mast cells	Asthma

Abbreviations: COPD, chronic obstructive pulmonary disease; IgE, immunoglobulin E.
Data from Bousquet J, Khaltaev N, Cruz AA, et al. Allergic rhinitis and its impact on asthma (ARIA) 2008 update (in collaboration with the World Health Organization, GA(2)LEN and AllerGen). Allergy 2008;63(Suppl 86):8–160; and Bousquet J, van Cauwenberge P, Ait Khaled N, et al. Pharmacologic and anti-IgE treatment of allergic rhinitis ARIA update (in collaboration with GA2LEN). Allergy 2006;61:1086–96.

before allergen exposure to prevent an allergic reaction. They have a short half-life and must be redosed multiple times daily. Advantages include a very limited side-effect profile.

Corticosteroids are anti-inflammatory agents that are primarily effective for the late-phase allergic reaction.[7] They do not prevent allergic reaction, but diminish the effects by mitigating effector cells and enzymes. Systemically administered, this class of medication has a side-effect profile list that is quite lengthy, often increased as dose and duration of treatment are increased. They can result in suppression of endogenous steroid production, central nervous system stimulation, gastrointestinal upset, exacerbation of hypertension and diabetes, and skeletal and tendon injury. Topical nasal or inhaled corticosteroids are a heavily relied upon class of agents for allergy and asthma symptom management, as they are the most potent nasal therapy and they diminish the need for systemic administration.[17] Topical administration results in very low systemic absorption, and has usually few side effects locally, including nasal crusting, epistaxis, hoarseness, oral candidiasis, and drying of the mucous membranes.

Anticholinergics were originally used systemically to counteract rhinorrhea present in allergy. They were poorly tolerated given the excessive mucosal drying effects, with nasal crusting and thickened mucous. Intranasal anticholinergics are effective at controlling rhinorrhea with very little systemic absorption and, therefore, limited side effects.[7]

Leukotriene modifiers were designed to modulate development of allergic reaction by inhibiting development of leukotrienes or barring their effects.[7] They were originally solely used for asthma and nasal polyposis, but have recently gained approval from the Food and Drug Administration for a role in treatment of allergic rhinitis as well.[7]

Immunotherapy

Systemic immunotherapy is offered to patients whose symptoms are not well controlled by simple pharmacotherapeutic measures, symptoms that are severe and prolonged, allergies to antigens that are not readily avoidable, and to patients who are capable of complying with the prolonged treatment time. Standard antigen-specific immunotherapy was developed in 1911 by Leonard Noon.[18] It entails injecting escalating doses of antigen until a maintenance dose is achieved, and then continuing injection treatments until the patient has been completely asymptomatic for perennial allergens for 1 to 5 years and seasonal allergens for 2 to 3 seasons. Injections are usually administered once weekly with increasing dose and potency of antigen until desired effects are noted, continued for a total of 1 year, and then maintenance doses are continued every 2 to 3 weeks for a total duration of 3 to 5 years. Patients are monitored in the treatment environment following each injection in the unlikely event that systemic reaction ensues. Multiple studies have been performed detailing efficacy of this regimen for treatment of multiple allergens in curing the patient of allergic symptoms with lasting efficacy after treatment has ceased.[19]

Alternative routes for administering immunotherapy have been explored and developed with the goal of creating a system of treatment that can be safely administered by the patient at home, decreasing cost and increasing convenience, while maintaining comparable results. Additional benefits that have been hypothesized are directly treating the reactive sites, namely airway mucosa. Oral administration of antigen concentrates was originally investigated in the 1920s; however, further pursuit was abandoned because of the perception of suboptimal efficacy.[19] An adaptation of oral immunotherapy is sublingual immunotherapy (SLIT), where the allergen extract is held under the tongue for 2 to 3 minutes before swallowing. Major investigations for this regimen have been pursued in Europe, and results from several studies demonstrate similar long-term results of symptom improvement with treatment for both seasonal and perennial allergens when compared with subcutaneous immuno-therapy.[19–25]

The concept of intranasal and intrabronchial immunotherapy has been suggested for many years. Initial trials from Europe revealed efficacy in local symptom control without development of a systemic effect, measured by a total decrease in serum IgE.[19,26–30] Further investigation has been abandoned given the superior efficacy and better tolerated side-effect profile of SLIT.

LOCAL IgE: INTRANASAL
Elevated IgE in Nasal Tissues

Local production of IgE was suspected as early as the 1950s when a higher concentration of IgE was detected in nasal secretions than in serum.[31] In 1970, Tse and colleagues demonstrated ragweed-specific IgE in nasal washings of ragweed-allergic patients with allergic rhinitis, providing additional evidence for local antigen-specific IgE in nasal mucosa.[31–33] In a 1974 study by Huggins and Brostoff,[34] patients with typical allergic rhinitis symptoms with both positive and negative systemic allergy tests, as well as patients free from any allergic symptoms, were exposed to grass-pollen extract intranasally. Subsequent nasal washings revealed elevated grass pollen–specific IgE in all patients with allergic rhinitis regardless of systemic allergy test status, when compared with nonallergic controls, suggesting local intranasal IgE production.[31,35] In a similar study by Merrett and colleagues,[36] nasal washings revealed specific IgE to grass, house-dust mite, animal dander, and mold without allergen provocation in patients with allergic rhinitis with both positive and negative systemic allergy tests.[19]

The role of local IgE has also been investigated in allergic fungal rhinosinusitis (AFRS). This disease process is classically defined by 5 criteria: type I hypersensitivity, nasal polyposis, characteristic radiologic findings, eosinophilic mucin without fungal invasion, and positive fungal stain.[35] Traditionally, systemic allergy testing is administered as an adjunct to diagnosis and treatment of this patient population. Patients with AFRS frequently exhibit positive reactions to multiple fungal and nonfungal antigens, guiding subsequent allergen-specific immunotherapy.[32,37–41] There is a subset of patients, however, who demonstrate the classic features of AFRS, but do not exhibit elevated systemic levels of total IgE.[32,42]

In a 2004 study, Collins and colleagues[43] investigated a phenomenon termed "entopy," or increased local IgE in the absence of systemic disease in AFRS.[32] These investigators identified fungus-specific IgE in paranasal sinus allergic mucin of patients with AFRS undergoing endoscopic sinus surgery in the absence of fungus-specific serum IgE. A study by Carney and colleagues[44] provided further support for local IgE in AFRS with the discovery of the highest concentrations of IgE-positive cells in sinus tissue biopsies from patients with AFRS when compared with samples from those with chronic rhinosinusitis (CRS) and with control subjects.[32] Wise and colleagues[45] further defined the role of local IgE production in paranasal sinus tissue of patients with AFRS by demonstrating profound elevation of IgE-secreting cells in the epithelium and subepithelium of tissue obtained from the osteomeatal complex from patients with AFRS as compared with samples evaluated at both levels from those with nonpolypoid CRS and controls. Specific IgE to both fungal and nonfungal antigens were also demonstrated in higher concentrations from patients with AFRS as opposed to controls.[45] A follow-up study by Ahn and colleagues[46] in 2009 affirmed previous findings of elevated levels of total and specific IgE in sinonasal tissue obtained from patients with AFRS relative to those with CRS and healthy controls. This group also demonstrated that elevated local tissue IgE appears to be a diffuse process throughout nose and paranasal sinuses, with similar amounts of IgE detectable in tissue from the paranasal sinuses as the inferior turbinate samples, despite the predisposition for polyps to form in the sinus cavity rather than on the inferior turbinates (**Figs. 1** and **2**).

The phenomenon of local IgE production has been used to speculate further on the etiology of nasal polyposis in disease processes other than classic AFRS. Since the 1930s, nasal polyps were presumed to have an allergic etiology because of the high concentration of eosinophils detectable in the polyp tissue,[47] but later evidence has disputed this hypothesis.[48–50] Early studies of nasal polyp tissue contributed to evidence for local production of IgE by revealing high concentrations of specific IgE in polyp tissue in subsets of patients both with and without systemic atopy.[51–55] Investigations to define the role of local IgE in nasal polyp tissue have described the significant contribution of *Staphylococcus aureus* superantigens.[32] *S aureus* is commonly found colonizing the upper respiratory tract; however, certain conditions can predispose the host to infection by the organism. These bacteria can cause infection via a variety of mechanisms, including coagulase enzymes, direct invasion, and enterotoxins with superantigenic properties. Superantigens differ from conventional antigens in that they are presented directly on antigen-presenting cells in an unprocessed state and are capable of activating up to 30% of circulating T cells, eliciting an extremely strong primary response.[56] To fully evaluate the role of *S aureus* superantigens in polyp formation, Bachert's[56] group used specific IgE antibodies to the *S aureus* enterotoxin (SAE) as a marker for current or former immune reaction to this entity. They described several different patterns of IgE antibodies in polyp samples. In 30% there is no evidence for the role of SAEs in nonallergic subjects, as there is no IgE to SAEs or to specific inhalant allergens and low total IgE. Approximately 50% demonstrate the situation of superantigen activity in an allergic patient with the presence of specific IgE to SAEs, high total IgE, and IgE to specific inhalant allergens. About 10% of subjects with nasal polyposis represent superantigen activity in a nonallergic subject with the presence of IgE to SAEs, moderate to high total IgE, and no

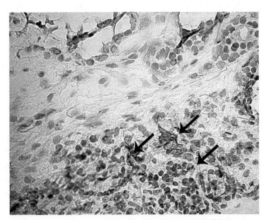

Fig. 1. Representative histologic section demonstrating IgE-positive staining (red-stained cells, *arrows*) in a biopsy from the osteomeatal complex of a patient with chronic rhinosinusitis.

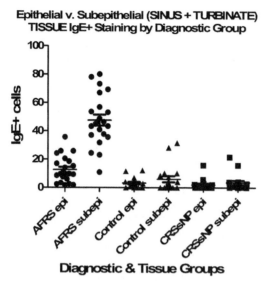

Fig. 2. Graph of local IgE staining by immunohistochemistry in AFRS, chronic rhinosinusitis without nasal polyps (CRSsNP), and control patients. Positive staining in osteomeatal complex sinus tissue and inferior turbinate (turb) tissue is compared between the epithelial (epi) and subepithelial (subepi) compartments. The largest number of IgE-positive cells was found in the subepithelium of AFRS patients. (*Data from* Wise S, Ahn C, Lathers D, et al. Antigen-specific IgE in sinus mucosa of allergic fungal rhinosinusitis patients. Am J Rhinol 2008;22:451–6; and Ahn CN, Wise SK, Lathers DMR, et al. Local production of antigen-specific IgE in different anatomic subsites of allergic fungal rhinosinusitis patients. Otolaryngol Head Neck Surg 2009;141:97–103.)

specific IgE to inhalant allergens. The final 10% of patients likely are allergic patients affected by superantigens other than classic SAE; nasal samples from this group show high total IgE and presence of IgE to specific inhalant allergens, but no IgE to SAEs.[57] Because asthma is frequently associated with nasal polyposis and because patients who have SAE-IgE–positive polyps more frequently have asthma compared with patients who have SAE-IgE–negative polyps, SAE investigation has delved into the lower airways as well.[56] Studies in mice provoked with SAE demonstrate recruitment of proinflammatory cells, including TCR Vβ(+) T cells, and release of cytokines associated with an increased airway responsiveness similar to asthma.[56] Bronchoalveolar lavage washings from humans demonstrate increased expression of TCR Vβ(+) T cells in human patients with poorly controlled asthma but not from those with well-controlled asthma or control subjects, potentiating the hypothesis that SAEs trigger T-cell activation in asthma.[56]

Local Production of Intranasal IgE

Some theorized that elevated intranasal IgE was attributable to immunoglobulin production by B cells in regional lymph nodes, binding to high-affinity receptors on cells such as mast cells, and subsequent migration to intranasal tissues. However, further research aspired to demonstrate that this concentrated intranasal IgE was indeed locally synthesized, rather than transported to nasal tissues.

The nasal mucosa has been shown to contain all of the elements necessary for synthesis of immunoglobulins, immunoglobulin heavy chain class switching, and for these elements to be inducible in response to allergen exposure.[58] Secondary lymphoid organization within nasal polyps was reported in a study by Gevaert and colleagues.[19,55] IgE was demonstrated in association with both follicular structures containing B and T cells as well as with plasma cells. Zurcher and colleagues[59] demonstrated that functional B cells from the nose cultured in an IL-4-rich medium with blocking antibodies of CD40 were capable of producing IgE. Kleinjan and colleagues[60] found the nasal mucosa of patients with allergic rhinitis to be a rich reposit of IgE-positive B cells and IgE-positive plasma cells. Further, this group observed that specific IgE-positive plasma cells were detected only in patients with allergic rhinitis and not found in healthy controls, and that specific IgE is the critical factor for a plasma cell to bind an allergen. No other immunoglobulin isotypes perform this function.

The necessary elements to promote synthesis of IgE and immunoglobulin heavy chain class switching, IL-4, IL-13, and CD40, were detected in sinonasal tissue, disputing previous theory that immunoglobulin class switching solely occurred within the large germinal centers comprising lymph nodes and splenic tissue.[31,32,55] Activation of these mediators following provocation by allergen was suggested in studies by Wise and colleagues[32] and Durham and colleagues.[61] Following exposure to grass pollen, inferior turbinate tissue in patients with known sensitivity were found to contain an increase in IL-4 RNA and germline ε gene exons, which are spliced out during immunoglobulin class–switching gene recombination. Further evidence that immunoglobulin class switching indeed occurs within sinonasal tissue was provided by the ex vivo study by Cameron and colleagues[62] in which similar findings were discovered after incubation of inferior turbinate biopsies from patients with ragweed allergy with the allergen.[32] Takhar and colleagues[63] demonstrated that both in vivo and in vitro exposure to grass pollen allergen in allergic patients stimulates production of circle transcripts, a marker of ongoing class switch recombination, and that class switch recombination to IgE from multiple other isotypes occurs in the nasal mucosa.

Marcucci and colleagues[64] demonstrated the increased sensitivity of nasal mucosa compared with serum in response to allergen provocation, suggesting that the production of IgE occurs first in the target organ induced by allergen exposure, and is later followed by a systemic response. After in situ incubation of timothy grass, serum and nasal mucosa IgE measurements detected a significant immediate increase in the nasal mucosal levels, most profound in patients with known allergy during the peak of the pollen season.

Future attention to local IgE production within the nose will likely be directed toward the clinical relevance of this important finding, including diagnostic and therapeutic options for allergy testing and local immunotherapy. This may include development of an ideal test that is sensitive to allergen-specific IgE within nasal mucosa, which can aid in diagnosis of allergy when traditional systemic testing fails. Therapeutic options may ultimately modify local production of IgE with the long-term goal of decreasing local tissue disease severity and improving quality of life.

LOCAL IgE: PULMONARY

Studies of elevated IgE in pulmonary tissues aimed to describe the patterns of expression and the relationship to asthma severity, with goals of improving asthma control by means of anti-IgE therapy. Balzar and colleagues[65] studied more than 90 lung specimens, including healthy controls and those from patients with a range of asthma severity with and without atopy, and described a pattern of IgE distribution limited to the submucosa and excluded from the lung parenchyma. Mast cells bound to IgE were found primarily in the proximal airways. The amount of mucosal IgE more directly correlated with eosinophilic and lymphocytic tissue inflammation, pulmonary function, and severity of asthma disease than did degree of systemic IgE. They proposed that an increase in serum IgE likely represents mucosal processes promoting an induction of the systemic IgE production mechanisms, and a high level of serum IgE occurs as a result of failure of immunologic process at the mucosal level.[65]

Murine models have been studied to delineate the cellular infiltrate present in asthma. Mice were sensitized using intratracheal instillation of ovalbumin, which has been shown to result in eosinophilia, mononuclear cell infiltration, and airway epithelial changes analogous to what is seen in asthma.[66] In the mice that had been sensitized, germinal centers were detected with the parenchyma of the inflamed lungs associated with follicular dendritic cells bearing ovalbumin on their plasma membranes and oval-bumin-specific IgE-producing plasma cells.[67] Germinal centers, or bronchial-associated lymphoid tissue, are constitutive structures in certain species such as rats and rabbits; however, are inducible in humans and mice via antigenic exposure.[67–71] These germinal centers are the likely local source of IgE-secreting plasma cells that contribute to release of inflammatory mediators in the lung during an allergic asthma exacerbation.

Given the correlation of local pulmonary IgE with degree of pathologic inflammation, degree of asthma severity, and pulmonary function, Soler and colleagues[72] tested the hypothesis that anti-IgE therapy would indeed improve asthma severity. Omalizu-mab is a recombinant humanized monoclonal antibody that binds free circulating IgE and thereby prevents its binding to mast cells, preemptively avoiding degranulation. Given to patients with moderate to severe asthma, it improved symptoms, improved quality of life, and permitted decrease in dosages of oral and inhaled corticosteroids.[72] Improving control of asthma and decreasing the number of exacerbations in patients with severe asthma will likely greatly decrease individual financial burden in addition to decreasing burden on the health care system.[73] A similar study undertaken in patients with allergic rhinitis revealed a less exuberant effect as an actual disease-modi-fying effector.[74] Although patients had improvement in nasal allergy symptoms while receiving the therapy, there was no correlating decrease in specific IgE or in ε mRNA, suggesting that therapy does not modulate synthesis of nasal IgE. Omalizumab therapy, therefore, is founded on local expression of IgE, but appears to be unrelated to local synthesis of IgE. Further, observations made by Corris and Dark[75] regarding transmission of asthma through lung transplantation from donors with mild asthma to recipients not previously afflicted, and cure of asthma by transplantation of healthy lungs into patients suffering with asthma gave strong support to the hypothesis that asthma was a local disease mediated by local production of chemical signals.

Much of the investigation into the matter of local production of IgE in the lungs parallels the steps that were addressed in the same phenomenon in nasal tissue. Durham and colleagues[8] and Ying and colleagues[9] showed that in asthmatic patients, irrespective of atopy, total number of CD20 + B cells present in bronchial mucosa was similar to the number found in healthy controls, however the number expressing ε germline gene transcript and mature mRNA for the ε heavy chain gene were elevated in asthmatic patients. It has been suggested that prior work evidencing local IgE synthesis in nasal tissue is applicable to the pulmonary system as well.[8,76,77]

ANTIGEN SPECIFICITY OR DISORDERED PRODUCTION?

Traditionally it has been assumed that the selective pressures shaping the immune repertoire through repeated cycles of finely tuned somatic mutation are the same for all immunoglobulin isotypes. Emerging evidence from studies focusing on the mutation rates and patterns observed in the variable region of the IgE gene suggest that IgE may develop along a distinct pathway. Recent studies have identified unusual mutation patterns in IgE from blood samples taken from individuals with allergic asthma, but few have investigated whether these patterns are also seen in IgE isolated from tissue.

Early B-cell development is a finely tuned process with multiple "check points" to eliminate self-reactive cells while ensuring the formation of functional immunoglobulin. Formation of the functional immunoglobulin gene requires a series of specialized tightly regulated somatic recombination events, known collectively as VDJ recombination, to occur early in B-cell development. Later, as mature naive B cells recirculate through the lymphatic system, they can be activated by encounters with antigen. During an immune challenge, the antigen specificity of activated cells is fine tuned within the germinal centers. Competition for antigen binding in the germinal centers results in selection of those B cells with the best existing binding affinity. Once selected, clonal expansion of these cells is initiated.[78] As the selected cells proliferate, they accumulate mutations with high frequency: approximately 1 mutation per generation.

These mutations are preferentially focused on hypervariable hotspots within the V region. Many of these hotspots fall within the complementarity-determining regions (CDRs) of the V gene, which correspond to the antigen-binding sites of an antibody.[79] The rate of mutations in the V region is a million times higher than the genome-wide rate, and negative selection eliminates cells with mutations that cause reduced antigen-binding affinity or loss of function.[78,80] Cells that accumulate mutations improving the antigen-binding affinity of the expressed immunoglobulin are selected to give a subset of highly antigen-specific B cells.

When a B cell has developed under the influence of pressure from antigen selection, a characteristic pattern of replacement mutations is seen in V region sequences. Antigen selection results in the accumulation of replacement mutations in the CDR of the V region (R_{CDR}) with higher frequency than in the surrounding framework regions (FR).[81] In our laboratory, seminested polymerase chain reaction (PCR) was used to amplify the entire V region of IgE sequences from individuals with CRS with nasal polyps (CRSwNP). IgE sequences were analyzed for evidence of antigen selection to see if the mutation pattern reported in other allergic and inflammatory disorders is reflected in sequences from CRS sufferers. IgE sequences were successfully amplified from 4 individuals. In total, 217 IgE sequences were amplified, of which 38 were unique, and VDJ gene usage and mutation rates were analyzed for these sequences.

Dahlke and colleagues[82] reported that there is a statistically significant difference in mutation frequency distribution among nonallergic IgE, allergic IgE, and IgG sequences. Although polyclonal IgE has been detected in nasal polyps, and it has been hypothesized that this is the result of stimulation by super-antigens.[83] Our studies have shown that there was no significant difference between the mean V region mutations of IgE sequences from individuals with CRSwNP and previously described nonallergic IgE sequences nor was there a difference with database-derived IgG (Richard J. Harvey, MD, unpublished data, 2009). Mutation analysis of 38 unique IgE sequences showed that only 6 were likely the product of IgE-expressing B cells that had developed under the influence of antigen selection (**Fig. 3**). Given that such IgE may have limited binding affinity for the proposed antigen and are unlikely to have undergone strong antigen selection, such findings have significant implications for the role of immunotherapy in chronic rhinosinusitis and the relevance of SAE or fungal IgE. Whether these IgE products and their production are tightly related to pathogenesis in chronic rhinosinusitis, merely a by-product of colonizing organisms

IgE sequence library

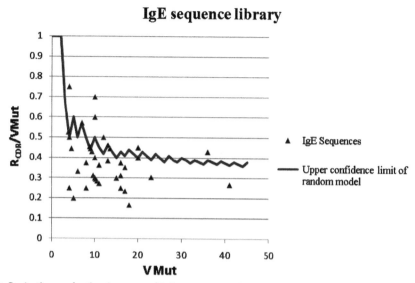

Fig. 3. Antigen selection in mucosal IgE sequences using R_{CDR}/VMut: VMut. Antigen selection results in the accumulation of replacement mutations in the CDR of the V region (R_{CDR}). VMut is the total mutations in the V region. Points falling on top of each other have been offset. Individual IgE sequences are represented by blue triangles. The red line shows the upper confidence limit of a random somatic mutation model. The lower confidence limit is not shown. Sequences above the red line suggest production under antigen selection.

(epiphenomenon), or part or a broader antigen-presenting cell disorder remains unresolved.

Implications for Research

Further research into the mechanisms that drive antigen presentation and then the subsequent immunologic response are more likely to procure future therapeutic targets. IgE production is likely to occur locally and under conditions of less antigen selectivity than previously believed. This significantly affects our current disease classifications and nomenclature, in particular for chronic rhinosinusitis. The concept of "AFRS-like" patient classification exemplifies this inability to match systemic markers with clinical findings. Likewise, research into SAE and fungal IgE may place too much assumption on the degree to which these antigens have influenced subsequent IgE production.

Implications for Clinical Practice

The blunt use of systemic IgE diagnostic testing may provide limited clinical insight to IgE-mediated disease in patients with sinonasal pathology. Immunotherapy, although effective for well-proven allergic IgE-mediated disease, is likely to have little role in chronic rhinosinusitis with polyps if highly selected antigen-specific IgE is not demonstrated in local mucosa.

SUMMARY

This is a review of local and systemic IgE as it relates to inflammatory conditions of the upper and lower airways. The potential exists for local IgE to enhance our identification and treatment of patients with airway inflammatory conditions in the absence of elevated systemic IgE. Development of disease-modifying agents capable of inhibiting local IgE production may ultimately decrease the symptomatic manifestations and socioeconomic burden of allergy.

REFERENCES

1. Derebery MJ, Berliner KI. Allergy and health-related quality of life. Otolaryngol Head Neck Surg 2000;123(4):393–9.
2. Arbes SJ, Gergen PJ, Elliott L. Prevalences of positive skin test responses to 10 common allergens in the U.S. population: results from the Third National Health and Nutrition Examination Survey. J Allergy Clin Immunol 2005;116(2):377–83.
3. Soni A. Allergic rhinitis: trends in use and expenditures, 2000 to 2005. Agency for Healthcare Research and Quality 2008. Statistical brief #204. Available at: http://www.aaaai.org/media/statistics/allergy-statistics.asp. Accessed October 27, 2009.
4. Orban NT, Saleh H, Durham SR. Allergic and non-allergic rhinitis. In: Adkinson NF, editor. Middleton's allergy: principles and practice. China: Mosby; 2008. Chapter 55.
5. Shah SB, Emanuel IA. Nonallergic and allergic rhinitis. In: Lalwani, editor. Current diagnosis & treatment in otolaryngology - head and neck surgery. New York: Lange; 2008. p. 264–72.
6. Canonica GW. Introduction to nasal and pulmonary allergy cascade. Allergy 2002;57(Suppl 75):8–12.
7. Mabry RL, Marple BF. Allergic rhinitis. In: Cummings. Otolaryngology: head and neck surgery. Philadelphia: Mosby; 2005. p. 981–89.
8. Durham SR, Smurthwaite L, Gould HJ. Local IgE production. Am J Rhinol 2000; 14:305–7.
9. Ying S, Humbert M, Meng Q, et al. Local expression of ε germline gene transcripts and RNA for the ε heavy chain of IgE in the bronchial mucosa in atopic and nonatopic asthma. J Allergy Clin Immunol 2001;107:686–92.
10. Nimmerjahn F, Ravetch JV. Divergent immunoglobulin g subclass activity through selective Fc receptor binding. Science 2005;310:1510–2.
11. Gould HJ, Sutton BJ, Beavil AJ, et al. The biology of IgE and the basis of allergic disease. Annu Rev Immunol 2003;21:579–628.
12. Demoly P, Bousquet J, Romano A. In vivo methods for the study of allergy. In: Adkinson NF, editor. Middleton's allergy: principles and practice. China: Mosby; 2008. Chapter 71.
13. Demoly P, Piette V, Bousquet J. In vivo methods for study of allergy: skin tests, techniques and interpretation. In: Adkinson NF, Yunginger JW, Busse WW, et al, editors. Allergy, principles and practice. New York: Mosby; 2003. p. 631–55.
14. Nalebuff DJ, Fadal RG. RAST-based immunotherapy. Rhinology 1984;22(1):11–9.
15. Tandy JR, Mabry RL, Mabry CS. Correlation of modified radioallergosorbent test scores and skin test results. Otolaryngol Head Neck Surg 1996;115(1):42–5.
16. van der Zee JS, de Groot H, van Swieten P, et al. Discrepancies between the skin test and IgE antibody assays: study of histamine release, complement activation in vitro, and occurrence of allergen-specific IgG. J Allergy Clin Immunol 1988;82: 270–81.
17. Weiner JM, Abramson MJ, Puy RM. Intranasal corticosteroids versus oral H1 receptor antagonists in allergic rhinitis: systematic review of randomised controlled trials. BMJ 1998;317:1624–9.

18. Noon L. Prophylactic inoculation against hay fever. Lancet 1911;1572–3.
19. Nelson HS. Immunotherapy for inhalant allergies. In: Adkinson NF, editor. Middleton's allergy: principles and practice. China: Mosby; 2008. Chapter 95.
20. Canonica GW, Passalacqua G. Sublingual immunotherapy in the treatment of adult allergic rhinitis patients. Allergy 2006;61(Suppl 81):20–3.
21. Giovane AL, Bardare M, Passalacqua G, et al. A three-year double-blind, placebo-controlled study with specific oral immunotherapy to Dermatophagoides: evidence of safety and efficacy in paediatric patients. Clin Exp Allergy 1994;24:53–9.
22. Wilson DR, Lima MT, Durham SR. Sublingual immunotherapy for allergic rhinitis: systematic review and meta-analysis. Allergy 2005;60:1–2.
23. Calderon MA, Alves B, Jacobson M, et al. Allergen injection immunotherapy for seasonal allergic rhinitis. Cochrane Database Syst Rev 2007;1:CD001936.
24. Marogna M, Spadlini I, Massolo A, et al. Effects of sublingual immunotherapy for multiple or single allergens in polysensitized patients. Ann Allergy Asthma Immunol 2007;98:274–80.
25. Khinchi MS, Poulsen LK, Carat F, et al. Clinical efficacy of sublingual and subcutaneous birch pollen allergen-specific immunotherapy: a randomized, placebo-controlled, double-blind, double-dummy study. Allergy 2004;59:45–53.
26. Welsh PW, Zimmermann EM, Yunginger JW, et al. Preseasonal intranasal immunotherapy with nebulized short ragweed extract. J Allergy Clin Immunol 1981;67:237–42.
27. Georgitis JW, Nickelsen JA, Wypych JI, et al. Local intranasal immunotherapy with high-dose polymerized ragweed extract. Int Arch Allergy Appl Immunol 1986;81:170–3.
28. Andri L, Senna G, Bettel C, et al. Local nasal immunotherapy for Dermatophagoides-induced rhinitis: efficacy of a powder inhaler. J Allergy Clin Immunol 1993;91:987–96.
29. Passalacqua G, Albano M, Ruffoni S, et al. Nasal immunotherapy to Parietaria: evidence of reduction of local allergic inflammation. Am J Respir Crit Care Med 1995;152:461–6.
30. Tari MG, Mancino M, Monti G. Immunotherapy by inhalation of allergen in powder in house dust allergic asthma—a double-blind study. J Investig Allergol Clin Immunol 1992;2:59–67.
31. Smurthwaite L, Durham SR. Local IgE synthesis in allergic rhinitis and asthma. Curr Allergy Asthma Rep 2002;2:231–8.
32. Wise SK, Ahn CN, Schlosser RJ. Localized immunoglobulin E expression in allergic rhinitis and nasal polyposis. Curr Opin Otolaryngol Head Neck Surg 2009;17:216–22.
33. Tse KS, Wicher K, Arbesman C. IgE antibodies in nasal secretions of ragweed allergic subjects. J Allergy 1970;46:352.
34. Huggins KG, Brostoff J. Local production of specific IgE antibodies in allergic-rhinitis patients with negative skin tests. Lancet 1975;2:148–50.
35. Bent J, Kuhn F. Diagnosis of allergic fungal sinusitis. Otolaryngol Head Neck Surg 1994;111:580–8.
36. Merret TG, Houri M, Mayer AL, et al. Measurement of specific IgE antibodies in nasal secretion—evidence for local production. Clin Allergy 1976;6:69–73.
37. Manning S, Mabry R, Schaefer S, et al. Evidence of IgE-mediated hypersensitivity in allergic fungal sinusitis. Laryngoscope 1993;103:717–21.
38. Braun J, Pauli G, Schultz P, et al. Allergic fungal sinusitis associated with allergic bronchopulmonary aspergillosis: an uncommon sinobronchial allergic mycosis. Am J Rhinol 2007;21:412–6.

39. Bartynski J, McCaffrey T, Frigas E. Allergic fungal sinusitis secondary to dermatiaceous fungi: *Curvularia lunata* and *Alternaria*. Otolaryngol Head Neck Surg 1990;103:32–9.
40. Gourley D, Whisman B, Jorgensen N, et al. Allergic bipolaris sinusitis: clinical and immunopathologic characteristics. J Allergy Clin Immunol 1990;85:583–91.
41. Stewart A, Hunsaker D. Fungus-specific IgG and IgE in allergic fungal rhinosinusitis. Otolaryngol Head Neck Surg 2002;127:324–32.
42. Kuhn F, Swain R. Allergic fungal sinusitis: diagnosis and treatment. Curr Opin Otolaryngol Head Neck Surg 2003;11:1–5.
43. Collins M, Nair S, Smith W, et al. Role of local immunoglobulin E production in the pathophysiology of noninvasive fungal sinusitis. Laryngoscope 2004;114: 1242–6.
44. Carney A, Tan L, Adams D, et al. Th2 immunological inflammation in allergic fungal sinusitis, nonallergic eosinophilic fungal sinusitis, and chronic rhinosinusitis. Am J Rhinol 2006;20:145–9.
45. Wise S, Ahn C, Lathers D, et al. Antigen-specific IgE in sinus mucosa of allergic fungal rhinosinusitis patients. Am J Rhinol 2008;22:451–6.
46. Ahn CN, Wise SK, Lathers DMR, et al. Local production of antigen-specific IgE in different anatomic subsites of allergic fungal rhinosinusitis patients. Otolaryngol Head Neck Surg 2009;141:97–103.
47. Kern RA, Schenck HP. Allergy, a constant factor in the etiology of so-called mucuous nasal polyps. J Allergy 1933;4:48597.
48. Settipane GA, Chaffe FH. Nasal polyps in asthma and rhinitis. A review of 6,037 patients. J Allergy Clin Immunol 1976;59:17–21.
49. Drake-Lee AB. Histamine and its release from nasal polyps: preliminary communication. J R Soc Med 1984;77:120–4.
50. Caplin I, Haynes T, Spahn J. Are nasal polyps an allergic phenomenon? Ann Allergy 1971;29:63–8.
51. Hirschberg A, Jokuti A, Darvas Z, et al. The pathogenesis of nasal polyposis by immunoglobulin E and interieukin-5 is completed by transforming growth factor beta-1. Laryngoscope 2003;113:120–4.
52. Wei C, Fang S. Tissue-specific immunoglobulin E in human nasal polyps. Ann Otol Rhinol Laryngol 2005;114:386–9.
53. Suh K, Park H, Nahm D, et al. Role of IgG, IgA, and IgE antibodies in nasal polyp tissue: their relationships with eosinophilic infiltration and degranulation. J Korean Med Sci 2002;17:375–80.
54. Sabirov A, Hamilton R, Jacobs J, et al. Role of local immunoglobulin E specific for *Alternaria alternata* in the pathogenesis of nasal polyposis. Laryngoscope 2008; 118:4–9.
55. Gevaert P, Holtappels G, Johansson SGO, et al. Organization of secondary lymphoid tissue and local IgE formation to *Staphylococcus aureus* enterotoxins in nasal polyp tissue. Allergy 2005;60:71–9.
56. Bachert C, van Zele T, Gevaert P, et al. Superantigens and nasal polyps. Curr Allergy Asthma Rep 2007;3:523–31.
57. Bachert C, Gevaert P, Holtappels G, et al. Total and specific IgE in nasal polyps is related to local eosinipholic inflammation. J Allergy Clin Immunol 2001;107:607–14.
58. Agresti A, Vercelli D. Molecular mechanisms of IgE regulation. In: Vercelli D, editor. New York: Wiley; 1997.
59. Zurcher AW, Derer T, Lang AB, et al. Culture and IgE synthesis of nasal B cells. Int Arch Allergy Immunol 1996;111:77–82.

60. Kleinjan A, Vinke J, Severijnen L. Local production and detection of (specific) IgE in nasal B-cells and plasma cells of allergic rhinitis patients. Eur Respir J 2000;15: 491–7.

61. Durham S, Gould H, Thiens C. Expression of the ε germ-line gene transcripts and mRNA for ε heavy chain of IgE in nasal B cells and the effects of topical corticosteroid. Eur J Immunol 1997;27:2899–906.

62. Cameron L, Gounni A, Frenkiel S. SεSμ and SεSγ switch circles in human nasal mucosa following ex vivo allergen challenge: evidence for direct as well as sequential class switch recombination. J Immunol 2003;171:3816–22.

63. Takhar P, Smurthwaite L, Coker H. Allergen drives class switching to IgE in the nasal mucosa of allergic rhinitis. J Immunol 2005;174:5024–32.

64. Marcucci F, Sensi LG, Migali E, et al. Eosinophil cationic protein and specific IgE in serum and nasal mucosa of patients with grass-pollen-allergic rhinitis and asthma. Allergy 2001;56:231–6.

65. Balzar S, Strand M, Rhodes D, et al. IgE expression pattern in lung: relation to systemic IgE and asthma phenotypes. J Allergy Clin Immunol 2007;119:855–62.

66. Blyth DI, Pedrick MS, Savage TJ, et al. Lung inflammation and epithelial changes in a murine model of atopic asthma. Am J Respir Cell Mol Biol 1996;14:425–38.

67. Chvatchko Y, Kosco-Vilbois MH, Herren S, et al. Germinal center formation and local immunoglobulin E (IgE) production in the lung after an airway antigenic challenge. J Exp Med 1996;184:2353–60.

68. Pabst R. Is BALT a major component of the human lung immune system? Immunol Today 1995;192:293–9.

69. Pabst R, Gehrke I. Is the bronchus-associated lymphoid tissue (BALT) an integral structure of the lung in normal mammals, including humans? Am J Respir Cell Mol Biol 1990;3:131–5.

70. Delventhal S, Hensel A, Petzoldt K, et al. Effects of microbial stimulation on the number, size and activity of bronchus-associated lymphoid tissue (BALT) structures in the pig. Int J Exp Pathol 1992;73:351–7.

71. Gould SJ, Isaacso PG. Bronchus-associated lymphoid tissue in human fetal and infant lung. J Pathol 1993;169:229–34.

72. Soler M, Matz J, Townley R, et al. The anti-IgE antibody omalizumab reduces exacerbations and steroid requirement in allergic asthmatics. Eur Respir J 2001;18:254–61.

73. Bousquet J, Cabrera P, Berkman N, et al. The effect of treatment with omalizumab, an anti-IgE antibody, on asthma exacerbations and emergency medical visits in patients with severe persistent asthma. Allergy 2005;60:302–8.

74. Corren J, Diaz-Sanchez D, Saxon A, et al. Effects of omalizumab, a humanized monoclonal anti-IgE antibody, on nasal reactivity to allergen and local IgE synthesis. Ann Allergy Asthma Immunol 2004;93:243–8.

75. Corris PA, Dark JH. Aetiology of asthma: lessons from lung transplantation. Lancet 1993;341(8857):1369–71.

76. Cameron LA, Durham SR, Jacobson MR, et al. Expression of IL-4, Cε RNA and Iε RNA in the nasal mucosa of patients with seasonal rhinitis: effect of topical corticosteroids. J Allergy Clin Immunol 1998;101:330–6.

77. Ghaffar O, Durham SR, Al-Ghamdi K, et al. Expression of IgE heavy chain transcripts in the sinus mucosa of atopic and nonatopic patients with chronic sinusitis. Am J Respir Cell Mol Biol 1998;18:706–11.

78. Honjo T, Kinoshita K, Muramatsu M. Molecular mechanism of class switch recombination: linkage with somatic hypermutation. Annu Rev Immunol 2002;20:165–96.

79. Delves PJ, Roitt IM. The immune system. Second of two parts. N Engl J Med 2000;343:108–17.
80. Davies JM, O'Hehir RE. Immunogenetic characteristics of immunoglobulin E in allergic disease. Clin Exp Allergy 2008;38:566–78.
81. Collins AM, Sewell WA, Edwards MR. Immunoglobulin gene rearrangement, repertoire diversity, and the allergic response. Pharmacol Ther 2003;100:157–70.
82. Dahlke I, Nott DJ, Ruhno J, et al. Antigen selection in the IgE response of allergic and nonallergic individuals. J Allergy Clin Immunol 2006;117:1477–83.
83. Kern RC, Conley DB, Walsh W, et al. Perspectives on the etiology of chronic rhinosinusitis: an immune barrier hypothesis. Am J Rhinol 2008;22:549–59.

Biofilms

Jeffrey D. Suh, MD, Vijay Ramakrishnan, MD,
James N. Palmer, MD*

KEYWORDS

• Biofilm • Chronic sinusitis • Rhinosinusitis

Chronic rhinosinusitis (CRS) is one of the most common chronic medical conditions, affecting between 14% and 16% of the US population. Direct health care costs are significant and are estimated to be more than $5.8 billion per year. According to the most recent data from the National Health Interview Survey (2007), rhinosinusitis continues to be one of the top 10 leading diagnoses of office visits in the United States. Patients with CRS demonstrate lower quality-of-life scores than those suffering from chronic obstructive pulmonary disease, congestive heart failure, back pain, or angina.[1] However, some patients with CRS suffer from persistent and recurrent infections despite maximal medical management and surgery. Since the initial description of biofilms on the sinonasal mucosa of patients with CRS, there has been a growing body of evidence supporting the contributory role of biofilms in poor disease progression and persistent sinonasal inflammation.

BIOFILMS OVERVIEW

It is currently estimated that at least 65% of all human bacterial infections may involve biofilm formation. These include a diverse range of infectious processes, including dental caries, periodontitis, musculoskeletal infections, osteomyelitis, bacterial prostatitis, endocarditis, and cystic fibrosis pneumonia. Biofilms have also been implicated in several conditions seen in an otolaryngology practice, including otitis media, chronic sinusitis, chronic tonsillitis, adenoiditis, and device infections (such as in cochlear implants, tympanostomy tubes, and tracheostomy tubes).[2] Bacterial biofilms are described as surface-associated communities of microorganisms encased in a protective extracellular matrix. The life cycle of bacterial biofilms can be divided into 5 parts (**Fig. 1**). Biofilms are initiated when free-floating, planktonic bacteria anchor to biologic or inert surfaces. The attached bacteria multiply and progress from a state of monolayer to a microcolony and then to a critical mass, in which interbacterial crosstalk occurs, triggering a phenomenon known as quorum sensing that leads to the biofilm phenotype. The bacteria respond collectively to express factors

No financial disclosures.
Department of Otorhinolaryngology–Head and Neck Surgery, Hospital of the University of Pennsylvania, Ravdin Building 5th Floor, 3400 Spruce Street, Philadelphia, PA 19104, USA
* Corresponding author.
E-mail address: james.palmer@uphs.upenn.edu

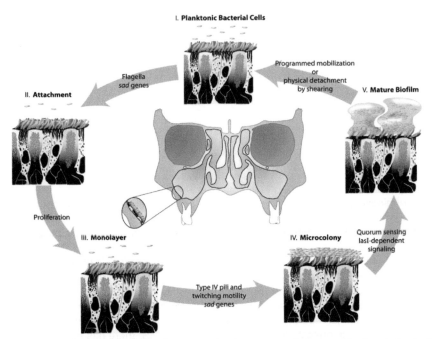

Fig. 1. Steps of bacterial biofilm formation in the paranasal sinuses. Planktonic bacterial cells (*I*) move from steps of attachment (*II*) to the formation of monolayers (*III*), microcolonies (*IV*), and a mature biofilm (*V*) through multiple progressions in gene expression.

that are specific to the biofilm phenotype, which lead to the secretion of an exopolysaccharide matrix. This biofilm phenotype is characterized morphologically by the formation of microbial towers, which are composed of layers of embedded, live bacteria with intervening water channels. Under the right environmental conditions, free-floating bacteria are released from the biofilms, and the cycle is continued at other surfaces. Approximately 80% of the world's microbial biomass resides in the biofilm state, and the National Institutes of Health estimates that more than 75% of microbial infections that occur in the human body are underpinned by the formation and persistence of biofilms.[3,4]

Biofilm formation is thought to provide a mechanism for enhanced bacterial survival. Bacteria in biofilms lack the antibiotic susceptibility of planktonic bacteria and can be up to 1000 times more resistant to antibiotic treatment.[5] Bacteria in biofilms are also more resistant to host defenses, because the extracellular matrix that makes up most of the biofilm serves to protect the bacteria against antibodies, immune-system phagocytosis, antibiotic penetration, and complement binding. There is also a decreased need for oxygen and nutrients when bacteria exist in the biofilm state, further reducing susceptibility to certain antimicrobials (**Box 1**).[6] This is especially true for bacteria within the core of the biofilm mass.[7] In addition, biofilms are environments where bacteria can share their DNA by transfer of genetic information via plasmids to encourage variability and adaptive mutations, such as antibiotic resistance. All of these properties encourage persistence of bacteria for extensive periods despite antibiotic treatment, resulting in chronic disease with intermittent acute infections. Biofilms also provide a source for recurrent infections by releasing planktonic bacteria, resulting in implantation and population of new anatomic locations.[8]

> **Box 1**
> **Biofilms in sinusitis**
>
> - Three-dimensional aggregates of bacteria encased in a secreted exopolysaccharide matrix
> - Increase evasion of host defenses
> - Increase resistance to antibiotic therapy
> - Release of planktonic bacteria can result in new or acute infections in the host

MUCOSAL BIOFILMS AND CRS

It is important to note that biofilms have a heterogeneous morphology because the biofilm phenotype is highly dependent on the surrounding environmental factors, including pH, nutrient availability, and oxidative potential.[9] Bacterial biofilms that have formed on mucosal surfaces are referred to as mucosal biofilms. Mucosal biofilms have a unique cascade of gene expression compared with biofilms on inert surfaces. Bacteria of mucosal biofilms must overcome the normal airway mucociliary clearance that usually protects the upper airways and sinonasal tract. With further detail in the sections to follow, multiple studies have visualized biofilms in an animal model of sinusitis,[10] on frontal sinus stents removed from patients with CRS,[11] and from the mucosa of patients undergoing sinus surgery.[12] **Fig. 2** depicts 3 separate methods of identifying bacterial biofilms from the same patient with CRS. Studies have shown that the presence of biofilms is associated with worse postoperative outcomes after endoscopic sinus surgery.[13,14] Treatments of biofilm-associated CRS are generally aimed at disrupting the biofilm life cycle and are described in the later sections.

VISUALIZATION OF BACTERIAL BIOFILMS

A variety of sophisticated assessment techniques have shown the presence of bacterial biofilms on sampled sinonasal mucosa from animals and patients with CRS. The classic approaches have included both scanning electron microscopy and transmission electron microscopy (SEM and TEM, respectively). These techniques provide detailed imaging of the intricate architecture, developmental stages, and polymicrobial nature of biofilms. However, both the techniques can be limited in clinical utility due to difficulty in fixation, the presence of artifacts in the fixation process, and

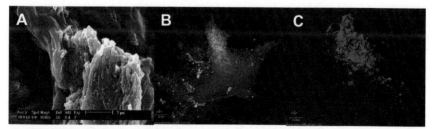

Fig. 2. Bacterial biofilms identified on the sinus mucosa in the same patient by 3 different imaging modalities. (*A*) Scanning electron microscopy (SEM), (*B*) confocal laser scanning microscopy (CLSM), and (*C*) fluorescence in situ hybridization (FISH). Note that only FISH can identify at least 1 of the bacterial species present in the biofilm. In this specimen, the biofilm was found to contain *Pseudomonas aeruginosa*.

difficulty in identifying individual bacterial species. SEM also has some limitations in differentiating between mucus, clot, and biofilm, whereas TEM only renders a 2-dimensional section of the biofilm.[15] Other techniques include fluorescence in situ hybridization (FISH) and confocal laser scanning microscopy (CLSM). FISH with CLSM provide both 3-dimensional biofilm structures and information regarding the polymicrobial nature of native biofilms.

MICROBIOLOGY OF BACTERIAL BIOFILMS

It is well known that one of the leading causes of medically refractory rhinosinusitis is the opportunistic gram-negative bacteria, *Pseudomonas aeruginosa*. A wealth of morphologic and physiologic evidence exists that biofilms enable *P aeruginosa* to persist in cystic fibrosis pulmonary infections.[16,17] Biofilm formation has been demonstrated by many other bacterial species including *Staphylococcus aureus*, *Streptococcus pneumoniae*, *Haemophilus influenzae*, and *Moraxella catarrhalis*. After sampling 157 consecutive patients with CRS over a 4-month period, Prince and colleagues[18] found that 28.6% of samples showed the potential for biofilm formation. *P aeruginosa* and *S aureus* composed 71% of the samples that showed biofilm growth. Polymicrobial samples with and without *P aeruginosa*, coagulase-negative staphylococci, and *H influenzae* made up the rest of the biofilm formers in their study. Sanderson and colleagues[19] used CLSM and FISH analyses to examine intraoperative samples taken from 18 patients with CRS and 5 controls undergoing septoplasty for the presence of biofilms. The analysis found 78% (14 out of 18) of patients with detectable bacteria in a biofilm matrix. The predominant biofilm forming species was *H influenzae* followed by *S pneumoniae* and *S aureus*, with *P aeruginosa* notably absent. They also found biofilms on 2 of 5 of the controls, underscoring the need to better clarify the connection between CRS and biofilms.

Increased antibiotic resistance is a trait common to biofilm bacteria. Bacteria in biofilms show 10- to 1000-fold less sensitivity to antibiotics than bacteria growing in culture. The mechanisms of biofilm antibiotic resistance are currently under study.[3] Theories include a combination of restricted antibiotic penetration through the biofilm extracellular matrix, reduced metabolic activity and growth rate, upregulation of efflux pumps, and subpopulations of phenotypically and genetically different bacteria. Another hypothesis proposes that the basal layers of the biofilm are composed of bacteria in a dormant state that is secondary to the accumulation of inhibitive waste products or the depletion of necessary substrate. The decrease in metabolic activity and growth rate may be explained by altered genetic expression in bacterial biofilms leading to a persister cell phenotype.[7] A recent study by May and colleagues[20] demonstrated that subinhibitory concentrations of antibiotics triggered biofilm formation in *Escherichia coli* and the induction of antibiotic efflux pumps. This study suggests that inadequate doses or courses of antibiotic treatment can trigger biofilm formation and lead to chronic infections.

FUNGAL BIOFILMS

A variety of fungal species have been demonstrated to form biofilms in vivo and in vitro.[21] *Candida* spp are among the most common causative agents of yeast biofilm infections; however, *Cryptococcus*, *Pneumocystis*, *Aspergillus*, *Coccidioides*, and other fungal species have been implicated as well. Among the pathogenic fungi, *Candida albicans* is most frequently associated with biofilm formation, especially with infection of indwelling medical devices. Chandra and colleagues[22] demonstrated that *C albicans* isolates in the form of biofilm exhibited increased resistance to amphotericin B, nystatin, chlorhexidine, and fluconazole when compared with plank-tonic cultures. Characterization of fungal biofilms is difficult, but studies have demon-strated that fungal biofilms, like bacterial biofilms, have defined developmental phases. The main phases of biofilm development are adhesion, filamentation, and hyphal and yeast proliferation with maturation and production of the extracellular matrix. In one study, it was demonstrated that *Candida* spp were able to form biofilms by directly attaching to bacteria that have already colonized a surface.[23] The extracel-lular matrix consists primarily of proteins, chitins, DNA, and carbohydrates. It covers the biofilm and is through to act as a protective barrier by preventing host immune factors, antifungals, and by impeding physical disruption of the underlying cells.

Fungal elements have been demonstrated within sinus mucosal biofilms in patients with CRS.[24] The investigators theorized that fungi may contribute to the chronic inflammation or fungi and bacteria may interact in a symbiotic way to increase resis-tance to host defenses and treatment. Foreman and colleagues[25] also identified mixed bacterial-fungal biofilms from intraoperative specimens in patients with CRS. In their study, 9 of 11 (82%) patients had mixed bacterial-fungal biofilms with either *S aureus* or *H influenzae*, whereas the remaining patients had only fungal biofilms. Further research is needed to determine what effects the presence of fungal biofilms has on sinus mucosa and in the pathophysiology of CRS.

HUMAN STUDIES

The senior author was the first to demonstrate bacterial biofilms on the sinus mucosa of patients with CRS[12] and in an animal model of pseudomonas sinusitis.[10] Multiple studies have since confirmed the presence of biofilms on the sinonasal mucosa of patients with CRS. Early work by Perloff and Palmer[11] involved the use of SEM to iden-tify the presence of biofilms on frontal sinus stents removed 6 weeks after endoscopic sinus surgery from 6 patients. These stents were considered to be analogous to pres-sure equalization tubes removed from children with biofilms. Biofilms were identified on all 6 stents but not in controls. Morphologic structures characterized on SEM of biofilm growth included water channels, glycocalyx coatings, and 3-dimensional structures.

Subsequently, sinonasal-mucosal specimens obtained at the time of surgery from 16 patients with CRS were examined for biofilms by SEM. The results were then compared with specimens from control subjects. All the patients showed signs of infection including cilia loss, whereas 25% (4 of 16) showed coverage of the mucosal surface with biofilms.[12] Other studies have also shown bacterial biofilms on sinus specimens. A study by Ferguson and Stolz[15] found biofilms on 50% (2 of 4) of intra-operative samples using TEM. A study by Ramadan and colleagues[26] analyzed tissue from the ethmoidal bulla in 5 patients with CRS who underwent endoscopic sinus surgery. Results showed that 100% (5 of 5) had morphologic features consistent with biofilm coating on SEM. A follow-up study by the same group analyzed 30 patients with CRS and 4 controls.[27] Eighty percent (24 of 30) of these patients revealed biofilm architecture on SEM, with none of the controls demonstrating biofilm forma-tion. Sanderson and colleagues[19] used CLSM and FISH analysis to examine intraoper-ative samples taken from 18 patients with CRS and 5 controls undergoing septoplasty. Fourteen of 18 (78%) patients were found to have biofilms with *H influenzae* being the most common species identified in the population. Healy and colleagues[24] showed mixed fungal-bacterial biofilms in patients with allergic fungal rhinosinusitis and eosin-ophilic mucin CRS compared with purely bacterial biofilm in patients with CRS.

ANIMAL MODELS

A variety of animal models have been used to demonstrate biofilm formation and to develop and test potential therapies. The authors conducted experiments using a rabbit model of sinusitis. The right maxillary sinuses of New Zealand white rabbits were occluded and instilled with P aeruginosa. The rabbits were analyzed at days 1, 5, 10, and 20 for biofilm formation. At day 5, evidence of biofilm formation on the epithelium was observed by SEM, whereas control animals did not demonstrate this finding. The structures seen on SEM included the characteristic structures of biofilms including water channels, glycocalyx coatings, and 3-dimensional structures. Chiu and colleagues[28] evaluated the in vivo effects of topical tobramycin against pseudomonas sinonasal biofilms in the rabbit model. The study found that topical tobramycin was effective in decreasing bacterial counts; however, biofilms were still present on the sinonasal mucosa after autopsy. Ha and colleagues[29] used an experimental sheep model and demonstrated the presence of bacterial biofilms in 100% of sheeps who had bacteria instilled in an obstructed frontal sinus. In another study using the sheep model, Le and colleagues[30] found that regular treatment with mupirocin produced a marked reduction in biofilm surface area coverage over an 8-day period.

EFFECTS ON OUTCOMES AFTER ENDOSCOPIC SINUS SURGERY

Bacterial biofilms are considered to be a potential cause of persistent symptoms in some patients after endoscopic sinus surgery. In a study by Zhang and colleagues,[31] 20 patients with intraoperative biofilms and 7 patients without intraoperative biofilms were followed postoperatively. Patients with intraoperative and postoperative biofilms had significantly higher preoperative Lund-Mackay CT scores and postoperative Lund-Kennedy endoscopic scores than patients without biofilms. In a retrospective study by Psaltis and colleagues,[13] specimens from 40 patients undergoing sinus surgery were analyzed for the presence of biofilms. In this study, the presence of biofilms on intraoperative mucosal samples was correlated with the persistence of postoperative symptoms and mucosal inflammation after functional endoscopic sinus surgery (FESS) for CRS. By studying sinonasal cultures from 157 consecutive patients over a 4-month period, the investigators found a statistically significant correlation between biofilm formation and the number of prior FESS procedures.[18] P aeruginosa, S aureus, and polymicrobial cultures composed 71% of the samples in the study. Bendouah and colleagues[14] followed up 19 patients for a minimum of 1 year after sinus surgery. Isolates from 14 patients demonstrated S aureus or P aeruginosa biofilms. Biofilm formation was associated with an unfavorable outcome after sinus surgery, suggesting a role for biofilms and the poor disease evolution.

CURRENT AND FUTURE TREATMENTS

A variety of techniques have been evaluated to manage and treat biofilms (**Table 1**). Treatments include surgery, topical antimicrobials, and other adjuvant therapies. Newer treatments are aimed at interfering with the biofilm life cycle and targeting bacterial attachment and quorum-sensing mechanisms. Surgical ventilation of the affected sinuses could be the optimal therapy for combating bacterial biofilms, eventually restoring normal sinus physiology.[31] Surgery is considered to be effective against biofilms because it increases oxygen tension, mechanically disrupts biofilms, and assists with the host's natural defenses to clear infections.

Use of topical medications is an alternative method aimed at delivering high concentrations of antibiotics directly to sinus mucosa and biofilms. The obvious

Table 1
Potential therapeutic options

Method	Description
Mechanical	Surgery
Surfactant	Baby shampoo irrigation[36]
	Citric acid/zwitterionic surfactant (CAZS)[37]
Antimicrobial	Mupirocin (Bactroban) irrigation for *S aureus* biofilm[32,33]
	Honey for *S aureus* and *P aeruginosa* biofilms[34]
	Innate immunity proteins[35]
Disrupt quorum sensing	Macrolide therapy[40,41]

advantage of topical preparations of antibiotics is that higher concentrations can be given with lower systemic side effects. Desrossiers and colleagues[32] examined mupirocin in vitro against various strains of *S aureus* to determine the effects on biofilm growth. After 24 hours, mupirocin at concentrations of 7.8 to 125 μg/mL eradicated 90% of biofilms in all isolates. The investigators noted that mupirocin's broad-spectrum activity makes it a potentially attractive treatment for many patients with CRS. Although not specifically addressing biofilms, a study from the Cleveland Clinic has shown encouraging data supporting the use of topical mupirocin nasal irrigations as an alternative to intravenous antibiotics in the treatment of acute exacerbations of CRS caused by methicillin-resistant *Staphylococcus aureus* (MRSA).[33] Patients using mupirocin in sinus irrigations showed improved symptoms and reduced MRSA recovery on subsequent cultures. Alandejani and coworkers[34] demonstrated that honey was effective against *S aureus* and *P aeruginosa* biofilms in vitro. They found that honey eradicated 73% of MRSA biofilms and 91% of pseudomonas biofilms. The clinical utility of honey for patients with biofilm-associated CRS has yet to be determined.

Chennupati and colleagues[35] demonstrated that the innate immunity protein LL-37 was able to eradicate *P aeruginosa* biofilms in a rabbit model of CRS. LL-37 is a peptide that is secreted in saliva and sweat and expressed in leukocytes that have been proposed to be a part of the innate defense system. It has been shown to be antibacterial against both gram-positive and gram-negative bacteria by attacking the cell membrane. In this study, high concentrations of topical tobramycin with 2.5 mg/mL of the peptide were effective in significantly lowering bacterial counts and biofilms; however, high concentrations of the peptide showed proinflammatory and ciliotoxic effects on sinus mucosa.

Surfactants have been proposed to be a method to break up biofilms and subsequently allow bacteria and debris to be irrigated from the sinuses. Chiu and colleagues[36] explored the use of baby shampoo as a chemical surfactant to disrupt biofilm integrity. In this prospective, nonrandomized study, post-FESS patients were irrigated with 1% baby shampoo in saline for 4 weeks. Of the 15 patients who completed the study, 46.6% had subjective improvement of the sinonasal outcome test 22 scores and 63% had improvements in olfaction as determined by the University of Pennsylvania Smell Identification Test. In addition, endoscopic appearance of the cavity after shampoo treatment showed decreased edema and polypoid degeneration. Desrosiers and colleagues[37] found that citric acid/zwitterionic surfactant solution by means of pressurized jet lavage was effective in breaking up biofilms in vitro. These results suggest that further development of surfactant-based therapies is warranted.

Using the *P aeruginosa* PA01 strain, Cross and colleagues[38] found that furosemide appeared to destabilize preformed biofilms at pH-dependent concentrations. Using the in vitro Calgary biofilm detection assay, the loop diuretic reduced pseudomonal biofilm size by half at concentrations of 10 mg/mL. The investigators concluded that furosemide appeared to destabilize pseudomonal biofilms, suggesting that it might be useful as an adjunctive therapy.

The use of long-term macrolide therapy has been shown to improve sinus symptoms in selected patients with CRS.[39] Investigators have demonstrated that treatment with low-dose macrolides, far below the established minimal inhibitory concentration for *Pseudomonas*, has some success in decreasing biofilm formation. Tré-Hardy and colleagues[40] found that the combination of clarithromycin and tobramycin had marked synergistic effects on in vitro biofilms of *P aeruginosa* strain PA01 than when either of the 2 drugs were used individually. In a study by Tateda and colleagues,[41] azithromycin was shown to decrease quorum sensing in *P aeruginosa* wild-type strain PA01. These studies show that the use of subminimum inhibitory concentrations of macrolides may become a useful adjuvant strategy to treat biofilm-associated CRS. More research will be necessary to further elucidate the clinical benefits of these therapies against biofilms.

SUMMARY
Implications for Clinical Practice

This article aims to highlight the history of the findings of bacterial and fungal biofilms and their association with worse clinical outcomes when identified. The authors believe that patients who have biofilm-associated sinusitis will have a more recalcitrant form of the disease, and therefore they should be counseled as such. As new therapies become available, it is hoped that this form of CRS will be more amenable to treatment.

Implications for Research

Since the authors' initial description of biofilms in patients with CRS in 2004, the literature supports the contribution of biofilms to poor disease progression and postoperative outcomes. Antimicrobial and nonantimicrobial therapies may have clinical applications to prevent biofilm formation, interfere with quorum sensing, and destabilize established biofilms. Further research will determine if these and other novel adjuvant treatments will be used to treat biofilm-associated CRS.

REFERENCES

1. Gliklich RE, Metson R. The health impact of chronic sinusitis in patients seeking otolaryngologic care. Otolaryngol Head Neck Surg 1995;113(1):104–9.
2. Solomon DH, Wobb J, Buttaro BA, et al. Characterization of bacterial biofilms on tracheostomy tubes. Laryngoscope 2009;119(8):1633–8.
3. Davies D. Understanding biofilm resistance to antibacterial agents. Nat Rev Drug Discov 2003;2(2):114–22.
4. Richards JJ, Melander C. Controlling bacterial biofilms. Chembiochem 2009. [Epub ahead of print].
5. Hoyle BD, Costerton WJ. Bacterial resistance to antibiotics: the role of biofilms. Prog Durg Res 1991;37:91–105.
6. Lewis K. Multidrug tolerance of biofilms and persister cells. Curr Top Microbiol Immunol 2008;322:107–31.

7. Lewis K. Persister cells, dormancy and infectious disease. Nat Rev Microbiol 2007;5:48–56.
8. Palmer JN. Bacterial biofilms. Do they play a role in chronic sinusitis? Otolaryngol Clin North Am 2005;38:1193–201, viii.
9. Post JC, Hiller NL, Nistico L, et al. The role of biofilms in otolaryngologic infections: update 2007. Curr Opin Otolaryngol Head Neck Surg 2007;15(5): 347–51.
10. Perloff JR, Palmer JN. Evidence of bacterial biofilms in a rabbit model of sinusitis. Am J Rhinol 2005;19(1):1–6.
11. Perloff JR, Palmer JN. Evidence of bacterial biofilms on frontal recess stents in patients with chronic rhinosinusitis. Am J Rhinol 2004;18(6):377–80.
12. Cryer J, Schipor I, Perloff JR, et al. Evidence of bacterial biofilms in human chronic sinusitis. ORL J Otorhinolaryngol Relat Spec 2004;66(3):155–8.
13. Psaltis AJ, Weitzel EK, Ha KR, et al. The effect of bacterial biofilms on post-sinus surgical outcomes. Am J Rhinol 2008;22(1):1–6.
14. Bendouah Z, Barbeau J, Hamad WA, et al. Biofilm formation by Staphylococcus aureus and *Pseudomonas aeruginosa* is associated with an unfavorable evolution after surgery for chronic sinusitis and nasal polyposis. Otolaryngol Head Neck Surg 2006;134(6):991–6.
15. Ferguson BJ, Stolz DB. Demonstration of biofilm in human bacterial chronic rhinosinusitis. Am J Rhinol 2005;19(5):452–7.
16. Parsek MR, Greenberg EP. Quorum sensing signals in development of Pseudomonas aeruginosa biofilms. Methods Enzymol 1999;10:43–55.
17. Singh PK, Schaefer AL, Parsek MR, et al. Quorum-sensing signals indicate that cystic fibrosis lungs are infected with bacterial biofilms. Nature 2000;407:762–4.
18. Prince AA, Steiger JD, Khalid AN, et al. Prevalence of biofilm-forming bacteria in chronic rhinosinusitis. Am J Rhinol 2008;22(3):239–45.
19. Sanderson AR, Leid JG, Hunsaker D. Bacterial biofilms on the sinus mucosa of human subjects with chronic rhinosinusitis. Laryngoscope 2006;116:1121–6.
20. May T, Ito A, Okabe S. Induction of multidrug resistance mechanism in Escherichia coli biofilms by interplay between tetracycline and ampicillin resistance genes. Antimicrob Agents Chemother 2009;53(11):4628–39.
21. Ramage G, Mowat E, Jones B. Our current understanding of fungal biofilms. Crit Rev Microbiol 2009;35(4):340–55.
22. Chandra J, Mukherjee PK, Leidich SD, et al. Antifungal resitance of candidal biofilms formed on denture acrylic in vitro. J Dent Res 2001;80(3):903–8.
23. El-Azizi MA, Starks SE, Khardori N. Interactions of *Candida albicans* with other *Candida* spp and bacteria in the biofilms. J Appl Microbiol 2004;96:1067–73.
24. Healy DY, Leid JG, Sanderson AR, et al. Biofilms in chronic rhinosinusitis. Otolaryngol Head Neck Surg 2008;138(5):641–7.
25. Foreman A, Psaltis AJ, Tan LW, et al. Characterization of bacterial and fungal biofilms in chronic rhinosinusitis. Am J Rhinol Allergy 2009;23(6):556–61.
26. Ramadan HH, Sanclement JA, Thomas JG. Chronic rhinosinusitis and biofilms. Otolaryngol Head Neck Surg 2005;132(3):414–7.
27. Sanclement JA, Webster P, Thomas J, et al. Bacterial biofilms in surgical specimens of patients with chronic rhinosinusitis. Laryngoscope 2005;115(4):578–82.
28. Chiu AG, Antunes MB, Palmer JN, et al. Evaluation of the in vivo efficacy of topical tobramycin against pseudomonas sinonasal biofilms. J Antimicrob Chemother 2007;59(6):1130–4.
29. Ha KR, Psaltis AJ, Tan L, et al. A sheep model for the study of biofilms in rhinosinusitis. Am J Rhinol 2007;21(3):339–45.

30. Le T, Psaltis A, Tan LW, et al. The efficacy of topical antibiofilm agents in a sheep model of rhinosinusitis. Am J Rhinol 2008;22(6):560–7.

31. Zhang Z, Han D, Zhang S, et al. Biofilms and mucosal healing in postsurgical patients with chronic rhinosinusitis. Am J Rhinol Allergy 2009;23(5):506–11.

32. Desrosiers M, Bendouah Z, Barbeau J. Effectiveness of topical antibiotics on Staphylococcus aureus biofilm in vitro. Am J Rhinol 2007;21(2):149–53.

33. Solares CA, Batra PS, Hall GS, et al. Treatment of chronic rhinosinusitis exacerbations due to methicillin-resistant *Staphylococcus aureus* with mupirocin irrigations. Am J Otolaryngol 2006;27(3):161–5.

34. Alandejani T, Marsan J, Ferris W, et al. Effectiveness of honey on Staphylococcus aureus and Pseudomonas aeruginosa biofilms. Otolaryngol Head Neck Surg 2009;141(1):114–8.

35. Chennupati SK, Chiu AG, Tamashiro E, et al. Effects of an LL-37 derived antimicrobial peptide in an animal model of biofilm pseudomonas sinusitis. Am J Rhinol Allergy 2009;23(1):46–51.

36. Chiu AG, Palmer JN, Woodworth BA, et al. Baby shampoo nasal irrigations for the symptomatic post-functional endoscopic sinus surgery patient. Am J Rhinol 2008;22(1):34–7.

37. Desrosiers M, Myntti M, James G. Methods for removing bacterial biofilms: in vitro study using clinical chronic rhinosinusitis specimens. Am J Rhinol 2007;21(5):527–32.

38. Cross JL, Ramadan HH, Thomas JG. The impact of a cation channel blocker (furosemide) on Pseudomonas aeruginosa PAO1 biofilm architecture. Otolaryngol Head Neck Surg 2007;137(1):21–6.

39. Wallwork B, Coman W, Mackay-Sim A, et al. A double-blind, randomized, placebo-controlled trial of macrolide in the treatment of chronic rhinosinusitis. Laryngoscope 2006;116:189–93.

40. Tré-Hardy M, Vanderbist F, Traore H, et al. In vitro activity of antibiotic combinations against Pseudomonas aeruginosa biofilm and planktonic cultures. Int J Antimicrob Agents 2008;31(4):329–36.

41. Tateda K, Comte R, Pechere JC, et al. Suppression of Pseudomonas aeruginosa quorum-sensing systems by macrolides: a promising strategy or an oriental mystery? J Infect Chemother 2007;13(6):357–67.

The Role of Fungus in Chronic Rhinosinusitis

Richard R. Orlandi, MD[a],*, Bradley F. Marple, MD[b]

KEYWORDS

- Chronic rhinosinusitis • Fungus • *Alternaria*
- Amphotericin B • Etiology • Pathogenesis

A unifying etiology of chronic rhinosinusitis (CRS) remains elusive. Patients and their physicians are understandably frustrated with a condition that is prevalent, generates large medical expenditures, and significantly affects quality of life. This frustration is further compounded by not knowing what causes CRS. Allergy (both systemic and localized), viruses, bacteria (both aerobic and anaerobic), superantigens, gastroesophageal reflux, osteitis, biofilms, and impaired mucosal barriers have all been touted as etiologic factors, and evidence exists to support each of these claims.

Fungus, or more specifically an immunologic reaction to ubiquitous fungi, has also been suggested as an etiologic factor. The role of fungi is well established in a few subtypes of rhinosinusitis, such as acute invasive fungal rhinosinusitis, allergic fungal rhinosinusitis, and fungal balls.[1] However, in more commonly seen cases of CRS (either with or without polyps), the role of fungi is less clear. Evidence has come to light during the last decade that supports this role, and some have touted fungus as not only *an* etiology, but have claimed it to be *the* etiology of CRS. Additional data have cast doubt on this claim.

Multiple possible pathophysiologic pathways involving fungus in CRS exist (**Box 1**). These possible pathways may be interrelated. For instance, fungi have recently been shown to be present in biofilms, which could perpetuate their presence at the epithelial surface and prolong the effect of proteases such as major basic protein.[2] Another example is the finding of localized IgE in greater amounts within the subepithelium than the epithelium, supporting the concept of a deficient innate mucosal barrier that may allow foreign antigens to penetrate the epithelium and cause an immunologic reaction in CRS patients.[3,4]

Fungus may have a minor role in CRS as part of a more complex interplay among multiple factors. Alternatively, it may be the principal factor as some have claimed. Its

---

Conflicts of interest: None.
[a] Division of Otolaryngology – Head and Neck Surgery, University of Utah, 50 North Medical Drive, 3C120, Salt Lake City, UT 84132, USA
[b] Department of Otolaryngology – Head and Neck Surgery, University of Texas-Southwestern Medical Center at Dallas, 5323 Harry Hines Boulevard, Dallas, TX 75390-9035, USA
* Corresponding author.
E-mail address: richard.orlandi@hsc.utah.edu

Otolaryngol Clin N Am 43 (2010) 531–537
doi:10.1016/j.otc.2010.02.011
0030-6665/10/$ – see front matter © 2010 Elsevier Inc. All rights reserved.

> **Box 1**
> **Possible pathophysiologic mechanisms involving fungus in CRS**
>
> –Systemic IgE-mediated reaction to fungi
>
> –Localized IgE-mediated reaction to fungi
>
> –Fulminant invasive infectious (eg, acute invasive fungal rhinosinusitis)
>
> –Chronic invasive infectious (eg, chronic invasive fungal rhinosinusitis, granulomatous fungal rhinosinusitis)
>
> –Epithelial damage at mucosal surface from eosinophilic proteases (eg, major basic protein)
>
> –Impaired epithelial barrier, leading to immunologic reaction following subepithelial entry
>
> –Biofilms containing fungi

relative importance and the exact pathophysiologic mechanism are crucial to understand, in order to determine whether it should be targeted in potential CRS treatments and, if so, how it should be addressed. In this article, evidence for and against fungus as a *principal* etiology in CRS is presented and weighed, to better understand its role.

EVIDENCE SUPPORTING THE ROLE OF FUNGUS IN CRS

Fungus has been found in the sinuses and/or nasal cavities of CRS patients as well as controls. An initial report described highly sensitive fungal culture techniques that demonstrated fungi in nearly all CRS patients—and in all controls.[5] The methods and results were subsequently duplicated in Europe,[6] and staining of fungal-specific chitin again demonstrated the presence of fungi in all CRS patients.[7] Others have shown the presence of *Alternaria* DNA in 100% of CRS patients' sinuses and in 67% of healthy controls' sinuses.[8] Inasmuch as these reports documented the presence of fungi in the sinuses not only in CRS patients but also in controls, fungi themselves do not appear to be the causative factor.

Much attention has focused on the *reaction* to fungus, especially the eosinophil and its relationship to fungus and local cytokines. Eosinophils are present in the late phase of allergic rhinitis and are also seen in many forms of CRS, particularly CRS with polyps. Eosinophils are also prominent in the reaction to parasitic infections. The mucin from CRS patients has been found to be more chemotactic for eosinophils compared with the mucin of healthy controls.[9] Mucin from CRS patients has been further found to heterogeneously contain clusters of eosinophils with high levels of eosinophilic granule major basic protein, a cationic protein toxic to extracellular microorganisms but also to respiratory mucosa.[10] Eosinophils are known to migrate into respiratory mucosa by interleukin (IL)-13–induced expression of adhesion molecules in the microvasculature, with subsequent migration out of the vessels and into the tissues. Another cytokine, IL-5, promotes eosinophil differentiation, activation, and survival in the tissues by inhibiting apoptosis. Shin and colleagues[11] exposed peripheral blood mononuclear cells (PBMCs) to fungal antigens in vitro, and reported increased IL-5 and IL-13 production in 89% of CRS patients but not controls. The response was particularly brisk with exposure to *Alternaria*. The IL-5 production was found to be independent of fungal-specific IgE and instead correlated with fungal-specific IgG, implying a nonallergic mechanism.

These findings have led to a hypothesis wherein fungi on the sinus mucosal surface induce production of cytokines, which promote eosinophil migration through the epithelium toward the mucin. These eosinophils arrive at the fungal-containing mucin and release cationic proteins to destroy the fungi, but in so doing perpetuate and potentially worsen the mucosal inflammation seen in CRS.[12] Some have even described this fungal-driven paradigm as the universal explanation for CRS, stating that "most, if not all, chronic rhinosinusitis conditions have a fungal etiology."[13]

EVIDENCE QUESTIONING THE ROLE OF FUNGUS IN CRS

With initial in vitro evidence showing fungus as a potential etiologic agent in CRS, clinical trials with antifungal therapy soon followed. In 2002, 2 nonblinded uncontrolled studies were published examining topical amphotericin B in the treatment of CRS. Ponikau and colleagues[14] noted symptomatic improvement in 75% of 51 CRS patients treated with amphotericin B irrigations. Endoscopic and radiologic improvements were also reported. Ricchetti and colleagues[15] similarly treated 74 nasal polyposis patients with amphotericin B nasal irrigations and reported resolution of polyps in 39%.

To minimize the potential for patient and observer bias, these open-label pilot studies were followed by randomized, double-blind, placebo-controlled trials of antifungal irrigation. Unfortunately, all of these studies failed to show a substantial clinical effect. Weschta and colleagues[16] compared amphotericin B spray to saline spray, and failed to see an effect in multiple patient parameters including symptom scores, endoscopy, radiologic evaluation, and overall quality of life. Presence of fungus in nasal lavage before or after treatment did not correlate with any outcome parameters. Subsequent work demonstrated that amphotericin B treatment had no effect on the eosinophilic markers tryptase and eosinophil cationic protein, and that these markers did not correlate with the success of fungal eradication.[17]

Ponikau and colleagues[18] examined amphotericin B irrigation, and reported an improvement in radiologic and endoscopic scores. The improvement was statistically significant but the clinical significance was questionable. Moreover, there were no significant improvements in symptom scoring, presence of *Alternaria*, IL-5 concentration in mucus, or blood eosinophil levels. In this study, 2 of 15 patients (13%) treated with amphotericin B experienced an adverse effect with the medication and discontinued it.

Ebbens and colleagues[19] exhaustively examined numerous symptom parameters and endoscopy scores in patients treated with amphotericin B, and found it to have no effect compared with placebo saline irrigation. A follow-up study examined 24 cytokines, chemokines, and growth factors in CRS nasal lavage samples, and found 13 weeks of topical amphotericin B treatment to affect none of them.[20] Shin and Ye[21] also failed to demonstrate an effect of amphotericin B on proinflammatory markers in patients with nasal polyps as compared with saline.

While these studies cast serious doubt on the fungal hypothesis, it is possible that lack of sufficient delivery could explain the failure of topical therapy. It is known that topical treatments have limited ability to access the sinuses and are instead predominantly delivered to the nasal cavity, even in patients who have previously undergone sinus surgery.[22,23] Unfortunately, systemic therapy has not been shown to be effective either. Kennedy and colleagues[24] examined the effect of oral systemic terbinafine and found no radiologic improvement in CRS patients compared with untreated controls, even in patients who were positive for fungus in pretreatment cultures. Nevertheless, with this study the possibility remained of inadequate systemic delivery to the sinus mucin. With systemic antifungal therapy, the risk of hepatic complications with systemic therapy must always be borne in mind.

Amphotericin B irrigations, though initially promising in nonblinded pilot studies, have failed to show clinical efficacy in more rigorous trials. Even in those instances where a small effect was noted, an immunomodulatory or cell-permeability effect seems to be just as likely or more likely to be the explanation. Amphotericin B works by binding ergosterol in the fungal cell wall, increasing its permeability to the point of cell death. Amphotericin B also binds cholesterol in the mammalian cell membrane and alters the cells' permeability, though to a lesser degree. It is therefore possible that the very limited clinical effect seen in one of these studies can be attributed to a direct reduction in mucosal edema, irrespective of the solution's antifungal activity.[15,25] Kanda and colleagues[26] further demonstrated that azole antifungals, such as itraconazole, suppress IL-4 and IL-5 expression by T lymphocytes, again questioning the relative importance of the antifungal versus an immunomodulatory effect of these oral medications. Additional in vitro work questions the importance of the antifungal effect in any of these studies. Shirazi and colleagues[27] examined the antifungal efficacy of the amphotericin B concentration commonly used in nasal lavage and found it to be ineffective, whereas 2- and 3-fold increases were effective. Unfortunately, these higher doses are poorly tolerated in the nasal cavity.

How does one reconcile the rather persuasive in vitro data with the paucity of evidence of antifungals' clinical effectiveness? Can the failure of antifungal medication simply be due to lack of sufficient delivery? Is fungus truly an appropriate universal target for therapy in CRS patients?

With the in vitro data appearing to be at odds with a large number of negative clinical reports, it is important to take a closer look at these laboratory data and, where possible, attempt to replicate them. Specifically, the finding of Shin and colleagues[11] that 89% of CRS patients had non-IgE–mediated elevated IL-5 responses to *Alternaria alternata* extract has remained compelling evidence that fungus may indeed be an etiologic factor in CRS. By painstakingly replicating the methods as far as possible, Orlandi and colleagues[28] recently examined this relationship in a more heterogeneous group of CRS patients. Patients at multiple points on the disease severity spectrum and residing in different areas of the United States (with sharply differing climates) were purposely chosen to test the universality of the fungal hypothesis. Not only did this subsequent study fail to produce the results of Shin and colleagues in more heterogeneous patients, but some of these results were directly opposite of the original findings.

Orlandi and colleagues[28] found that IL-5 was produced following *Alternaria* exposure by PBMCs of patients but also by those of controls, and the response was heterogeneous and did not correlate with the presence of CRS. In addition, *Alternaria*-induced levels of IL-13, the principal chemoattractant for eosinophils, did not differ between CRS patients and controls. Moreover, IL-5 levels correlated strongly with fungal-specific IgE and did not correlate with fungal-specific IgG, contrary to the results seen by Shin and colleagues.[11]

SUMMARY OF EVIDENCE

These in vitro data must now be viewed in the context of the clinical data on antifungal therapy presented to this point. While additional work needs to be completed to effectively settle the difference between the results of Shin and colleagues and Orlandi and colleagues, these new findings nonetheless add further weight to the argument against fungus as a universal etiologic factor. CRS has many manifestations, raising the question of whether it is one disease or a syndrome of multiple diseases—with differing etiologic factors—manifesting commonly as impaired mucociliary clearance and inflammation.[29] Fungal colonization may therefore be an epiphenomenon, with delayed mucociliary clearance resulting from a nonfungal cause, allowing ubiquitous fungal spores to subsequently germinate into hyphae. It is possible that in some cases of CRS these fungal hyphae may indeed intensify and/or perpetuate the inflammatory reaction that was already present and which impaired the mucociliary clearance to begin with. Nevertheless, the preponderance of the currently published evidence questions the role of fungus as a (the?) primary etiologic agent in CRS. In weighing the evidence over the last decade for and against fungus as a major etiological factor in CRS, the scales seem to be increasingly tipping against this hypothesis.

IMPLICATIONS FOR FUTURE RESEARCH

The scientific method requires research results, especially those thought to shift long-standing paradigms, to be confirmed by additional independent researchers. Where opposing data are present, additional work must be done to understand and resolve that difference. The currently published in vitro data on the role of fungus as a primary or even secondary etiologic agent in CRS are in such a conflict. The opposing findings of Shin and colleagues in their patients and Orlandi and colleagues in their more heterogeneous patients clearly call for additional studies. Both studies had relatively small sample sizes and looked at potentially different subsets of CRS patients. Additional work must be done to understand whether fungus indeed does have a role and, if so, in which types of patients.

It is likely that fungus will be found to have a role in at least some subclassifications of CRS, for example, allergic fungal rhinosinusitis. In the cases where it plays a role, the nature of that role must be further elucidated. The pathophysiologic mechanisms whereby fungus initiates or perpetuates inflammation will need to be worked out to determine appropriate therapeutic strategies. For instance, is the reaction mediated by IgE, IgG, or more nonspecific surface immunity? The nature of fungal interactions with the mucosal surface (eg, as part of a biofilm or as a nonspecific invader of impaired epithelial barriers) will also need to be addressed in order to create more effective therapies. Determining the optimal delivery method will maximize therapeutic effectiveness while minimizing side effects. Lastly, inasmuch as fungal spores are ubiquitously and constantly inhaled into the nasal cavity, an end point of therapy must be addressed.

IMPLICATIONS FOR CLINICAL TREATMENT

While additional research will be needed to clarify the exact etiologic role of fungus in CRS and potential treatment strategies, the current role of antifungal therapy appears to be much clearer. It has been claimed that for amphotericin B, "intranasal topical antifungal treatment can be considered as an early line of therapy to safely relieve the symptoms of CRS and, in the post-surgical patient, to prevent or delay recurrence."[30] The preponderance of the double-blind, randomized, placebo-controlled data published to date would strongly oppose such a view. Systemic therapy has significant side effects and the limited data published thus far indicate no improvement. Topical therapy avoids the hepatic toxicity but does not appear to be effective either. Amphotericin B nasal lavage is not effective in vitro in the concentrations tolerated by patients, and does not appear to alter any inflammatory indicator measured thus far. Indeed, it appears that amphotericin B is "not a solution for patients with chronic rhinosinusitis."[19]

REFERENCES

1. Chakrabarti A, Denning DW, Ferguson BJ, et al. Fungal rhinosinusitis: a categorization and definitional schema addressing current controversies. Laryngoscope 2009;119:1809–18.
2. Healy DY, Leid JG, Sanderson AR, et al. Biofilms with fungi in chronic rhinosinusitis. Otolaryngol Head Neck Surg 2008;138:641–7.
3. Ahn CN, Wise SK, Lathers DM, et al. Local production of antigen-specific IgE in different anatomic subsites of allergic fungal rhinosinusitis patients. Otolaryngol Head Neck Surg 2009;141:97–103.
4. Tieu DD, Kern RC, Schleimer RP. Alterations in epithelial barrier function and host defense responses in chronic rhinosinusitis. J Allergy Clin Immunol 2009;124: 37–42.
5. Ponikau JU, Sherris DA, Kern EB, et al. The diagnosis and incidence of allergic fungal sinusitis. Mayo Clin Proc 1999;74:877–84.
6. Braun H, Buzina W, Freudenschuss K, et al. "Eosinophilic fungal rhinosinusitis": a common disorder in Europe? Laryngoscope 2003;113:264–9.
7. Taylor MJ, Ponikau JU, Sherris DA, et al. Detection of fungal organisms in eosinophilic mucin using a fluorescein-labeled chitin-specific binding protein. Otolaryngol Head Neck Surg 2002;127:377–83.
8. Gosepath J, Brieger J, Vlachtsis K, et al. Fungal DNA is present in tissue specimens of patients with chronic rhinosinusitis. Am J Rhinol 2004;18:9–13.
9. Wei JL, Kita H, Sherris DA, et al. The chemotactic behavior of eosinophils in patients with chronic rhinosinusitis. Laryngoscope 2003;113:303–6.
10. Ponikau JU, Sherris DA, Kephart GM, et al. Striking deposition of toxic eosinophil major basic protein in mucus: implications for chronic rhinosinusitis. J Allergy Clin Immunol 2005;116:362–9.
11. Shin SH, Ponikau JU, Sherris DA, et al. Chronic rhinosinusitis: an enhanced immune response to ubiquitous airborne fungi. J Allergy Clin Immunol 2004; 114:1369–75.
12. Sasama J, Sherris DA, Shin SH, et al. New paradigm for the roles of fungi and eosinophils in chronic rhinosinusitis. Curr Opin Otolaryngol Head Neck Surg 2005;13:2–8.
13. Ponikau JU. Methods and materials for treating and preventing inflammation of mucosal tissue. 2001; Patent # 6,207,703.
14. Ponikau JU, Sherris DA, Kita H, et al. Intranasal antifungal treatment in 51 patients with chronic rhinosinusitis. J Allergy Clin Immunol 2002;110:862–6.
15. Ricchetti A, Landis BN, Maffioli A, et al. Effect of anti-fungal nasal lavage with amphotericin B on nasal polyposis. J Laryngol Otol 2002;116:261–3.
16. Weschta M, Rimek D, Formanek M, et al. Topical antifungal treatment of chronic rhinosinusitis with nasal polyps: a randomized, double-blind clinical trial. J Allergy Clin Immunol 2004;113:1122–8.
17. Weschta M, Rimek D, Formanek M, et al. Effect of nasal antifungal therapy on nasal cell activation markers in chronic rhinosinusitis. Arch Otolaryngol Head Neck Surg 2006;132:743–7.
18. Ponikau JU, Sherris DA, Weaver A, et al. Treatment of chronic rhinosinusitis with intranasal amphotericin B: a randomized, placebo-controlled, double-blind pilot trial. J Allergy Clin Immunol 2005;115:125–31.
19. Ebbens FA, Scadding GK, Badia L, et al. Amphotericin B nasal lavages: not a solution for patients with chronic rhinosinusitis. J Allergy Clin Immunol 2006; 118:1149–56.

20. Ebbens FA, Georgalas C, Luiten S, et al. The effect of topical amphotericin B on inflammatory markers in patients with chronic rhinosinusitis: a multicenter randomized controlled study. Laryngoscope 2009;119:401–8.
21. Shin SH, Ye MK. Effects of topical amphotericin B on expression of cytokines in nasal polyps. Acta Otolaryngol 2004;124:1174–7.
22. Miller TR, Muntz HR, Gilbert ME, et al. Comparison of topical medication delivery systems after sinus surgery. Laryngoscope 2004;114:201–4.
23. Olson DE, Rasgon BM, Hilsinger RL Jr. Radiographic comparison of three methods for nasal saline irrigation. Laryngoscope 2002;112:1394–8.
24. Kennedy DW, Kuhn FA, Hamilos DL, et al. Treatment of chronic rhinosinusitis with high-dose oral terbinafine: a double blind, placebo-controlled study. Laryngoscope 2005;115:1793–9.
25. Jornot L, Rochat T, Lacroix JS. Nasal polyps and middle turbinates epithelial cells sensitivity to amphotericin B. Rhinology 2003;41:201–5.
26. Kanda N, Enomoto U, Watanabe S. Anti-mycotics suppress interleukin-4 and interleukin-5 production in anti-CD3 plus anti-CD28-stimulated T cells from patients with a topic dermatitis. J Invest Dermatol 2001;117:1635–46.
27. Shirazi MA, Stankiewicz JA, Kammeyer P. Activity of nasal amphotericin B irrigation against fungal organisms in vitro. Am J Rhinol 2007;21:145–8.
28. Orlandi RR, Marple BF, Georgelas A, et al. Immunologic response to fungus is not universally associated with rhinosinusitis. Otolaryngol Head Neck Surg 2009;141: 750–6 e1–2.
29. Lanza DC, Kennedy DW. Adult rhinosinusitis defined. Otolaryngol Head Neck Surg 1997;117:S1–7.
30. Kern EB, Sherris D, Stergiou AM, et al. Diagnosis and treatment of chronic rhinosinusitis: focus on intranasal Amphotericin B. Ther Clin Risk Manag 2007; 3:319–25.

Novel Topical Therapeutics

Benjamin S. Bleier, MD

KEYWORDS

- Topical therapy • Implantable therapeutics • Drug-eluting stent
- Drug absorption • Drug-eluting polymer

Intranasal drug delivery is a rapidly expanding field with great potential for the management of local and systemic disease. A growing body of literature has focused on the use of topical therapies for the treatment of allergic and inflammatory sinusitis. These treatments offer the potential for the delivery of high concentrations of therapeutic agent directly to the effected area. Intranasal drug administration for systemic delivery has also gained attention because it offers an easily accessible, highly vascularized mucosal surface area coupled to a porous endothelial basement membrane with a high total blood flow per volume of tissue. These attributes allow for direct absorption into the blood stream with decreased enzymatic degradation relative to the gut or liver, avoidance of the first-pass effect, and the potential for enhanced patient compliance.[1] Although the goal of each of these strategies is fundamentally different, they must overcome a similar set of anatomic and physiologic obstacles to be successful. Current techniques include optimization of traditional delivery devices and physiochemical modulation of pharmaceuticals to improve absorption. However, novel drug delivery strategies that have the potential to dramatically alter the transnasal management of a host of local and systemic pathologies are currently in development.

DISTRIBUTION STRATEGIES: INTRANASAL CAVITY

Regardless of the choice of agent, the mechanism of action of all intranasal pharmaceuticals is predicated on successful delivery to the respiratory mucosa. Because of the complex geometry and dynamic air flow patterns of the sinonasal labyrinth, efficient and predictable drug delivery in an unoperated patient is a challenge. Multiple variables including particle size, flow rate volume, pressure, and spray angle have all been shown to have a significant effect on delivery.[2] The major mechanism of

Financial disclosure: The chitosan glycerophosphate (CGP) drug-eluting polymer referenced in this content is protected under a nonprovisional US patent application on which the author is a coinventor.

Division of Rhinology, Department of Otolaryngology-Head and Neck Surgery, Medical University of South Carolina, 135 Rutledge Avenue, MSC 550, Charleston, SC 29425, USA

E-mail address: bleierb@gmail.com

drug deposition relies on inertial impaction on the nasal mucosa while gravitational sedimentation and Brownian diffusion play secondary roles. As a result, particulate size and density affect the degree and site of deposition. Particles greater than 10 μm will tend to remain within the nasal vault whereas those smaller than 5 μm remain aerosolized and are absorbed in the lower airways.[1] Using a cast model, Saijo and colleagues[3] demonstrated that efficiency of intranasal particle deposition could be further increased not only by altering the size but also the flow rate of the application. As a result, most commercial nasal delivery sprays use a monodroplet dispersion system with particle sizes of 50 to 70 μm and flow rates between 7 and 20 L/min.[4] Despite these strategies, a significant volume of each dose is deposited in the anterior nasal vault where it is rapidly cleared, severely limiting its systemic or local pharmacologic efficacy (**Fig. 1**).

DISTRIBUTION STRATEGIES: PARANASAL SINUS

This significant drug loss confounds efforts to determine optimal dosing regimens for systemic distribution because the percentage of medication actually reaching the respiratory mucosa is variable and difficult to predict. The problem is further compounded when addressing intraluminal sinus disease, because the treatment may never reach the intended site of action even if it does penetrate the nasal cavity. Olson and colleagues[5] looked at the distribution of 40 mL of radiopaque contrast by computed tomography (CT) in 8 unoperated patients using a range of delivery methods, and found that contrast reached the sphenoid in only 1 of 8 patients. While contrast was seen in the frontal recess in 2 patients, there was no penetration seen within the frontal sinus itself. Regardless of the mechanism of delivery, estimates of luminal delivery in an unoperated patient are less than 5% of the total volume

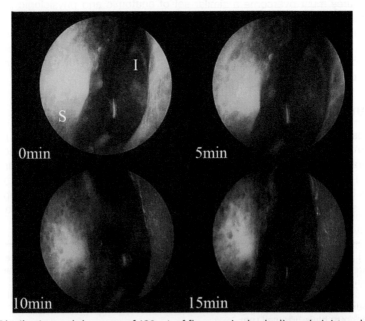

Fig. 1. Distribution and clearance of 120 mL of fluorescein-dyed saline administered by positive pressure irrigation bottle (S, septum; I, inferior turbinate). Note the predominant accumulation in the squamous portion of the vestibule and almost complete clearance of fluorescein from the inferior turbinate within 10 minutes.

administered.[6,7] In fact, Grobler and colleagues[8] demonstrated that an ostial diameter of at least 3.95 mm is required to achieve any significant luminal penetration. However, following functional endoscopic sinus surgery, high-volume pressurized irrigations have been shown to be superior to other methods in achieving intraluminal delivery. Miller and colleagues[9] compared the degree of deposition of several delivery methods in postsurgical patients with chronic rhinosinusitis using a blinded endoscopic grading system, and found that while the bulb syringe offered the greatest distribution, all methods produced significant deposition in the anterior nasal vault.

RADIOLOGIC DISTRIBUTION STUDIES

These findings suggest that the full potential of self-administered intranasal drug delivery is yet to be achieved. The advent of nuclear emission imaging has offered new insights into the mechanism of drug distribution and has led to novel delivery devices that seek to overcome the limitations of current techniques.[10] Technetium-99m is the most commonly used radiotracer for planar imaging; however, radionuclides are not commonly found in the drugs themselves and therefore it is not possible to label the drug. Validation of the tracer is important because it must not independently affect the behavior or distribution of the drug. Therefore, these tracers typically provide an accurate representation of the distribution of the drug until absorption into the tissue, binding, and evaporation result in uncoupling of the drug and the tracer. Thus only the initial deposition can be accurately measured, although this may be the most important aspect. Particulate tracers for dry powder formulations also exist and may include polystyrene, albumin microspheres, and technetium-iron oxide.[10] While useful, one critique of planar imaging is that the data are acquired in only 2 dimensions and while there are algorithms that can create 3-dimensional reconstructions, there are important attenuation effects by the intervening soft tissue that must be taken into account.

Positron emission tomography (PET) scanning represents a superior imaging modality, as isotropic substitution may be used to make the drug the tracer. These images may be acquired in 3 dimensions and can be coregistered with CT or magnetic resonance imaging to create precise anatomic correlations. Furthermore, PET imaging uses positron emitting radionuclides which, when annihilated, give off 2 511-keV gamma rays thereby allowing PET to quantify the volume of drug distribution. PET imaging has already been used to aid in the development of delivery techniques to the lower airways and has great potential in intranasal drug administration.[11] Several novel nasal delivery techniques have been designed using knowledge gleaned from these imaging modalities, including controlled air-particle streams and bidirectional vortical airflow devices, although their clinical utility is yet to be fully elucidated.[4]

MUCUS BARRIER AND MUCOCILIARY CLEARANCE

Even if adequate nasal penetration is achieved, various physiologic obstacles remain that may impair the therapeutic efficacy (**Fig. 2**). The nasal cavity can be divided into the vestibule ($0.6-1$ cm^2), respiratory epithelium (150 cm^2), and olfactory epithelium ($20-40$ cm^2). The vestibule is composed of stratified squamous epithelium and while it is resistant to dehydration and noxious substances, its permeability to drugs is very poor. The respiratory epithelium is composed of pseudostratified columnar epithelial cells with cilia, goblet cells, basal cells, and seromucinous ducts. Each ciliated cell contains approximately 100 cilia and all cells contain about 300 microvilli, which serve to further increase the absorptive surface area. The secretory glands operate under autonomic control, and parasympathetic input leads to dilation of the capacitance vessels and increased seromucinous secretion.[12]

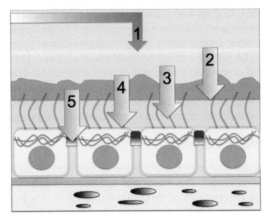

Fig. 2. Multiple sequential obstacles to topical drug delivery. 1, distribution to mucosal surface to enable inertial impaction; 2, mucus layer demonstrating superficial gel and periciliary sol layer; 3, ciliary beat driving mucociliary transit with subsequent drug clearance; 4, cellular lipid bilayer comprising the principal transcellular transport barrier; 5, intercellular TJ (bound to cytoskeleton) comprising the principal paracellular transport barrier.

Following nasal deposition, the mucus blanket is the first obstacle encountered by a pharmaceutical agent. Daily, 1.5 to 2 L of mucus is secreted by approximately 100,000 submucosal glands in a 5-μm blanket. While most mucus is composed of hydrated mucin, it also contains a host of proteins including albumin, immunoglobulins, lysozymes, and lactoferrin. Mucin is a high molecular weight glycoprotein cross-linked with disulfide bridges and ionic bonds, which contains a large number of reactive free hydroxyl groups.[1] Although this mucus blanket is over 100 times thinner than the equivalent layer in the lower gastrointestinal tract, it still represents a significant size-dependent barrier to diffusion. For smaller molecules, the degree of lipophilicity largely governs the permeability whereas for larger molecules, such as peptides, hydrogen bonding and ionic interactions between the molecule and the mucus glycopeptide chains can limit diffusion.[13] Several strategies to enhance epithelial drug deposition have focused on disruption of the mucus barrier. Dornase alfa, an rhDNase, acts to decrease mucus viscosity through selective hydrolysis of entangled DNA, and is commonly used in the cystic fibrosis population.[14] Despite its mucolytic effects, high-resolution multiple particle tracking in sputum of patients with cystic fibrosis treated with Dornase alfa failed to show a significant enhancement in average particle diffusion rates.[15] Alternatively, N-acetylcysteine (NAC), another mucolytic that functions through hydrogen and disulfide bond disruption, has been shown to improve transmucosal cationic molecular delivery to the epithelial surface.[16]

The mucus barrier effect is further enhanced by the relatively rapid clearance of xenobiotics because of gravity and mucociliary clearance, which has a half-life of approximately 15 to 20 minutes.[17] One strategy that has been investigated to circumvent this effect is the use of bioadhesive pharmaceutical carriers. The use of bioadhesive carriers has been shown to prolong nasal residence for more than a week.[18] Following hydration, bioadhesive polymers swell, leading to interpenetration between the polymer chains and those of the mucus. Factors influencing mucoadhesion include type of functional group, cross-linking density, spatial orientation, and environmental pH. Spatial orientation becomes important when structures such as helices result in the shielding of active sites, leading to a reduction in bioadhesive strength.[1]

In addition to its role as a physical barrier, the mucus layer acts to prolong drug exposure to various degrading enzymes present in the mucus and at the epithelial surface. These drugs may be subjected to hydrolysis, oxidation, isomerization, photo-chemical decomposition, or polymerization. As a result, chemical and physical stability of the compound play an important role. Cytochrome P450 has a broad ability to oxidize lipophilic xenobiotics in a nicotinamide adenine dinucleotide phosphate (NADPH)-dependent manner, and is present in the nasal mucosa at levels second only to those in the liver. In addition, multiple proteases capable of cleaving the N and C termini such as exopeptidases, mono/diaminopeptidases, and endopeptidases including serine, cysteine, and aspartic proteinases are found within the mucosa. As a result, peptides and protein-based drugs tend to be more fragile than lower molec-ular weight compounds. These effects can be countered by the coadministration of protease inhibitors and moieties that resist oxidation, such as bestatin and L-aspar-tase, respectively.[13]

EPITHELIAL PERMEABILITY

Once an agent has successfully traversed the mucus layer, it must then be absorbed through the epithelial surface. The epithelial barrier comprises the cell wall and inter-cellular tight junctions (TJ) that bind the cells together. TJ represent an elaborate series of integral membrane proteins that connect directly to the actin cytoskeleton and allow for dynamic regulation of paracellular transport. Claudins represent a large gene family that makes up a significant component of TJ and has been shown to participate in charge and size selectivity of the paracellular barrier.[19]

The cell wall is composed of a phospholipid bilayer and thus transcellular absorption favors lipophilic, low molecular weight compounds of less than 1000 Da. As a result, the permeability of acids and bases will be affected by the microenvironment of the respiratory epithelium. Weak acids and bases will be most highly absorbed in their nonionized state; however, there will still be some baseline level of absorption even when ionized.[13]

Several strategies have been explored that seek to maximize transcellular delivery. Prodrugs function to enhance the lipophilic profile, thereby allowing for greater absorption across the epithelium. Hussain and colleagues[20] found that the lipophilic testosterone 17β-N,N-dimethylglycinate hydrochloride prodrug had a solubility that is 10^5 times greater than testosterone alone. Following absorption, these prodrugs are metabolized into their active state.[13] Another strategy has been to directly modify the lipid bilayer using permeability enhancers. Molecules such as sodium glycocho-late, sodium lauryl sulfate, and polyoxyethylene-9-lauryl ether improves absorption in a concentration-dependent manner, although their effect is directly related to molecular weight. These enhancers must be used with caution as they can also act as detergents, resulting in permanent disruption of the lipid bilayer.[13]

A third strategy focuses on enhanced drug delivery to the epithelial surface rather than drug or membrane modification. The nasal cavity has a limited volume, and thus the poor solubility of lipophilic drugs results in suboptimal dosing concentrations within a given amount of solvent. One solution to this problem rests in a family of cyclic oligosaccharides known as cyclodextrins. These hydrophilic molecules contain a hydrophobic central cavity capable of forming noncovalent water-soluble inclusion complexes with lipophilic molecules. The cyclodextrins therefore act as an aqueous vehicle delivering higher concentrations of lipophilic drugs to the epithelial surface. The complexed form may then equilibrate with the unbound form and is subsequently free to diffuse across the cell membrane.[21]

Despite these strategies, hydrophilic and higher molecular weight molecules are almost exclusively absorbed through the paracellular route. TJ have a resting pore size of approximately 10 Å and thus the rate of transport for large polar drugs is highly dependent on molecular weight and size. This pathway represents a potential area for modulation, as TJ may be dynamically regulated through various mechanisms including protein kinase C–dependent pathways.[13] Certain cationic polymers such as poly-L-lysines and polyethyleneimine have been shown to be capable of inducing protein kinase C–dependent TJ dilation in several epithelial cell models.[19]

A further complication of nasal drug delivery is the effect of the agent or vehicle on the physiologic function of the underlying mucosa. While multiple techniques are available to enhance drug delivery and absorption, these maneuvers may lead to disruption of the native epithelial architecture or lead to prolonged ciliary dysfunction or destruction. Furthermore, the impact of preexisting mucosal disease on baseline drug permeability and susceptibility to disruption remains unknown.

IN VITRO EXPERIMENTAL PLATFORMS TO STUDY TOPICAL DELIVERY

The air-liquid interface (ALI) cell culture is a technique that offers the potential to analyze drug-specific mucosal effects in an in vitro setting, thereby providing a powerful screening tool for potential nasally delivered compounds (**Fig. 3**).[22] Several well-described immortalized bronchial and nasal human epithelial cultures exist that have been used to establish normative ALI parameters, including the 16HBE14o-, Calu-3, and RPMI 2650 lines. These cell lines have been shown to form confluent ciliated monolayers with functional gap junctions and to express various transport proteins and efflux pumps.[23] Although phenotypic differences exist between these cell lines and native respiratory mucosa their basic epithelial physiologic function is preserved, and thus transepithelial electrical resistance, apparent permeability, and ciliary beat frequency may all be measured under a wide array of conditions. Furthermore, drug-specific absorption pathways may be selectively analyzed using known transcellular and paracellular markers such as dexamethasone and fluorescein, respectively.

Despite the benefits of these immortalized cell lines, disease-specific mucosal attributes such as phospholipid secretion, xenobiotic metabolism, interactions with extracellular matrices, morphology, polyamine uptake characteristics, and expression of major histocompatibility complex molecules may not be accurately reflected.[24] While techniques for the establishment of primary ALI cell cultures are in use, their utility in analyzing the relationship between underlying mucosal disease and drug delivery is yet to be explored.

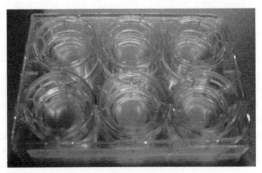

Fig. 3. ALI culture seen on a 6-well transwell permeable support.

MUCOADHESIVE DRUG-ELUTING POLYMERS

While the theoretical benefits of topical nasal therapy make it a highly attractive mode of drug delivery, the reality of the challenges of distribution and absorption reveal that its full potential remains elusive using current techniques. One potential solution may be found in the recent development of biocompatible drug-eluting polymers. These polymers could theoretically be loaded with a pharmaceutical agent and implanted in any desired location, including regions that are otherwise poorly accessed by nasal irrigations. The agent would be continuously eluted over a predetermined period and be distributed to adjacent mucosa using native mucociliary clearance mechanisms. Over time, the polymer would degrade in situ and either locally absorbed or mechanically cleared from the sinonasal cavity. The future success of implantable nasal therapeutics (INT) hinges on the choice of an appropriate carrier with optimal physicochemical characteristics. One polymer known as chitosan has been advanced as a particularly promising target, given its multiple attributes uniquely suited for nasal drug delivery.

Chitosan is an amino-polysaccharide derived from the alkaline deacetylation of chitin, a naturally occurring component of crustacean shells. As a cationic polymer, it is naturally mucoadherent, hemostatic, and has antimicrobial properties. Chitosan is dissolved following amine group protonation and may then be induced to form either a pH- or temperature-dependent hydrogel.[25] This hydrogel is biodegradable and functions as a spongelike polymer, which may be loaded with various therapeutic agents. These agents remain in dynamic equilibrium with the surrounding aqueous environment and may therefore be progressively released over time following implantation. This theory has been tested in various animal models that directly address the behavior of chitosan in respiratory mucosa. In one study, Paulson and colleagues[26] demonstrated continuous elution of steroid in a mouse middle ear model over a period of 5 days.

The chitosan hydrogel may also be manufactured as a flexible sheet, which may provide mechanical support as a drug-eluting implant or stent following sinus surgery. The authors' group has demonstrated that following implantation in a rabbit maxillary sinus model (see **Fig. 3**), a chitosan-based semirigid sheet is inert, biodegradable, and capable of continuous dexamethasone elution over 15 days (**Figs. 4** and **5**).[18] While steroids represent an important focus of interest in the treatment of inflammatory sinus disorders, the hydrogel is capable of eluting a wide variety of compounds, and thus the therapeutic potential of other agents represents an active area of investigation.

While these properties make chitosan a valuable tool in the treatment of primary sinus disorders, it also has attributes that may enhance systemic drug delivery. As a result of size and charge limitations, most pharmaceutical agents will be shunted toward the paracellular absorption route. Chitosan is among the group of molecules capable of active modulation of gap junctions[18] and can therefore enhance the paracellular permeability of various agents. For example, chitosan has been shown to enhance insulin absorption across the nasal mucosa in a rat model[27] and can produce a 6-fold increase in the bioavailability of intranasal morphine.[17]

NANOPARTICULATE DRUG CARRIERS

An alternative approach for enhancing drug delivery is complexing pharmacologically active agents to particulate carriers capable of selectively binding to mucus and cell surface proteins. These carriers can be manufactured on scales less than 200 nm, thereby allowing them to readily diffuse through the mucus glycoprotein matrix. After

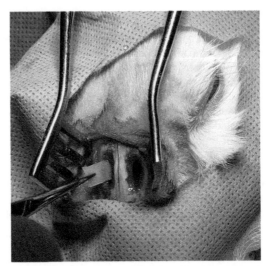

Fig. 4. Placement of chitosan glycerophosphate (CGP) implant in a New Zealand white rabbit maxillary sinus.

binding to their intended site of action, these particles may be able to sustain stable, prolonged drug delivery. Biodegradable polymers such as polylactic acid and poly(-lactic-coglycolic acid) have been shown to be well tolerated in vivo and may prove to function as optimal nanoparticulate carriers for various pharmaceutical agents (**Fig. 6**) (Schlosser RJ, personal communication, 2009).

IMPLICATIONS FOR RESEARCH

Recent radiologic, cadaveric, and clinical studies have contributed greatly to the evolving understanding of the impact of sinus surgery and high-volume irrigations on the degree of postoperative intraluminal drug distribution. In addition, a wide array of novel mucolytics, permeability enhancers, mucoadhesive agents, and

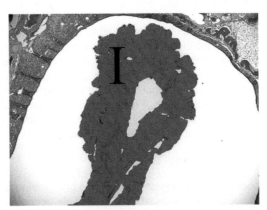

Fig. 5. CGP implant (I) within a rabbit maxillary sinus. Note the lack of inflammatory reaction to the inert biopolymer (hematoxylin-eosin stain ×25).

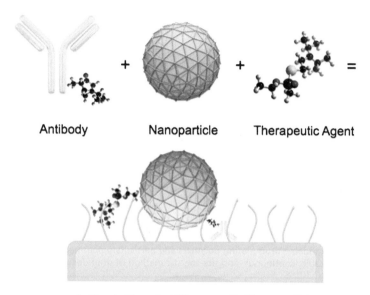

Antibody Targeted Therapeutic Nanoparticle

Fig. 6. Antibody-conjugated therapeutic nanoparticle.

nanoparticles are currently being investigated, which may prove to overcome many of the problems associated with current methods. The elaboration of in vitro models to study the effects of these interventions in an experimental setting may also serve to further accelerate the introduction of these techniques into clinical practice. While great strides in the understanding of the effects of topical drug delivery have been made, additional studies are required to further optimize drug distribution and efficacy at the target site.

IMPLICATIONS FOR CLINICAL PRACTICE

Intranasal drug delivery offers multiple benefits over traditional therapeutic interventions for local and systemic disease. The advantages include access to a large surface area, porous endothelium, high total blood flow, decreased enzymatic degradation, and avoidance of the first-pass effect. Despite the widespread availability of a range of delivery devices, it has become evident that in the setting of native anatomy, drug distribution beyond the internal valve is minimal. This limited efficacy is further compounded by rapid clearance of the solvent carrier found in most Food and Drug Administration–approved formulations. While novel drug formulations and delivery devices are on the horizon, practitioners are faced with the challenge of optimizing efficacy using currently available techniques. Multiple studies have supported the benefits of high-volume irrigations and the improved delivery in the postoperative nasal cavity. Consequently, these concepts have begun to be adopted by many clinicians. The varied yet synergistic lines of investigation surrounding local drug delivery have contributed greatly to the understanding of the distribution and effects of topical and INT, and may ultimately serve to fundamentally alter the way in which sinonasal disease is managed in the future.

REFERENCES

1. Ugwoke MI, Verbeke N, Kinget R. The biopharmaceutical aspects of nasal mucoadhesive drug delivery. J Pharm Pharmacol 2001;53(1):3–21.
2. Elliott KA, Stringer SP. Evidence-based recommendations for antimicrobial nasal washes in chronic rhinosinusitis. Am J Rhinol 2006;20(1):1–6.
3. Saijo R, Majima Y, Hyo N, et al. Particle deposition of therapeutic aerosols in the nose and paranasal sinuses after transnasal sinus surgery: a cast model study. Am J Rhinol 2004;18(1):1–7.
4. Kleinstreuer C, Zhang Z, Donohue JF. Targeted drug-aerosol delivery in the human respiratory system. Annu Rev Biomed Eng 2008;10:195–220.
5. Olson DE, Rasgon BM, Hilsinger RL Jr. Radiographic comparison of three methods for nasal saline irrigation. Laryngoscope 2002;112(8 Pt 1):1394–8.
6. Snidvongs K, Chaowanapanja P, Aeumjaturapat S, et al. Does nasal irrigation enter paranasal sinuses in chronic rhinosinusitis? Am J Rhinol 2008;22:483–6.
7. Hyo N, Takano H, Hyo Y. Particle deposition efficiency of therapeutic aerosols in the human maxillary sinus. Rhinology 1989;27:17–26.
8. Grobler A, Weitzel EK, Buele A, et al. Pre- and postoperative sinus penetration of nasal irrigation. Laryngoscope 2008;118:2078–81.
9. Miller TR, Muntz HR, Gilbert ME, et al. Comparison of topical medication delivery systems after sinus surgery. Laryngoscope 2004;114(2):201–4.
10. Berridge MS, Lee Z, Heald DL. Regional distribution and kinetics of inhaled pharmaceuticals. Curr Pharm Des 2000;6(16):1631–51.
11. Lee Z, Berridge MS. PET imaging-based evaluation of aerosol drugs and their delivery devices: nasal and pulmonary studies. IEEE Trans Med Imaging 2002;21(10):1324–31.
12. Türker S, Onur E, Ozer Y. Nasal route and drug delivery systems. Pharm World Sci 2004;26(3):137–42.
13. Costantino HR, Illum L, Brandt G, et al. Intranasal delivery: physicochemical and therapeutic aspects. Int J Pharm 2007;337(1–2):1–24.
14. Shah PL, Scott SF, Knight RA, et al. In vivo effects of recombinant human DNase I on sputum in patients with cystic fibrosis. Thorax 1996;51:119–25.

15. Dawson M, Wirtz D, Hanes J. Enhanced viscoelasticity of human cystic fibrotic sputum correlates with increasing microheterogeneity in particle transport. J Biol Chem 2003;278:50393–401.
16. Ferrari S, Kitson C, Farley R, et al. Mucus altering agents as adjuncts for nonviral gene transfer to airway epithelium. Gene Ther 2001;8:1380–6.
17. Illum L. Nasal drug delivery—possibilities, problems and solutions. J Control Release 2003;87(1–3):187–98.
18. Bleier BS, Paulson DP, O'Malley BW, et al. Chitosan glycerophosphate-based semirigid dexamethasone eluting biodegradable stent. Am J Rhinol Allergy 2009;23(1):76–9.
19. Deli MA. Potential use of tight junction modulators to reversibly open membranous barriers and improve drug delivery. Biochim Biophys Acta 2009;1788(4): 892–910.
20. Hussain AA, Al-Bayatti AA, Dakkuri A, et al. Testosterone 17B-N,N-dimethylglycinate hydrochloride: a pro-drug with a potential for nasal delivery of testosterone. J Pharm Sci 2002;91:785–9.
21. Loftsson T, Masson M. Cyclodextrins in topical drug formulations: theory and practice. Int J Pharm 2001;225(1–2):15–30.
22. Mallants R, Vlaeminck V, Jorissen M, et al. An improved primary human nasal cell culture for the simultaneous determination of transepithelial transport and ciliary beat frequency. J Pharm Pharmacol 2009;61(7):883–90.
23. Forbes B, Ehrhardt C. Human respiratory epithelial cell culture for drug delivery applications. Eur J Pharm Biopharm 2005;60(2):193–205.
24. Sakagami M. In vivo, in vitro and ex vivo models to assess pulmonary absorption and disposition of inhaled therapeutics for systemic delivery. Adv Drug Deliv Rev 2006;58(9–10):1030–60.
25. Chenite A, Chaput C, Wang D, et al. Novel injectable neutral solutions of chitosan form biodegradable gels in situ. Biomaterials 2000;21(21):2155–61.
26. Paulson DP, Abuzeid W, Jiang H, et al. A novel controlled local drug delivery system for inner ear disease. Laryngoscope 2008;118(4):706–11.
27. Di Colo G, Zambito Y, Zaino C. Polymeric enhancers of mucosal epithelia permeability: synthesis, transepithelial penetration-enhancing properties, mechanism of action, safety issues. J Pharm Sci 2008;97(5):1652–80.

Systemic Therapies in Managing Sinonasal Inflammation

Michael A. DeMarcantonio, MD, Joseph K. Han, MD*

KEYWORDS

- Sinusitis • Leukotriene • Aspirin desensitization • Steroid
- Inflammation • Polyp • Allergy • Immunotherapy

Despite affecting approximately 20 million Americans, chronic rhinosinusitis (CRS) remains a frustrating and controversial disease entity.[1] Traditional theories on the pathogenesis of CRS have centered on anatomic obstruction, resulting in bacterial infection. This convention has guided antimicrobial and surgical therapies for decades. Although this approach has yielded some success, many patients continue to suffer from CRS despite surgical and medical therapy. Such frustrations have resulted in a shift in focus toward further elucidating the pathogenesis and developing directed therapies. The cornerstone of this approach is the acknowledgment that allergy and inflammation may not only simply exacerbate CRS but also may play a role in its development. Such a paradigm shift allows researchers and clinicians to pursue systemic therapies that target mucosal inflammation and the allergic response as a new means of treating CRS.

CRS is a heterogeneous spectrum disorder that is constantly being further categorized and classified. Classically, patients with CRS can be divided by the presence or lack of polyps. Such a distinction between CRS with nasal polyps (CRSwNP) and CRS without nasal polyps (CRSsNP) demonstrates not only a clinical but also a pathologic difference. Although a poignant inflammatory response is seen in each subset of CRS, the features of each subset vary greatly. Nasal polyp inflammation is predominantly mediated by eosinophils, which constitute 60% of the mucosal cell population.[2] This presence of a large proportion of eosinophils points toward a mast cell– and histamine-associated response. This proposition is further supported by the demonstration of not only high levels of eosinophils in polypoid tissue but also of increased levels of histamine, interleukin (IL) 5, and IL-13.[3] Most of the systemic therapies

Disclosures: There is nothing to declare and no conflict of interest.
Department of Otolaryngology–Head and Neck Surgery, Eastern Virginia Medical School, 600 Gresham Drive, Suite 1100, Norfolk, VA 23507, USA
* Corresponding author.
E-mail address: hanjk@evms.edu

Otolaryngol Clin N Am 43 (2010) 551–563
doi:10.1016/j.otc.2010.02.013
0030-6665/10/$ – see front matter

currently in use seek to treat CRS by disruption of these cytokines and their associated inflammatory cascade.

CRSsNP at first glance seems to be a more straightforward process. Much like acute sinusitis, neutrophils dominate mucosal inflammation in CRSsNP.[4] However, this distinction proves an oversimplification. All CRSsNP are not created equal. Those affected by allergy or asthma may in fact have extensive infiltration by eosinophils, much like CRSwNP.[5] It is therefore possible to see mucosal hypereosinophilia separate from polypoid disease. Such a complex subset indicates the possibility for further categorization of CRS, which may allow for more patient-specific targeted therapy.

The diversity of CRS demands varied and new treatment approaches. Although the final role of systemic therapies remains unsettled, their development combined with the better understanding for the cause of CRS should present a new avenue for CRS therapy.

ANTILEUKOTRIENES

Leukotrienes are produced by the lipoxygenase pathway from the initial substrate of arachidonic acid. The pathway eventually results in 3 clinically significant leukotrienes: LTC4, LTD4, and LTE4. These products all contain cysteine and are therefore collectively known as cysteinyl leukotrienes, or cys-LTs. Cysteinyl leukotrienes are stored in many different cells, including mast cells. Mast cell release of leukotrienes seems to spur on inflammation and act as early- and late-phase mediators to the allergic response.[6,7]

As with most systemic therapies, mostof the research involving CRS and antileukotrienes centers on patients with nasal polyposis. As early as 1987, Jung and colleagues[8] had identified elevated levels of leukotrienes in patients with Samter triad. In further research, by challenging aspirin-sensitive patients, researchers observed mast cell activation. The resultant nasal tryptase, histamine, and leukotriene levels were deemed essential for the nasal symptoms experienced in these patients.[9]

Currently, 2 therapeutic approaches exist to control the inflammatory effect of cysteinyl leukotrienes. Medications named with the suffix -lukast, such as montelukast or zafirlukast, bind to cysteinyl leukotriene receptors, whereas the drug zileuton works in a different fashion by inhibiting the action of the enzyme 5-lipoxygenase. Initially, the ability of these medications to reduce nasal symptoms was observed anecdotally in asthmatic patients with nasal polyps undergoing therapy. In 1999, Parnes and Chuma[10] examined the acute effects of antileukotrienes in patients with CRSwNP. These patients were treated in a prospective manner with zafirlukast initially with crossover to zileuton for failure to respond to zafirlukast. Overall, the therapy resulted in reduction of polyps which was observed by endoscopy, decreased steroid use, and improvement in patient-reported symptoms. This study, however, was limited by open trial design and short follow-up. There have been other studies that have also demonstrated the benefit of the use of leukotriene modifiers in reducing polyp size and subjective improvement of patients with CRSwNP, but there remains a paucity of well-designed randomized controlled trials examining the effectiveness of antileukotrienes in patients with CRS.[7,11,12]

Although there is a scarcity of robust data to demonstrate that leukotriene modifiers may be beneficial for patients with CRS, this does not translate to lack of benefit. Cysteinyl leukotriene receptor antagonists are most likely to be helpful in patients with allergic rhinitis and asthma that have sinusitis because leukotrienes are responsible for the chronic inflammation in these patients. Patients with extremely elevated levels of cysteinyl leukotrienes such as in aspirin triad, also known as aspirin exacerbated respiratory disease (AERD), are less likely to benefit from cysteinyl leukotriene receptors antagonists and more likely to benefit from lipoxygenase inhibitors such as zileuton, which decrease cysteinyl leukotriene production higher upstream. However, the use of zileuton requires careful monitoring of the liver enzymes to monitor liver toxicity. Although patients with severe polyposis may benefit from this group of medications, further rigid investigation is necessary.

CORTICOSTEROIDS

The use of oral corticosteroids such as prednisone in CRS, particularly in patients with nasal polyps (CRSwNP), has been advocated for decades. Initial anecdotal evidence has been supported by years of successful clinical implementation. With further understanding of the role of eosinophils in CRS comes a possible explanation for the effect of corticosteroids. It is proposed that the benefit observed might stem from the ability of corticosteroids to limit the availability of IL-1, IL-3, and IL-5, all of which are necessary for eosinophil survival.[13] Effects of steroids on inflammatory cytokines were further examined by Lennard and colleagues[14] in 2000. This small study evaluated cytokine profiles in patients with CRS by nasal biopsy before and after a short course of systemic steroids. They noted a significant decrease in IL-6 levels with other cytokines, including tumor necrosis factor α trending toward significance. This research did not attempt to correlate their findings with symptom relief.

In an attempt to evaluate symptomatic relief, several open label trials have examined corticosteroid use in CRS. These studies have often combined oral with topical treatment and have demonstrated improvements in nasal symptoms including congestion and olfaction.[15] Despite the widespread use of this treatment modality, few randomized trials exist. A randomized, controlled, double-blind study demonstrated improved nasal symptom scores when comparing placebo with a 14-day treatment with 50 mg prednisolone.[16] In the same study, patients were found to have reduction of nasal polyp size on magnetic resonance imaging and endoscopy.

Years of clinical practice and some focused research have shown the possible benefits of systemic corticosteroids in CRS, particularly in patients with polyposis. With the available data it seems reasonable to recommend the use of corticosteroids in a multifaceted treatment plan including other systemic therapies and topical agents. Although further investigation into the mechanisms and extent of efficacy of corticosteroids in CRS is needed, their success, particularly in the treatment of nasal polyposis, is apparent. Less clear is the role, if any, of corticosteroids in patients with CRSsNP. There is currently no evidence to support the use of oral or topical steroids despite anecdotal clinical success.

Oral steroids should be used judiciously, understanding the potential complications associated with the long-term use of corticosteroid, such as adrenal suppression and bone density loss. In children, the risk for inhibition of the hypothalamic pituitary adrenal axis should be strongly considered, and therefore oral steroid use should be minimized as much as possible.

IMMUNOTHERAPY

The pathogenesis of CRS has been influenced by the unified airway theory.[17] This theory represents a movement to view allergic rhinitis, CRS, and asthma as similar entities resulting from generalized inflammation.[18] These previously separate conditions could variably affect the development of, or alter the course of, one another. Researchers and clinicians have noticed that therapies directed at one disease process often have benefits on other aspects of symptomatology.[19] Such interplay was demonstrated when management of sinusitis resulted in improvement of asthma symptoms.[20] In keeping with this trend, if one could prevent the inflammation associated with allergic rhinitis caused by seasonal allergies, perhaps patients would also experience improvement in their CRS symptoms.

Immunotherapy achieves its effects by modulating the immunoglobulin and T lymphocyte responses. After several months of immunotherapy, a shift in the circulating allergy-specific immunoglobulin occurs with an increase in IgG4 level, which may serve to block IgE-mediated release of histamine.[21] The response of T lymphocytes to allergens is also altered with a shift from T_H2 to T_H1 predominance. This alters the cytokines produced from T_H2 (IL-4, IL-5, and IL-13) to T_H1 cytokines (interferon gamma and IL-2). Such a transition away from the T_H2-driven inflammatory process involved in CRS could have therapeutic effects. One study compared the nasal eosinophil and cytokine profiles of patients treated with ragweed immunotherapy with placebo. After a course of therapy, nasal biopsies were performed on treatment and control groups after allergen challenge. Biopsy specimens demonstrated significantly decreased level of eosinophils and IL-4–mRNA positive cells in the treatment group.[22] Such findings support a shift from T_H2 to T_H1 cytokine production. In addition, after prolonged follow-up, treatment group patients experienced a significant reduction in chest symptoms and a trend toward improved nasal symptoms. This research points to the profound effect that treatment with immunotherapy can have a local tissue response to allergen. At least in theory some patients with CRS should benefit from the decreased inflammatory response offered by immunotherapy. Even though the cause-and-effect relationship between allergic rhinitis, asthma, and sinusitis is not completely clear, it is reasonable to evaluate patients with CRS for allergy in an attempt to remove an additional insulting inflammatory process.

Subcutaneous Immunotherapy and Sublingual Immunotherapy

There are no clinical trials examining the efficacy of subcutaneous (SCIT) or sublingual immunotherapy (SLIT) in CRS. Nevertheless, to successfully treat patients with CRS with coinciding atopy, an understanding of the practice of immunotherapy is crucial. Although not one article or review is likely to settle the debate between SCIT and SLIT, it is reasonable to delineate the efficacy, safety, and practical considerations associated with both. With the increasing involvement of otolaryngologists in allergy and immunotherapy, these basic tenets are important to understand even though one may perform either SCIT or SLIT.

The efficacy of SCIT has been evaluated in multiple trials over the past several decades with typically positive results. A Cochrane review was undertaken by Calderon and colleagues[23] to assess the available randomized data. This review included a total of 2871 patients. Although the studies included were found to be somewhat heterogeneous, meta-analysis did reveal significant improvements in symptom scores and medication use.

It has long been accepted that there is a small but real risk associated with SCIT. In surveys of allergy practitioners, fatal reactions are estimated to occur in 1 in every 2 to 2.8 million injections.[24] Until recently there was little quantification of nonfatal but severe reactions. Near-fatal reactions are defined as severe respiratory compromise, hypotension, or both, requiring emergency epinephrine treatment.[24] A large survey by Amin and colleagues[24] determined that serious near-fatal reactions were 2.5 times more likely than fatal reactions, with 1 event per million doses. This rate would result in 5 such reactions per year in the United States. Asthma was found to be an important risk factor for a reaction. Eighty-eight percent of fatal reactions and 46% of near-fatal reactions were found in asthmatic patients. With regard to severity of reaction, 88% of reported incidents involved hypotension, whereas only 10% of patients developed severe respiratory distress. All of those patients experiencing severe respiratory symptoms were known to have asthma. It must also be realized that dosing error was found to be at fault in 25% of cases in which cause could be determined. These results should give some guidance toward identifying those rare patients who may have a serious or fatal reaction to SCIT, allowing for refinement and improvement of practice.

With the limited availability of SLIT in the United States most clinical trials have taken place in Europe or Asia. In 2005, Wilson and colleagues[25] sought to review the available research in a large meta-analysis study. As in the review by Calderon and colleagues[23] a significant improvement and reduction in the need for medication was once again demonstrated. In general, the safety profile of SLIT is considered to be better than that of SCIT. To date there have been no reported deaths and only 3 case reports of anaphylaxis.[26] However, as the use of SLIT increases over the next few decades, these numbers may change.

At this time in the United States, immunotherapy is an underused tool. Although there are approximately 55 million Americans with allergy in the United States, only 2 to 3 million patients are currently receiving immunotherapy.[27] The benefits of SLIT including home dosing and decreased risk of systemic reactions seem to offer practical means to increase the number of patients treated. However, more investigation is needed to fully understand the exact dosing and potential amount of extract required in determining evidence-based approach for the guideline of SLIT antigen or extract. It is even possible that the doses required may be too high to practically treat millions of patients with SLIT. Clearly, more research is needed. The effect of allergy on CRS is indisputable, but how they are exactly related remains unclear. The heterogeneous nature of CRS still requires further delineation because it relates to atopy; however, early identification and treatment of patients in whom allergic rhinitis effects CRS may minimize further disease progression of CRS and provide an early-preventative and cost-effective intervention.

IMMUNOMODULATORS

With the recognition that certain cytokines and mediators play a role in allergic rhinitis and CRS, inevitably came the strategy to target and disable these propagators of inflammation. The interrelationship of IL-5 with eosinophils and mast cells made it an ideal initial target for the creation of a monoclonal antibody. Early research focused on treatment of asthma with mepolizumab. Initial in vitro studies showed promising results, demonstrating decreased tissue eosinophilia and apoptosis.[28] Although Leckie and colleagues[29] were able to show an 80% to 90% reduction of circulating eosinophils with a one time dose, their study was underpowered for efficacy.[6] Later, a pilot study examining a competitor's product SCH55700 failed to effect lung function in controlled clinical trials.[30]

The use of IL-5 monoclonal antibodies in CRS was initially spurred on by the role of IL-5 in the recruitment, maturation, and activation of eosinophils in nasal polyposis.[31] Randomized data for IL-5 therapy in nasal polyposis have thus far been limited to a few small studies.[32] For example, Gevaert and colleagues[33] evaluated patients with CRSwNP who were treated with a one time dose of placebo, 1 mg/kg or 3 mg/kg of anti-IL-5 and monitored for change in blood eosinophil levels as well as levels of serum and nasal eosinophil cationic protein. Although their results pointed toward an improvement in the treatment group, there was no statistical difference among the control and treatment groups. One possible explanation for the lack of statistical significance is that the CRSwNP groups are a mixture of different diseases. When the subjects in the treatment arms were divided into responders and nonresponders, those demonstrating a measurable response were significantly more likely to have a higher baseline IL-5 level. The treatment appeared safe with no increase in adverse events compared with placebo.

In 2009, 2 research groups published randomized controlled studies describing the effective use of mepolizumab in a subset of severe asthmatic patients with sputum eosinophilia. Parameswaran and colleagues[34] worked on 20 patients with prednisone-dependent asthma and were able to show a significant reduction of asthma exacerbations as well as improvement in level of serum eosinophils, asthma control, and forced expiratory volume in the first second of expiration (FEV_1). Similarly, Halder and colleagues[35] also demonstrated a reduced number of exacerbations in 61 patients with refractory eosinophilic asthma. However, no significant change was found in FEV_1, bronchodilator use, airway hyperresponsiveness, or asthma symptoms. These trials are limited by their size and seem to be applicable to a small subset of patients with asthma. However, the successful use of anti-IL-5 in a particular type of asthmatic patient may provide a guiding influence for further research in CRS.

IL-5 has not stood alone as the only target of monoclonal antibody therapy. Omalizumab, a monoclonal antibody against IgE, has received approval for treatment of severe asthma. In particular, patients with severe persistent allergic asthma have been shown to benefit from omalizumab.[36] Most notably, the Investigation of Omalizumab in Severe Asthma Treatment trial showed a 26% reduction in exacerbations compared with placebo when more than 400 such patients were treated in a randomized fashion.[37]

Success in the treatment of allergic asthma has led to several studies investigating the efficacy of anti-IgE therapy in allergic rhinitis. Two such studies have found improvements in symptoms and quality of life.[36] Success in asthma and rhinitis has prompted some limited use of anti-IgE therapy in patients with CRSwNP. A pilot study analyzing the treatment of nasal polyposis with anti-IgE has shown promising, although limited, results. Another small study with 8 patients treated with omalizumab was found to have improvement in nasal polyp scores when compared with a control group of similar untreated patients.[38]

Immunomodulators offer an interesting new frontier in the treatment of CRS. Further research involving well-designed and well-selected randomized trials is necessary. It is important not to ignore the practical issues involved in these therapies. Whereas mepolizumab has yet to become commercially available, omalizumab currently costs $694 for a 150-mg dose.[39] Because of their cost, their use must be rationed to those patients refractory to other treatments in which clinical benefit seems likely. With this possible limitation in mind, focus in immunomodulation should be placed on determining the cytokine characteristics and specific patient populations that will allow for effective targeted therapy. Again a cornerstone to providing the correct medical treatment is to better define the different pathophysiology of CRS with specific cytokine profiles so that the benefit from immunomodulation can be reaped. Studies so far appear to point toward the future of immunomodulator therapy in CRS, but much research and treatment outcomes still need to be addressed.

ASPIRIN DESENSITIZATION

A small subset of patients with CRS will have the diagnosis of Samter triad, also known as aspirin triad and AERD. The classic triad to diagnose aspirin triad includes aspirin (acetylsalicylic acid [ASA]) sensitivity, nasal polyposis, and asthma. These patients with aspirin triad or AERD also have a fourth element: extensive eosinophilia in the sinus mucosa. The pathogenesis in this disease involves an abnormal metabolic shift of arachidonic acid toward the lipoxygenase pathway and increased reactivity to the increased level of cysteinyl leukotrienes. The resultant excess level of cysteinyl leukotrienes has severe inflammatory consequences.[40] Although diagnosis for AERD can be easily determined by history and physical examination alone, one can challenge these patients to confirm the diagnosis.

Although variability exists with regard to specific aspirin challenge and desensitization techniques, standard precautions do exist.[41] Before densensitization, patients should have an assessment of FEV_1, pretreatment with leukotriene modifiers, and elimination of antihistamines 2 to 3 days before treatment. The importance of eliminating antihistamines must be stressed to the patient, because their effects may mask the early nasoocular symptoms that indicate a positive response. Also patients with poor pulmonary function, meaning a FEV_1 less than 70% of baseline or absolute number of 1.5 L in an adult, will not tolerate stress of the aspirin exposure. Patients should also be evaluated by their pulmonary physician to ensure optimized asthma therapy and should remain on corticosteroids, if required, for control of symptoms.

The general treatment approach in these patients involves typical CRSwNP therapy including oral or topical corticosteroids, leukotriene modifiers, and surgical intervention. In addition to these treatments, there is strong evidence that supports the efficacy of aspirin desensitization with multiple clinical trials demonstrating benefit.[41] In 1984, Stevenson and colleagues[42] performed a randomized, double-blind, controlled trial. Patients in the treatment arm reported improved nasal symptoms and reduced nasal corticosteroid use, although there was no significant effect on asthma symptoms or systemic corticosteroid use. However, another study demonstrated improved nasal symptoms, asthma symptoms, sinus infections, and less need for sinus surgery compared with baseline, when evaluating several doses of aspirin in a prospective manner.[43]

Typical aspirin desensitization procedure involves the administration of low-dose aspirin and then increasing the amount given over 2 to 3 days. The initial amount of aspirin given is 30 mg, which is then increased by 30 mg 3 hours later. The increase of aspirin is done twice in the first day. If the patient tolerates the desensitization on the first day, the patient should have reached 90 mg at the end of the first day. On the second day, 100 mg is given to start. Then 325 mg is given after 3 hours of the 100-mg dose. Then 650 mg is given 3 hours later. If the patient tolerates the 650-mg dose then the patient is sent home with a maintenance dose of 650 mg of aspirin twice a day. Patients are observed for nasal, ocular, and bronchoalveolar reactions during the desensitization.

Hope and colleagues examined their experience with 420 patients in an attempt to identify the most likely inciting dose and risk factors for severe reaction. They found 9% of reactions at the first dose of 30 mg, 75% at a dose between 45 and 60 mg, 3% from 150 to 325 mg, and no reactions at 650 mg. The identified risk factors for bronchopulmonary reactions to aspirin include the lack of use of leukotriene modifier, a baseline FEV_1 less than 80% of expected, and previous asthma related visit to the emergency room. With these results, this group recommended starting patients without significant risk factors with 40 to 60 mg initial dose and complete omission of the 650-mg dose.[44]

There remain differing opinions about where such procedures should occur, with recommendations ranging from the outpatient setting to the intensive care unit

(ICU). It is clearly prudent that patients with risk factors for significant respiratory reaction should be admitted to a level of care where intubation, if required, would be safe and quickly available. However, large allergy centers have achieved excellent safety results in the outpatient setting with 1 group reporting no deaths or intubations in 1375 patients.[45] Nevertheless, it is important to realize that such institutions have a wealth of experience with aspirin desensitization. At instititutions where both physician and nursing staff have limited experience with this procedure, the ICU may be the most prudent and safest location for desensitization.

After desensitization patients will require long-term aspirin therapy. Although variability in dosing exists, many practitioners use a regimen of 650 mg ASA twice a day for 6 months followed by a decrease in dosing to 325 or 650 mg/d.[44] With the inherent side effects associated with prolonged aspirin use there is a reasonable desire to determine the lowest possible effective dose. A small randomized prospective study evaluated patients with AERD for 1 year comparing a dosage of 100 mg/d with 300 mg/d. Results showed the 300-mg dose to be significantly superior in reducing the need for asthma medications and the incidence of recurrent nasal polyps. This study's effect on clinical practice, however, is limited by the small number of participants involved (N = 14).[46] The future of aspirin desensitization research will involve further refinement of the process to a streamlined and standardized technique that can comfortably be performed in a non-ICU setting on low- to moderate-risk patients. This allows for safe expansion of the practice beyond large academic allergy centers. A large randomized trial comparing 650 mg, 325 mg, and perhaps 100 mg long-term dosing would also serve to establish an indisputable standard for maintenance therapy. Until such data are available aspirin desensitization should continue to be performed taking all possible precautions and treating with established high-dose long-term therapy.

POSSIBLE ROLE OF STATINS

In reviewing the possible systemic therapies available for the treatment of CRS, it seems prudent to acknowledge the role that other unrelated systemic medications may affect the pathogenesis of CRS. Statins or HMG-CoA (3-hydroxy-3-methylglutaryl coenzyme A) reductase inhibitors have been suggested as a possible instigator in the development of nasal polyposis. Bucca and colleagues[47] reported 3 cases of asthma or chronic obstructive pulmonary disease that developed new-onset CRSwNP associated with a decrease in FEV_1 and worsening of symptoms. All 3 patients were found to have recently started statin therapy and experienced relief of symptoms with cessation of statins. New research has shed light on a possible mechanism for enhanced polyp development with statin use. In a scenario opposite of immunotherapy, statins have been linked to increase T_H1 to T_H2 polarization.[48] As previously demonstrated such a shift results in increased levels of inflammatory cytokines and eosinophilia.

Data supporting a connection between statins and nasal polyposis are thus far limited. Research in this topic will be difficult, given the ubiquitous use of statins in the United States and relatively low number of patients complaining of CRSwNP. Although this complication is intriguing, the incidence may be so small it would be difficult to detect. Possible study outlines could involve prospective enrollment and symptom evaluation of patients with asthma being treated for hypercholesterolemia or even a randomized controlled trial initiating statins in asthmatic patients with as yet untreated elevated cholesterol levels. Further study is also needed to delineate a clear immunologic side effect for the use of statin. Regardless, the limited available data does allow physicians to be aware of, and to monitor for a possible association between, statin use and chronic sinus disease.

MACROLIDES

In the field of CRS, macrolides have received great interest not only for their effect on bacteria but also for their previously unknown antiinflammatory properties. Research in this area has been spurred by the dramatic treatment of the previously deadly airway inflammatory disorder, diffuse panbronchiolitis.[49] Although definitive answers regarding the mechanism remain elusive, years of in vitro and in vivo studies have served to clarify the likely mechanisms of action. In macrolide therapy, the primary targets appear to be neutrophils and their associated cytokines. Research has demonstrated in vitro macrolide suppression of IL-8, IL-6, and granulocyte-macrophage colony-stimulating factor as well as inhibition of neutrophil adhesion to epithelial cells.[50] Other investigators have noted that macrolides and prednisolone similarly suppress IL-5, IL-8, and granulocyte-macrophage colony-stimulating factor in ex vivo studies of the nasal mucosa from patients with CRS. These findings have been further correlated with reduced IL-8 levels on lavage and reduction of nasal polyps after macrolide therapy.[51]

Until recently there existed few randomized well-controlled trials examining the effects of macrolide therapy in CRS. In 2006, Wallwork and colleagues[52] randomized 64 patients to receive roxithromycin or placebo for 3 months. The study demonstrated a statistically significant improvement in sinonasal outcome test 20 score, nasal endoscopy, saccharine transit time, and IL-8 levels.

Like many other vanguard CRS therapies the nonantimicrobial activity of macrolides seems to stem from immunomodulation[49]; however, the tendency to influence a primarily neutrophil-dominated inflammation presents a unique opportunity. Unlike other systemic therapies, such as use of immunomodulators, leukotriene inhibitors, and immunotherapy, macrolides seem unlikely to be effective in diseases dominated by atopy and eosinophilia. A correlation has even been noted between effective macrolide therapy and low-IgE levels.[53] It is therefore reasonable to assume that careful patient selection will allow for further enlightening research and future selective employment of macrolide therapy.

SUMMARY
Implications for Research

There exist 2 primary areas where research in this field should be directed. The first involves further quantifying and comparing the effectiveness of various systemic therapies for CRS. Additional large, well-designed randomized controlled trials are needed to compare the effectiveness of antileukotrienes, corticosteroids, and macrolides in CRS. Similarly, randomized trials are further required to assess the value of immunomodulators, such as mepolizumab and omalizumab, in treating CRS. It is essential to remember that these therapies are unlikely to benefit all patients with CRS. It is therefore important to select the appropriate patients to include in clinical research, lest real effects be underestimated.

This selective approach is thought to form the core foundation for future research in the field of CRS. The key to future therapies will involve further delineation of this heterogeneous disorder. By identifying the specific inflammatory processes and cytokines involved in separate subsets of CRS, individualized therapies can be implemented. A thorough classification of CRS will not be a simple endeavor and will involve the collection of huge amounts of prospective, pathologic, and clinical data.

Table 1
Systemic treatments of rhinosinusitis

Treatment	Proposed Mechanism of Action	Patient Population
Corticosteroids	• Inhibition of arachidonic acid synthesis • Decrease in the levels of IL-1, IL-3, IL-5, and IL-6	• Patients with aspirin triad • CRSwNP
Immunotherapy	• Shift T_H2 (IL-4, IL-5, and IL-13) to T_H1 products (interferon gamma and IL-2) • Increase IgG4 level, decrease IgE level	CRS with atopy
Mepolizumab	Anti-IL-5 monoclonal antibody	Eosinophilic asthma
Omalizumab	Anti-IgE monoclonal antibody	Allergic asthma
Aspirin Desensitization	Desensitization to cysteinyl leukotrienes	Patients with aspirin triad
Macrolides	Antiinflammatory: neutrophil cytokines (ie, IL-8)	CRSsNP

Nevertheless, by further understanding the problem one may more effectively implement the solution.

Implications for Clinical Practice

Although current research indicates a promising future role for new systemic therapies in CRS, it is obvious that leukotriene inhibitors, corticosteroids, macrolides, and aspirin desensitization will continue to be the cornerstones of treatment. Immunomodulators and allergy therapy may offer additional weapons in the arsenal against CRS, if applied appropriately. The key to the effectiveness of systemic medical treatment lies in its use in the treatment of specific CRS subtypes and patterns of inflammation. Understanding the mechanisms of applied systemic therapies also allows for correct and appropriate implementation (**Table 1**). With such patient selection and directed therapy it is not impossible to envision a future in which patients will be classified and treated based on their specific disease pathology. Such targeted therapy represents the future of medicine in general as well as in CRS.

REFERENCES

1. Benson V, Marano M. Current estimates from the national health interview survey, 1995. Hyattsville (MD): National Center for Health Statistics; 1998. Vital Health Stat 10, No. 199.
2. Pawanker R. Nasal polyposis: an update. Curr Opin Allergy Clin Immunol 2003;3: 1–6.
3. Drake-Lee AB, McLaughlan P. Clinical symptoms, free histamine and IgE in patients with nasal polyposis. Int Arch Allergy Appl Immunol 1982;69(3):268–71.
4. Pawankar R, Nanoka M. Inflammatory mechanisms and remodeling in chronic rhinosinusitis and nasal polyps. Curr Allergy Asthma Rep 2007;7:202–8.
5. Georgitis JW, Matthews BL, Stone B. Chronic sinusitis: characterization of cellular influx and inflammatory mediators in sinus lavage. Int Arch Allergy Immunol 1995; 106:416–21.

6. Statham MM, Seiden A. Potential new avenues of treatment for chronic rhinosinusitis: an anti-inflammatory approach. Otolaryngol Clin North Am 2005;38:1351–65.
7. Parnes SM. The role of leukotriene inhibitors in patients with paranasal sinus disease. Curr Opin Otolaryngol Head Neck Surg 2003;11:184–91.
8. Jung TT, Juhn SK, Hwang D, et al. Prostaglandins, leukotrienes, and other arachidonic acid metabolites in nasal polyps and nasal mucosa. Laryngoscope 1987; 97(2):184–9.
9. Fischer AR, Rosenberg MA, Lilly CM, et al. Direct evidence for a role of the mast cell in the nasal response to aspirin in aspirin-sensitive asthma. J Allergy Clin Immunol 1994;94(6 Pt 1):1046–56.
10. Parnes SM, Chuma AV. Acute effects of antileukotrienes on sinonasal polyposis and sinusitis. Ear Nose Throat J 2000;79(1):18–20, 24.
11. Ragab S, Parikh A, Darby YC, et al. An open audit of montelukast, a leukotriene receptor antagonist, in nasal polyposis associated with asthma. Clin Exp Allergy 2001;31(9):1385–91.
12. Ulualp SO, Sterman BM, Toohill RJ. Antileukotriene therapy for the relief of sinus symptoms in aspirin triad disease. Ear Nose Throat J 1999;78(8):604–6, 608, 613, passim.
13. Cox G, Ohtoshi T, Vancheri C, et al. Promotion of eosinophil survival by human bronchial epithelial cells and its modulation by steroids. Am J Respir Cell Mol Biol 1991;4(6):525–31.
14. Lennard C, Mann E, Sun L, et al. Interleukin-1B, interleukin-5, interleukin-6, interleukin-8, and tumor necrosis factor-α in chronic sinusitis: response to systemic corticosteroids. Am J Rhinol 2000;14(6):367–73.
15. Van Camp C, Clement PA. Results of oral steroid treatment in nasal polyposis. Rhinology 1994;32(1):5–9.
16. Hissaria P, Smith W, Wormald P, et al. Short course of systemic corticosteroids in sinonasal polyposis: a double blind, randomized, placebo controlled trial with evaluation of outcome measures. J Allergy Clin Immunol 2006;118(1):128–33.
17. Krouse JH, Brown RW, Fineman SM, et al. Asthma and the unified airway [review]. Otolaryngol Head Neck Surg 2007;136(Suppl 5):S75–106.
18. Krouse JH, Veling MC, Ryan MW, et al. Executive summary: asthma and the unified airway. Otolaryngol Head Neck Surg 2007;136(5):699–706.
19. Ahmad N, Zacharek M. Allergic rhinitis and rhinosinusitis. Otolaryngol Clin North Am 2008;41:267–81.
20. Batra PS, Kern RC, Tripathi A, et al. Outcome analysis of endoscopic sinus surgery in patients with nasal polyps and asthma. Laryngoscope 2003;113(10): 1703–6.
21. Till SJ, Francis JN, Nouri-Aria K, et al. Mechanisms of immunotherapy. J Allergy Clin Immunol 2004;113:1025–34.
22. Tulic MK, Fiset PO, Christodoulopoulos P, et al. Amb a 1-immunostimulatory oligodeoxynucleotide conjugate immunotherapy decreases the nasal inflammatory response. J Allergy Clin Immunol 2004;113(2):235–41.
23. Calderon MA, Alves B, Jacobson M, et al. Allergen injection immunotherapy for seasonal allergic rhinitis. Cochrane Database Syst Rev 2007;1:CD001936.
24. Amin HS, Llss GM, Bernstein DI. Evaluation of near-fatal reactions to allergen immunotherapy injections. J Allergy Clin Immunol 2006;117:169–75.
25. Wilson DR, Lima MT, Durham SR. Sublingual immunotherapy for allergic rhinitis: systematic review and meta-analysis. Allergy 2005;60(1):4–12.
26. Leatherman B. Injection and sublingual immunotherapy in the management of allergies affecting the unified airway. Otolaryngol Clin North Am 2008;41:359–74.

27. Cox LS, Linnemann DL, Nolte H, et al. Sublingual immunotherapy: a comprehensive review. J Allergy Clin Immunol 2006;117:1021–35.

28. Simon HU, Yousefi S, Schranz C, et al. Direct demonstration of delayed eosinophil apoptosis as a mechanism causing tissue eosinophilia. J Immunol 1997; 158(8):3902–8.

29. Leckie MJ, ten Brinke A, Khan J, et al. Effects of an interleukin-5 blocking monoclonal antibody on eosinophils, airway hyper-responsiveness, and the late asthmatic response. Lancet 2000;356(9248):2144–8.

30. Kips JC, O'Connor BJ, Langley SJ, et al. Effect of SCH55700, a humanized antihuman interleukin-5 antibody, in severe persistent asthma: a pilot study. Am J Respir Crit Care Med 2003;167(12):1655–9.

31. Bachert C, Wagenmann M, Hauser U, et al. IL-5 synthesis is upregulated in human nasal polyp tissue. J Allergy Clin Immunol 1997;99(6 Pt 1):837–42.

32. Nelson HS. Advances in upper airway diseases and allergen immunotherapy. J Allergy Clin Immunol 2007;119:872–80.

33. Gevaert P, Lang-Loidolt D, Lackner A, et al. Nasal IL-5 levels determine the response to anti-IL-5 treatment in patients with nasal polyps. J Allergy Clin Immunol 2006;118:1133–41.

34. Parameswaran N, Pizzichini M, Kjarsgaard M, et al. Mepolizumab for prednisonedependent asthma with sputum eosinophilia. N Engl J Med 2009;360(10): 985–93.

35. Halder P, Brightling C, Hargadon B, et al. Mepolizumab and exacerbations of refractory eosinophilic asthma. N Engl J Med 2009;360(10):973–83.

36. Nowak D. Management of asthma with anti-immunoglobulin E: a review of clinical trials of omalizumab. Respir Med 2006;100:1907–17.

37. Humbert M, Beasley R, Ayres J, et al. Benefits of omalziumab as add-on therapy in patients with severe persistent asthma who are inadequately controlled despite available therapy (GINA 2002 step 4 treatment), INNOVATE. Allergy 2005;60:309–16.

38. Penn R, Mikula S. The role of anti-IgE immunoglobulin therapy in nasal polyposis: a pilot study. Am J Rhinol 2007;21:428–33.

39. Neil Mason. Correspondence; Source: Amerisourcebergen prescription wholesaler, Sentara pharmacy department, Hospital directory for pricing. October 22, 2009.

40. Szczeklik A, Stevenson DD. Aspirin- induced asthma: advances in pathogenesis, diagnosis, and management. J Allergy Clin Immunol 2003;111(5):913–21 [quiz: 922].

41. Williams AN, Woessner KM. The clinical effectiveness of aspirin desensitization in chronic rhinosinusitis. Curr Allergy Asthma Rep 2008;8(3):245–52.

42. Stevenson DD, Pleskow WW, Simon RA, et al. Aspirin-sensitive rhinosinusitis asthma: a double-blind crossover study of treatment with aspirin. J Allergy Clin Immunol 1984;73(4):500–7.

43. Lee JY, Simon RA, Stevenson DD. Selection of aspirin dosages for aspirin desensitization treatment in patients with aspirin-exacerbated respiratory disease. J Allergy Clin Immunol 2007;119(1):157–64.

44. Hope AP, Woessner KA, Simon RA, et al. Rational approach to aspirin dosing during oral challenges and desensitization of patients with aspirin-exacerated respiratory disease. J Allergy Clin Immunol 2009;123:406–10.

45. Stevenson DD. Aspirin sensitivity and desensitization for asthma and sinusitis. Curr Allergy Asthma Rep 2009;9:155–63.

46. Rozsasi A, Polzehl D, Deutschle T, et al. Long-term treatment with aspirin desensitization: a prospective clinical trial comparing 100 and 300 mg aspirin daily. Allergy 2008;63:1228–34.

47. Bucca C, Marsico A, Panaro E, et al. Statins and nasal polyps. Ann Intern Med 2005;142(4):310–1.
48. Hakamada-Taguchi R, Uehara Y, Kuribayashi K, et al. Inhibition of hydroxymethyl-glutaryl-coenzyme a reductase reduces Th1 development and promotes Th2 development. Circ Res 2003;93:948–56.
49. Harvey R, Wallwork B, Lund V. Anti-inflammatory effects of macrolides: applications in chronic rhinosinusitis. Immunol Allergy Clin North Am 2009;29:689–703.
50. Kawasaki S, Takizawa H, Ohtoshi T, et al. Roxithromycin inhibits cytokine production by and neutrophil attachment to human bronchial epithelial cells in vitro. Antimicrob Agents Chemother 1998;42:1499–502.
51. Yamada T, Fujieda S, Mori S, et al. Macrolide treatment decreased size of nasal polyps and IL-8 levels in nasal lavage. Am J Rhinol 2000;14:143–8.
52. Wallwork B, Coman W, Feron F, et al. Clarithromycin and prednisolone inhibit cytokine production in chronic rhinosinusitis. Laryngoscope 2002;112:1827–30.
53. Wallwork B, Coman W, Mackay-Sim A, et al. A double-blind, randomized, placebo-controlled trial of macrolide in the treatment of chronic rhinosinusitis. Laryngoscope 2006;116:189–93.

Application of Minimally Invasive Endoscopic Sinus Surgery Techniques

Kevin C. Welch, MD*, James A. Stankiewicz, MD

KEYWORDS

- Surgical techniques • Minimally invasive surgery
- Endoscopic sinus surgery • Chronic rhinosinusitis treatment

Since the early 1980s, endoscopic sinus surgery (ESS) has been widely used to treat recalcitrant chronic rhinosinusitis (CRS). Over the last 10 years, techniques and tools have emerged that offer targeted, minimally invasive therapy aimed at standardizing endoscopic sinus surgery, reducing operative time, and improving patient outcomes.

The minimally invasive sinus technique (MIST) was the first such effort designed to provide minimally invasive, targeted intervention to key areas within the sinuses. The basis of this minimally invasive technique is work done early by Messerklinger[1,2] and his studies regarding mucociliary clearance. Minimally invasive sinus technique sought to standardize ESS by defining starting and ending points, minimizing mucosal trauma, and addressing four key areas within the sinuses.

More recent developments in the minimally invasive treatment of the sinuses include the use of balloon catheters that dilate the sinus ostia. Balloon catheter dilatation can be performed via two routes, transnasal or transantral, the later being more limited in capability. Both instruments, however, can be used to deliver minimally invasive targeted therapy to diseased sinuses.

MINIMALLY INVASIVE SINUS TECHNIQUE

The minimally invasive sinus technique was originally described by Ruben Setliff[3] and Peter Catalano[4,5] as a means of surgically addressing CRS while at the same time fulfilling several of the supposed shortcomings of conventional endoscopic sinus surgery. Catalano describes MIST as a "targeted intervention"[5] that is designed to address not the sinus ostia themselves but rather the transition spaces surrounding the sinus ostia. Fundamental to the philosophy of MIST is that the transition spaces

Department of Otolaryngology – Head & Neck Surgery, Loyola University Medical Center, 2160 South First Avenue, Magquire Building, Maywood, IL 60153, USA
* Corresponding author.
E-mail address: kwelch1@lumc.edu

Otolaryngol Clin N Am 43 (2010) 565–578
doi:10.1016/j.otc.2010.02.021
0030-6665/10/$ – see front matter © 2010 Elsevier Inc. All rights reserved.

oto.theclinics.com

are sources of CRS caused by mucosal contact when tissues become edematous, come into contact, and subsequently disrupt mucociliary transportation.[3-5] The observations of Stammberger[6] confirm that when these diseased transition spaces are cleared surgically, the more dependent sinuses (eg, maxillary, frontal) do demonstrate the capability of recovering function. This observation is the central tenant of MIST philosophy; therefore, the procedure is considered minimally invasive because of its specific intervention style. According to the authors,[3-5] targeted intervention leads to less mucosal disruption, decreased discomfort, and decreased debridement requirements.

A second principle of MIST is the establishment of four landmarks, which reveal the key four transition spaces that need to be addressed during surgery. It is thought that these four transition spaces represent the contact points from where obstruction originates.

The first landmark is the uncinate process. The uncinate process, together with the hiatus semilunaris, leads to the first transition space, which is the infundibulum. During the MIST procedure, the uncinate process is removed using a technique described by Parsons.[7,8] The uncinate process is fractured with a probe (**Fig. 1**) and removed using a backbiting instrument (**Fig. 2**) until the lacrimal bone is reached. The microdebrider, which is thought to be an atraumatic device because of its oscillating sharp teeth, is also used to resect the uncinate process. The agger nasi is exposed and the infundibulum is opened during this maneuver. The maxillary sinus ostium is not addressed, because opening the first transition space permits ventilation of the maxillary sinus and eventual recovery.

Ethmoid dissection is limited to the second landmark, which is the medial wall of the ethmoid bulla and the second space, or superior semilunar hiatus.[3-5] Again, the microdebrider is used to remove the landmark and expose completely the second transition space (**Fig. 3**). The lamina papyracea is identified as is the basal lamella. No further ethmoid dissection is performed at this point. The basal lamella is not perforated, and the posterior ethmoid sinuses are not dissected. The sphenoethmoidal recess is left unaddressed, and the sphenoid is not entered.

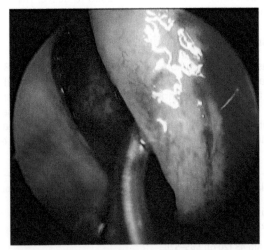

Fig. 1. Endoscopic view of the left uncinate process. A maxillary seeker is used to distract the uncinate process from the lamina papyracea.

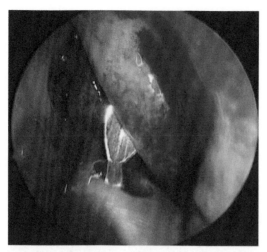

Fig. 2. Endoscopic view of the left uncinate process during the creation of the inferior uncinate window with a back-biting instrument. The surgeon must monitor the working ends of
the instrument to ensure that the middle turbinate and inferior turbinate are not lacerated
or abraded with this instrument while the uncinate window is fashioned.

The completion of the procedure is performed by opening the third and fourth transition spaces. The third landmark (posteromedial wall of the agger nasi) and third
space (frontal recess) are inspected (**Fig. 4**). After this the fourth landmark (basal
lamella) and fourth space (retrobulbar space) are identified and inspected. Catalano
advocates that the agger nasi be taken down to improve frontal recess patency
when required because clearance of the first, second, and third spaces in theory
permit ventilation of the frontal sinus and improve mucociliary transport out of the

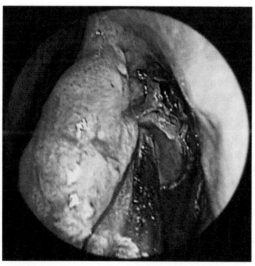

Fig. 3. Endoscopic view of the left middle meatus with the microdebrider being used to
resect the ethmoid bulla.

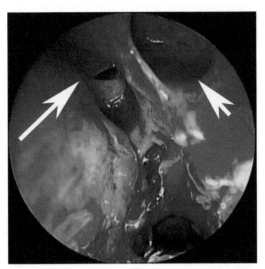

Fig. 4. Endoscopic views of the left third landmark (agger nasi) and third transition space (frontal recess). In this patient, the agger nasi is not diseased and the frontal recess is clear.

frontal sinus. No specific manipulation of the frontal sinus is undertaken. When the procedure is completed, the middle meatus is not stented, or if necessary is filled with a bioabsorbable gel.

There are few studies that demonstrate outcomes when this technique is used. Quality-of-life surveys issued in early studies[9,10] demonstrated improvements over baseline assessments. Elderly subjects undergoing this procedure reported an average of 84% improvement in quality of life.[10] Catalano and Roffman[9] prospectively treated subjects with the MIST protocol and assessed quality-of-life outcomes via the Chronic Sinusitis Survey over a period of 23 months. Significant improvements were noted in several domains, notably symptom scores, medication usage, mean total score. Forty percent of subjects reported quality-of-life levels that were comparable to control subjects. The Glasgow benefit inventory was used by Salama and coworkers[11] to evaluate 143 subjects undergoing the MIST procedure. At 6 weeks, 12 weeks, 1 year, and 3 years following the procedure, significant reductions in nasal symptom scores and increases in total quality-of life scores were demonstrated.

There are no studies comparing outcomes of MIST with those of conventional functional endoscopic sinus surgery; therefore, no real conclusions can be drawn regarding the efficacy of one technique over the other. The only study that appears to compare on some level MIST and conventional endoscopic sinus surgery was one performed by Kuehnemund and colleagues.[12] Sixty-five disease-matched subjects underwent limited (infundibulotomy, anterior ethmoidectomy, and maxillary antrostomy) or extended (sphenoethmoidectomy, frontal recess dissection, and partial middle turbinate resection) endoscopic sinus surgeries. The authors found identical outcomes in subjects when symptoms were assessed and saccharin transit times in both groups. The authors proposed that more conservative surgical approaches could produce adequate treatment results.

In clinical practice, MIST presents the surgeon with a limited and defined surgical intervention. The technique is easy to accomplish, has defined endpoints, and is easily tolerated by patients. Perhaps a significant drawback of conventional endoscopic sinus surgery is the lack of standardization. From another perspective, the limitations of MIST reveal its potential shortcomings. Ultimately, questions may arise regarding the treatment of a sphenoid sinus lesion or the posterior ethmoid sinuses if neither the superior meatus nor the sphenoethmoidal recess are manipulated. Additionally, in the treatment of diffuse hyperplastic disease, host factors and biofilms are not specifically addressed with this intervention. Nevertheless, the standardized technique presents the surgeon with a means of easily reproducing their approach and assessing personal outcomes. Additionally, patients can be offered clear expectations related to the extent of surgery.

The lack of outcomes data for MIST presents clinicians with a sizable challenge. All outcomes data in patients undergoing MIST is based on prospective, nonrandomized studies. Because a randomized prospective study between patients undergoing MIST and patients undergoing conventional endoscopic sinus surgery has not been performed to date, the knowledge gained from such a study would ultimately help to determine whether patients would be better served by one technique over the other.

BALLOON CATHETER DILATATION
History

In 2005, Acclarent, Inc (Melrose Park, CA, USA) introduced a transnasal balloon catheter dilatation system that could be used during endoscopic sinus surgery for the minimally invasive treatment of chronic sinus disease. More recently, ENTellus Medical (Maple Grove, MN, USA) introduced a balloon catheter system for treating the maxillary sinus and infundibulum via a canine fossa puncture that can be performed under local anesthesia or with minimal sedation. Although these devices have widely been considered novel instruments for the treatment of sinus ostia during endoscopic sinus surgery, the concept of balloon dilatation for the treatment of sinus disease is not new.

In 1947, Janse and Houser reported on the use of a "carefully lubricated and sterile finger cot" that was attached to a sphygmomanometer that was used to "distend the sinus openings into the meatus" to relieve the patient of several cranial neuralgias.[13] Since that time, balloon catheters have been put to use for purposes with more sound medical bases: the repair of orbital floor fractures,[14,15] the treatment of choanal atresia,[16] and even the reduction and repair of a sphenoid sinus encephalocele and cerebrospinal fluid leak.[17]

Newer forms of balloon catheters exist for the treatment of inflammatory sinus disease and treat the sinuses via two routes: transnasal and transantral. Although the routes of deployment differ, the principles underlying their benefit are the same.

Transnasal Balloon Catheter Dilatation

Since 2005, transnasal balloon catheter dilatation of the sinuses has been widely performed to surgically treat CRS. The system has three components: (1) guide, (2) guidewire, and (3) balloon catheter. The vehicle through which balloon catheter dilates the sinuses is the sinus guide catheter, which is a rigid translucent tube that is either curved (maxillary and frontal sinuses) or straight (sphenoid sinus) at the tip. After the catheter guide is chosen, a transillumination guidewire is threaded into the sinus. In the past, confirmation of entry into the sinus was exclusively performed with fluoroscopy. Studies[18,19] have demonstrated that radiation dose to the patient and surgeon is low during use of fluoroscopy; however, transillumination removes these risks and can be performed in all three sinuses to confirm proper placement (**Fig. 5**). A balloon catheter is inserted over the guidewire into the sinus. The balloon is inflated with saline or contrast material (if fluoroscopy is used). Inflation of the balloon results in fracture and

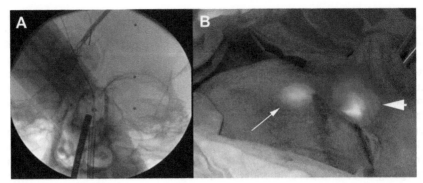

Fig. 5. Confirmation of the proper placement of the guidewire can be performed via fluoroscopy (*A*) or via transillumination (*B*). When transillumination catheter is used, transillumination of the catheter tip (*arrow*) and endoscope tip (*arrowhead*) can be seen. Removal of the endoscope and dimming the operating room lights can help facilitate transillumination when necessary.

dilation of the sinus ostia. Studies performed by Brown and Bolger[20,21] confirm the feasibility of this technique.

Balloon dilation of the maxillary sinus is typically performed while using the 0-degree telescope. The middle turbinate is gently medialized to facilitate placement of the instrumentation. The uncinate process does not need to be removed; however, resection can facilitate proper placement of the sinus catheter guide. The catheter guide is inserted into the middle meatus at the junction of the superior two thirds and inferior one third of the maxillary line to accommodate the anatomic position of the maxillary sinus os (**Fig. 6**). The guidewire is placed into the maxillary sinus where transillumination or fluoroscopy can be used to confirm entry. The ostium is then dilated using the balloon catheter. It is critically important to subsequently visualize the dilated ostium

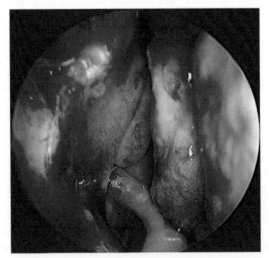

Fig. 6. Endoscopic view of the right middle meatus during the placement of the maxillary sinus guide catheter. The catheter is directed toward the natural os, which is located at the junction of the superior twp thirds and inferior one third of the maxillary line.

with a 45-degree or 70-degree telescope to confirm that the true ostium and not an accessory ostium was dilated to avoid a recirculation phenomenon,[7,22,23] especially if the uncinate is preserved.

Balloon catheter treatment of the ethmoid sinuses is limited to deployment of a drug-eluting reservoir. The anterior ethmoid is punctured with a trocar and the reservoir is deployed (**Fig. 7**). Currently, this reservoir is approved by the US Food and Drug Administration for use with saline only; however, trials are under way that are evaluating the effectiveness of passive delivery of triamcinolone acetate 40 mg/mL for chronic ethmoidal disease. If the ethmoid sinuses require surgical treatment for significant disease, either a limited or complete ethmoidectomy must be performed with conventional instruments. Balloon catheter dilation of the frontal sinus (**Fig. 8**) can be done with or without previous ethmoidectomy. Similarly, a reservoir with triamcinolone acetate 40 mg/mL can be deployed within the frontal sinus to deliver topical therapy.

Surgical treatment of the sphenoid sinus is done under endoscopic visualization and confirmation of the illumination catheter in the floor of the sphenoid sinus. Using the straight catheter guide, the balloon is threaded through the sphenoethmoidal recess and is used to dilate the sphenoid sinus ostium.

Patient-selection criteria for transnasal balloon catheter dilation of the sinuses are not established. However, Friedman and Schlach[24] detailed their experience with balloon catheter dilation of the sinuses and suggest the following: failed medical management including antibiotics, topical steroid sprays and allergy evaluation; persistently abnormal CT after treatment of 4 weeks; three or more episodes of recurrent sinus disease in 1 year; and critically ill patients for whom endoscopically derived cultures for fever of unknown origin are necessary. In their series, subjects had Lund-McKay scores less than 10. The authors suggest that patients who need revision surgery, have sustained significant trauma, have primary ciliary disorders, or extensive polyposis are less ideal candidates for transnasal balloon catheter dilation and would likely benefit more from conventional endoscopic sinus surgery with hand instruments.

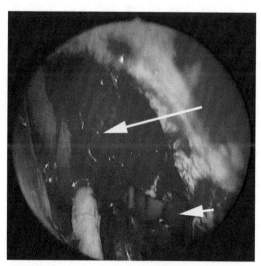

Fig. 7. Endoscopic view of the left middle meatus during the placement of the passive eluting reservoir (lower left corner). The ethmoid bulla (*arrow*) and maxillary antrostomy (*arrowhead*) can be visualized.

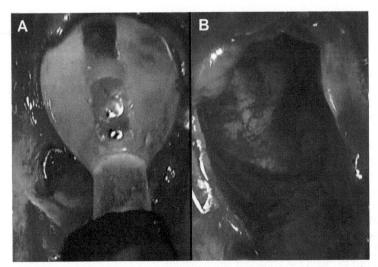

Fig. 8. Endoscopic visualization of the frontal recess during transnasal balloon catheter dilatation during (*A*) and after (*B*). The mucosa of the frontal recess is undisturbed while the bony recess is remodeled by the expansion of the balloon.

Given its recent deployment, the outcomes following transnasal balloon catheter dilatation of the sinuses are limited to a few prospective, nonrandomized studies.[25–28] Specific outcomes measured have included the ostial patency, Sino-nasal Outcomes Test 20 (SNOT-20) quality-of-life indices, endoscopic examination, and CT scores. Outcomes are reported primarily on a series of 109 subjects who underwent transnasal balloon dilatation of 307 sinuses and were followed over a period of 2 years. Outcomes were broken down into three follow-up studies. Initial reports from Bolger and colleagues[25] revealed a patency rate of 80.5% (247 out of 307) with reductions in SNOT-20 scores from 2.25 down to 1.09. Kuhn and colleagues[27] performed endoscopy on 66 of the original 109 subjects and noted that 172 out of 202 sinus ostia remained patent. Together with the 56 that underwent CT imaging, functional patency was determined to be 93.5% (86 out of 92) in the maxillary sinus; 86.1% (31 out of 36) in the sphenoid sinus; and 91.9% (68 out of 74) in the frontal sinus. After 2 years, SNOT-20 scores stabilized at 0.87 (2.17 at baseline) and Lund-MacKay scores changed from 9.66 preoperatively to 2.69 during this follow-up period.[28] There is some dropout in this series; therefore, outcomes on several subjects and sinuses are unavailable for review.

The minimally invasive treatment of CRS with transnasal balloon catheters has several clinical and research implications. From a clinical standpoint, the use of transnasal balloon catheters presents an interesting option for patients with chronic or recurrent rhinosinusitis who desire surgical treatment but are concerned about having, or may not be candidates for, conventional endoscopic sinus surgery. For physicians, balloon catheters represent tools that can be used to potentially decrease operative time, decrease blood loss, and improve outcomes for patients. Furthermore, the ease by which balloon catheter dilatation can be performed raises the question of whether transnasal balloon catheter dilatation is suitable as an office-based procedure, either in the primary or in the revision setting. An example would be the completely stenosed sinus in patients who are symptomatic for whom dilatation could be performed in the office without requiring a general anesthetic.

The indications for use of transnasal balloon catheters, whether in the operating room or within the office, have yet to be clarified. Despite seemingly straightforward criteria proposed by Friedman and Schalch,[24] transnasal balloon catheters may in fact be indicated in more severe disease. Catalano and Payne[26] have recently published data regarding the efficacy of balloon dilatation of the severely diseased (eg, diffuse hyperplastic disease, frontal opacification, and Samter's triad) to determine the utility of these tools in this patient subset. Subjects were not treated preoperatively with systemic corticosteroids and were excluded from the study if there was no postoperative follow-up or postoperative imaging. Overall, 14 out of 29 frontal sinuses demonstrated improvement in Lund-MacKay scores: 1.48 to 1.10. Of the remaining 15 frontal sinuses, three worsened. Subjects were followed for a minimum of 6 months and a maximum of 9 months. The short-term follow-up, uncertain dropout rate, and limited results do not help us determine whether the balloon is a useful instrument in severe disease, but it in some fashion does offer the potential to treat severe disease. Studies establishing patient criteria are, therefore, indicated.

Several unanswered questions present potential areas for clinical research. Although 2-year data is available regarding patients treated with transnasal balloon catheters, the long-term benefit of this technology is not yet known. There was a considerable dropout rate of the original cohort studied by Bolger and colleagues[25] and data on missing subjects is not known. Long-term outcomes present the first consideration for long-term clinical research where balloon catheters are concerned.

Another issue to be considered is the cost of endoscopic sinus surgery with and without the use of the transnasal balloon catheters. Friedman and coworkers[29] retrospectively reviewed the cost of transnasal balloon catheter dilatation compared with conventional endoscopic sinus surgery. In their analysis, the cost of using transnasal balloon catheters was compared with conventional endoscopic sinus surgery; however, when comparing revision endoscopic sinus surgery, data indicated a cost advantage to using balloon catheters. By their own criteria,[24] subjects who were severely diseased were not included in the study, so it is unclear what the extent of disease was that required revision and why transnasal balloon catheter dilatation cost less in revision cases. This study could be expanded to be done in a prospective fashion, and incorporate the expense of postoperative debridement or cost of revision surgery. Furthermore, the cost of using balloon catheters in the outpatient setting and how reimbursement weighs against this cost would also be useful for clinical decision making.

There has been much research and discussion about the influence of osteitis in the pathogenesis of CRS. If osteitis were to play a significant role in the pathogenesis, a reasonable assumption would be that the osteitis needs to be addressed. The manner in which the osteitic bone needs to be addressed has not been clarified. Some advocate removal of as much osteitic bone as possible; however, others[30] note that removal of certain osteitic bone is impractical. How well does balloon catheter dilatation succeed in patients with osteitis of the frontal recess or sphenoid sinus? If concomitant hybrid ethmoidectomies are performed, does osteitis of the anterior ethmoid and frontal recess occur in the long term?

Perhaps the biggest determinant of whether the use of balloon catheters represents an emerging technology that will survive the test of time is a yet-to-be-performed prospective study comparing ESS with transnasal balloon catheters to ESS with strictly conventional handheld or powered instruments. The randomized enrollment of patients who are similarly diseased into two treatment arms and comparing quality of life and surgical outcomes are the most effective means of demonstrating whether there has been selection bias in either group,. Comparison of outcomes with transnasal balloon catheters to historical outcomes of ESS with handheld or powered instruments.

Transantral Balloon Catheter Dilatation

The idea of the transantral canine fossa approach to dilate the maxillary antrostomy was developed by Entellus Medical (Maple Grove, MN) as the FinESS[31,32] system (**Fig. 9**).

A trocar with a cutting tip is screwed into the anterior wall of the maxillary sinus through the canine fossa, avoiding the infraorbital nerve.[33] Once inside the maxillary sinus, a small flexible or rigid endoscope is placed to permit visualization of the natural ostia of the maxillary sinus (**Fig. 10**). The balloon catheter is inserted through a separate portal on the cannula and placed into the natural ostium. The ostium is dilated with the balloon and the uncinate is displaced (**Fig. 11**). At present, no instrumentation is available with the FinESS system to allow for disease removal.

The system is designed for use in the operating room or in the clinic. The cost of clinic surgery at this time is dependent on individual insurance companies honoring a facility or practice fee to pay for the FinESS kit along with the surgical procedure fee.

Only two studies are available evaluating safety and efficacy of the FinESS system. A multicenter study[31] of 30 subjects showed no safety issues with excellent results over a 6-month period of post-procedure observation. Ostial patency with disease improvement was 96% at 3 months on postoperative CT scan. Ninety seven percent of the procedures were under local anesthesia. The only complications of note were three cases of facial or tooth numbness, one resolved. The second study[32] reflected the above subjects at a 1-year follow-up with a follow-up compliance of 97%. SNOT-20 score results were reduced at 12 months to 1.06 from a preoperative score of 2.9. All subjects maintained ostia patency.

The transantral approach to the maxillary ostia with balloon dilation is a viable, safe, and efficacious procedure for the treatment of limited sinusitis of the infundibulum and the maxillary sinus ostia with good 1-year outcomes. The tool and approach is especially geared for use either in an outpatient clinic under local anesthesia with good patient tolerance or in an operating room. If coupled with an office-practice fee to

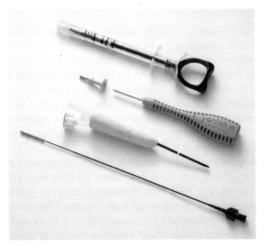

Fig. 9. The transantral balloon catheter dilatation system.

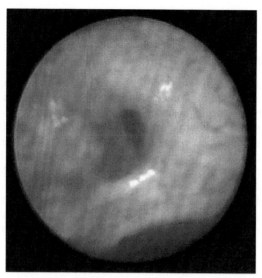

Fig. 10. Endoscopic view through the canine fossa puncture using the transantral port. The maxillary ostium can be seen along the right medial maxillary wall.

support the cost of this tool, outpatient transantral balloon dilation may become a staple of cost-effective sinus surgery.

IMPLICATIONS FOR RESEARCH

The application of minimally invasive sinus surgery techniques has the potential to rapidly change the way sinus surgery is performed. However, more research needs to be performed to determine whether these newer techniques translate to better outcomes. Long-term follow-up and randomized prospective trials will help physicians determine the true benefit, if any, of these minimally invasive techniques. The potential to reduce operating room time and operating costs are attractive features of these minimally invasive techniques, but there are few data to support these claims at

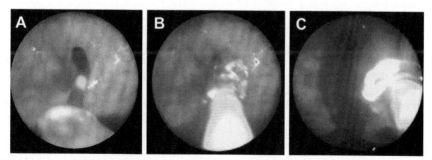

Fig. 11. Endoscopic view of a transantral balloon catheter dilatation sequence. The guide-wire is threaded through the maxillary os into the infundibulum (*A*). The balloon catheter is subsequently placed over the guidewire through the maxillary sinus os (*B*). Finally, the balloon is inflated to dilate the os (*C*).

present. Assessment of the financial impact of minimally invasive sinus surgery techniques should also be explored.

IMPLICATIONS FOR CLINICAL PRACTICE

The use of minimally invasive sinus surgery techniques at present should be reserved for patients with mild chronic inflammatory disease that is refractory to medical management. If the physician believes that a patient is an excellent candidate for a minimally invasive technique, that patient should be made aware of potential limitations of these procedures and what, if any, additional medical therapy and surgical therapy would be required in the long-term. Because candidacy for these procedures is not yet established, physicians will continue to have inexact criteria for inclusion. Lastly, if these minimally invasive sinus surgery techniques, especially transnasal and transantral balloon catheter dilatation, can be useful for patients in the outpatient office setting, they may prove to be invaluable additions to the surgical armamentarium of the otolaryngologist as we move into an era of increased financial conservation and medical scrutiny.

SUMMARY

Endoscopic sinus surgery is evolving. Although we tend to view conventional endoscopic sinus surgery as minimally invasive, new instrumentation and techniques are presently available that offer the potential of successfully treating recalcitrant CRS in a manner that minimizes operative times, sinus-mucosal trauma, and operative costs. Newer minimally invasive techniques also offer the potential of surgically treating sinus disease in the office using local anesthesia. In a changing medical climate, this may open new avenues for surgeons to treat patients. However, much work needs to be done to determine whether these treatments will be effective in the long run.

REFERENCES

1. Messerklinger W. On the drainage of the normal frontal sinus of man. Acta Otolaryngol 1967;63:176–81.
2. Messerklinger W. Endoscopy of the nose. Baltimore (MD): Urban & Schwarzenberg; 1978.
3. Setliff RC 3rd. Minimally invasive sinus surgery: the rationale and the technique. Otolaryngol Clin North Am 1996;29:115–24.
4. Catalano PJ. Minimally invasive sinus technique: what is it? Should we consider it? Curr Opin Otolaryngol Head Neck Surg 2004;12:34–7.
5. Catalano PJ, Strouch M. The minimally invasive sinus technique: theory and practice. Otolaryngol Clin North Am 2004;37:401–9, viii.
6. Stammberger H. Endoscopic endonasal surgery–concepts in treatment of recurring rhinosinusitis. Part I. Anatomic and pathophysiologic considerations. Otolaryngol Head Neck Surg 1986;94:143–7.
7. Parsons DS, Setliff RC 3rd, Chambers DW. Special considerations in pediatric functional endoscopic sinus surgery. Operat Tech Otolaryngol Head Neck Surg 1994;5:40–2.
8. Parsons DS, Stivers FE, Talbot AR. The missed ostium sequence and the surgical approach to revision functional endoscopic sinus surgery. Otolaryngol Clin North Am 1996;29:169–83.
9. Catalano P, Roffman E. Outcome in patients with chronic sinusitis after the minimally invasive sinus technique. Am J Rhinol 2003;17:17–22.

10. Catalano P, Setliff RC 3rd, Catalano L. Minimally invasive sinus surgery in the geriatric patient. Operat Tech Otolaryngol Head Neck Surg 2001;12:85–90.
11. Salama N, Oakley RJ, Skilbeck CJ, et al. Benefit from the minimally invasive sinus technique. J Laryngol Otol 2009;123:186–90.
12. Kuehnemund M, Lopatin A, Amedee RG, et al. Endonasal sinus surgery: extended versus limited approach. Am J Rhinol 2002;16:187–92.
13. Janse J, Houser R, Wells B. Chiropractic principles and technique. Chicago (IL): National College of Chiropractic; 1947.
14. Moore C, Conlin A. Endoscopic transnasal repair of a medial wall orbital blow-out fracture using a balloon catheter. J Otolaryngol Head Neck Surg 2008;37:E22–5.
15. Maran AG, Gover GW. The use of the Foley balloon catheter in the tripod fracture. J Laryngol Otol 1971;85:897–902.
16. Goettmann D, Strohm M, Strecker EP. Treatment of a recurrent choanal atresia by balloon dilatation. Cardiovasc Intervent Radiol 2000;23:480–1.
17. Alfieri A, Schettino R, Taborelli A, et al. Endoscopic endonasal treatment of a spontaneous temporosphenoidal encephalocele with a detachable silicone balloon. Case report. J Neurosurg 2002;97:1212–6.
18. Chandra RK. Estimate of radiation dose to the lens in balloon sinuplasty. Otolaryngol Head Neck Surg 2007;137:953–5.
19. Church CA, Kuhn FA, Mikhail J, et al. Patient and surgeon radiation exposure in balloon catheter sinus ostial dilation. Otolaryngol Head Neck Surg 2008;138:187–91.
20. Brown CL, Bolger WE. Safety and feasibility of balloon catheter dilation of paranasal sinus ostia: a preliminary investigation. Ann Otol Rhinol Laryngol 2006;115:293–9 [discussion: 300–1].
21. Bolger WE, Vaughan WC. Catheter-based dilation of the sinus ostia: initial safety and feasibility analysis in a cadaver model. Am J Rhinol 2006;20:290–4.
22. Gutman M, Houser S. Iatrogenic maxillary sinus recirculation and beyond. Ear Nose Throat J 2003;82:61–3.
23. Matthews BL, Burke AJ. Recirculation of mucus via accessory ostia causing chronic maxillary sinus disease. Otolaryngol Head Neck Surg 1997;117:422–3.
24. Friedman M, Schalch P. Functional endoscopic dilatation of the sinuses (FEDS): Patient selection and surgical technique. Operat Tech Otolaryngol Head Neck Surg 2006;17:126–34.
25. Bolger WE, Brown CL, Church CA, et al. Safety and outcomes of balloon catheter sinusotomy: a multicenter 24-week analysis in 115 patients. Otolaryngol Head Neck Surg 2007;137:10–20.
26. Catalano PJ, Payne SC. Balloon dilation of the frontal recess in patients with chronic frontal sinusitis and advanced sinus disease: an initial report. Ann Otol Rhinol Laryngol 2009;118:107–12.
27. Kuhn FA, Church CA, Goldberg AN, et al. Balloon catheter sinusotomy: one-year follow-up—outcomes and role in functional endoscopic sinus surgery. Otolaryngol Head Neck Surg 2008;139:S27–37.
28. Weiss RL, Church CA, Kuhn FA, et al. Long-term outcome analysis of balloon catheter sinusotomy: two-year follow-up. Otolaryngol Head Neck Surg 2008;139:S38–46.
29. Friedman M, Schalch P, Lin HC, et al. Functional endoscopic dilatation of the sinuses: patient satisfaction, postoperative pain, and cost. Am J Rhinol 2008;22:204–9.
30. Melroy CT. The balloon dilating catheter as an instrument in sinus surgery. Otolaryngol Head Neck Surg 2008;139:S23–6.

31. Stankiewicz J, Tami T, Truitt T, et al. Transantral, endoscopically guided balloon dilatation of the ostiomeatal complex for chronic rhinosinusitis under local anesthesia. Am J Rhinol 2009;23:321–7.

32. Stankiewicz J, Truitt T, Atkins J. One-year results: trans-antral balloon dilatation of the ethmoid infundibulum. Academy of Otolaryngology, Head and Neck Surgery Annual Meeting. San Diego (CA), October 4–7, 2009.

33. Robinson S, Wormald PJ. Patterns of innervation of the anterior maxilla: a cadaver study with relevance to canine fossa puncture of the maxillary sinus. Laryngoscope 2005;115:1785–8.

Role of Maximal Endoscopic Sinus Surgery Techniques in Chronic Rhinosinusitis

John M. Lee, MD, FRCSC[a],*, Alexander G. Chiu, MD[b]

KEYWORDS

- Maximum techniques • Topical irrigations
- Wide maxillary antrostomy • Endoscopic modified Lothrop
- Intraoperative computed tomography • Nasalization

Since its introduction into North America in the mid-1980s, techniques of endoscopic sinus surgery (ESS) have continued to evolve as further understanding is gained in the pathogenesis of chronic rhinosinusitis (CRS). Although the fundamental concepts of improving sinus ventilation and mucociliary function remain paramount in treatment efforts, there remains a continued debate regarding the extent of ESS required for patients. Various studies have shown that ESS achieves symptomatic success rates ranging from 74% to 97.5%.[1–5] This, however, leaves upward of 26% of patients with persistent disease despite surgical treatment, with approximately 10% of patients requiring revision surgery within 3 years.[6] Patient symptoms recalcitrant to primary surgery is often secondary to persistent mucosal disease, such as polypoid edema, biofilm colonization, and the pooling of thick, allergic mucin. To minimize these failures as well as to offer a surgical alternative to the treatment of CRS recalcitrant to primary surgery, this article aims to highlight some of the reasons for performing maximal techniques in ESS. In addition, the authors hope to expand this concept in various surgical maneuvers that may help in the long-term management of patients with CRS.

REASONS FOR MAXIMAL TECHNIQUE

Although this article emphasizes the utility of maximal techniques in ESS, it should be mentioned that normal nasal physiology and mucociliary clearance mechanisms are not neglected. Instead, the indications for maximal surgery reflect the reasons why

Disclosures: J.M.L.: None. A.G.C.: BrainLAB, Gyrus, Medtronic.
[a] Department of Otolaryngology-Head & Neck Surgery, University of Toronto, St Michael's Hospital, 30 Bond Street, 8C-118, Toronto, ON, Canada M5B 1W8
[b] Division of Rhinology, Department of Otorhinolaryngology-Head and Neck Surgery, University of Pennsylvania, 3400 Spruce Street, Philadelphia, PA 19104, USA
* Corresponding author.
E-mail address: jlee.ut@gmail.com

Otolaryngol Clin N Am 43 (2010) 579–589
doi:10.1016/j.otc.2010.02.014
0030-6665/10/$ – see front matter © 2010 Elsevier Inc. All rights reserved.

patients fail primary ESS and ultimately have recalcitrant CRS. These reasons can be divided in 3 main categories: anatomic, etiologic, and postoperative factors.

ANATOMIC FACTORS

There have been numerous studies that have evaluated anatomic findings in patients who require revision surgery. Musy and Kountakis[7] evaluated a prospective series of patients undergoing revision ESS and reported that the most common postsurgical alterations include lateralization of the middle turbinate (78%), incomplete anterior ethmoidectomy (64%), scarred frontal recess (50%), retained agger nasi cell (49%), incomplete posterior ethmoidectomy (41%), middle meatal antrostomy stenosis (39%), and a retained uncinate process (37%). These findings are further substantiated in a case series by Chiu and Vaughan,[8] which demonstrated that patients requiring revision frontal sinus surgery often have residual agger nasi cell or ethmoidal bulla remnants, retained uncinate process, lateralized middle turbinate, and unopened frontal recess cells. With the exception of a destabilized middle turbinate, all these anatomic findings are suggestive of incomplete surgery that has led to persistent sinus obstruction and surgical failure. Hence, one of the basic tenets of maximal technique is to ensure complete removal of all obstructing bony partitions and to maximally enlarge diseased sinus ostia to help reduce this risk of scarring and stenosis.

ETIOLOGIC FACTORS

Maximal techniques in ESS are also supported by an increased understanding of the pathogenesis of recalcitrant CRS. Kennedy and colleagues[9–12] have previously described histologic and endoscopic evidence of underlying bony inflammation in patients with persistent mucosal disease. These features can be appreciated on computed tomography (CT) scans where there is increased bone density or thickening in the paranasal sinuses. Both animal and clinical experiments have shown increased bone remodeling in these regions. Although bacteria have never been demonstrated within the bone itself, these areas of bony osteitis may be a significant source of persistent mucosal inflammation. Although areas of bony thickening along the skull base and medial orbital wall should be left intact, one should attempt to remove all osteitic bony partitions in the ethmoid labyrinth or in the frontal recess to help prevent disease recurrence. Minimal techniques aimed at only opening transition spaces do not address this potential contributing factor in recalcitrant CRS.

More recently, there have been numerous studies that have implicated biofilms as a potential etiologic factor in CRS.[13] Biofilms are a "structured community of bacterial cells enclosed in a self-produced polymeric matrix."[14] One of their unique and challenging characteristics is their adherent nature on sinus mucosa and their ability to resist systemic antibiotics and evade host defenses.[15] Consequently, new strategies including delivery of topical antibiotics to achieve high local minimum inhibitory concentrations as well as surfactants to increase mucociliary clearance have been employed, with promising results both in in vitro and limited clinical studies.[16–20] Most of these medications are delivered to the nasal cavity as an irrigation wash with topical saline. However, the effectiveness of these treatments is based on the premise that irrigations efficiently reach and coat the paranasal sinuses. This concept has recently been investigated by a cadaver study performed by Harvey and colleagues.[21] In this experiment, the effectiveness of sinus irrigation was studied in the nonoperated state and also following complete ESS (including uncinectomy, maxillary antrostomy, total ethmoidectomy, sphenoidotomy, and wide frontal sinusotomy). Using 3 different delivery devices filled with Gastroview contrast (pressured spray, neti pot, and squeeze bottle), the investigators found that there was limited penetration into the paranasal sinuses in the nonoperated state. However, following ESS there was a statistically significant improvement in total sinus distribution for all delivery devices, with the frontal and sphenoid sinus most affected by surgery. Extrapolating these results, these findings clearly demonstrate that a major advantage of maximal ESS techniques would be an improved delivery of topical medications. Whether or not biofilms continue to be implicated in CRS, complete ESS with wide sinus openings will have the advantage of facilitating optimum local therapy including anti-inflammatories and antibiotics. In addition, the role of mechanical debridement with high-volume saline irrigations should not be underestimated.

POSTOPERATIVE FACTORS

One final consideration when deciding on the extent of sinus surgery should be the ability to provide adequate postoperative monitoring and care. It is during this crucial period that the sinus surgeon can continue to endoscopically monitor and adjust the medical therapy required for resolution of disease. Important findings may include areas of mucosal swelling, purulent discharge, and the presence of allergic mucin (**Fig. 1**). Without adequate openings, endoscopic visualization of sinus cavities and in-office debridement can be cumbersome and often impossible despite topical anesthesia. Similarly, widely opened sinuses may decrease the need for repeat imaging, as direct endoscopic examinations can provide objective evidence for recurrent or persistent infections. Ultimately, maximum technique in ESS is a concept of providing the most complete surgery required for long-term disease resolution. The following sections describe individual "maximum" techniques that may be a useful adjunct in the treatment of CRS.

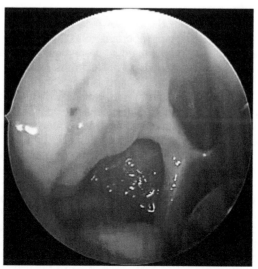

Fig. 1. Postoperative endoscopic view of right maxillary sinus filled with allergic mucin.

WIDE MAXILLARY ANTROSTOMY TECHNIQUE

Chronic maxillary sinusitis was one of the first diseases to be effectively addressed and treated by endoscopic surgical technique.[22] Rather than the Caldwell-Luc procedure whereby the diseased sinus mucosa is stripped, endoscopic middle meatal antrostomy aims to restore mucociliary clearance at the natural ostium while preserving the sinus mucosa. For the majority of their patients with chronic maxillary disease requiring ESS, the authors believe that a wide maxillary antrostomy technique is often appropriate. This procedure involves the following steps:

1. Complete uncinectomy
2. Visualizing the natural sinus ostium (usually with an angled 30° endoscope)
3. Enlarging the ostium posteriorly to include the posterior fontanelle and any accessory ostia
4. Enlarging the ostium inferiorly to the insertion of the inferior turbinate
5. Removal of any obstructing infraorbital (Haller) cells
6. If the maxillary sinus bulges medially into the nasal airway, the antrostomy should be extended posteriorly to the pterygoid plate to prevent deflection of airflow into the maxillary sinus.

There has been much debate recently over the optimum size of the maxillary antrostomy. In fact, some surgeons only advocate an uncinectomy alone as they believe its proximity to the natural ostium is the limiting factor in maxillary sinus disease.[23,24] The authors certainly acknowledge that mild mucosal disease may require minimal manipulation of the sinus ostia. In fact, this level of disease may respond to medical therapy alone.[25] However, patients requiring surgical intervention often have edematous mucosa with polyps, purulent discharge, allergic mucin or, possibly, biofilms. Without an adequate antrostomy, endoscopic inspection and clearance of disease may be limited. Perhaps most importantly, topical penetration into the maxillary sinus is significantly improved following antrostomy, regardless of the delivery device used,[21,26,27] This single factor may underscore the need for an adequate maxillary sinus opening, especially as new topical therapies emerge for the treatment of CRS.

The primary concern over a large antrostomy often centers on the role of nitric oxide (NO) in the maxillary sinus. NO is known to be produced in the paranasal sinuses, and is thought to play an important role in ciliary function as well as providing antibacterial, antiviral, and antifungal properties.[28] The fear is that a large antrostomy would lead to decreased levels of NO in the maxillary sinus resulting in ciliary stasis and persistent infections. Although there has been a study that has shown decreased levels of NO in the maxillary sinus with an ostium greater than 5×5 mm, investigators also note there is no scientific evidence linking low NO levels and recurrent maxillary sinusitis.[29] In one clinical study, Albu and Tomescu[30] attempted to evaluate the size of middle meatal antrostomies in the treatment of chronic maxillary disease. These investigators found no symptomatic difference in treatment outcomes between patients who had antrostomy sizes of 16 mm versus 6 mm. However, there were no data showing that subjects were adequately matched preoperatively for disease severity based on either objective radiographic or endoscopic findings. In addition, Albu and Tomescu note that the study was significantly underpowered to detect a difference between the 2 treatment groups.

Based on current research available, the overall principle of wide maxillary antrostomy reflects the nature of inflammatory disease requiring surgical intervention and adequate postoperative care. In fact, for severe disease, 2 clinical studies have shown a benefit through extending the antrostomy to the maxillary sinus floor ("modified medial maxillectomy" or "mega-antrostomy") in patients who fail the initial surgical approach.[31,32] However, in the absence of a nonfunctional maxillary sinus, a wide middle meatal antrostomy is often adequate for the majority of chronic maxillary sinusitis.

MAXIMAL ENDOSCOPIC TECHNIQUES IN FRONTAL SINUS SURGERY

Chronic frontal sinusitis remains a difficult disease to manage despite advances in medical and surgical therapy. Even in the context of maximal techniques for ESS, inflammatory frontal sinus disease should be managed along a spectrum of graduated surgical procedures. If surgical dissection is warranted, the authors believe that a complete Draf IIa dissection should be the first procedure performed, as it successfully manages the majority of frontal sinus disease. This technique involves the removal of the agger nasi cell and any obstructing frontal recess or supraorbital cells to maximize the anterior-posterior and medial-lateral dimensions of the frontal recess (**Fig. 2**). In a review of more than 717 frontal sinus procedures for inflammatory disease performed at the University of Pennsylvania, Draf IIa dissection was effective in managing more than 92% of cases in a tertiary sinus center.[33] Even when faced with revision cases, the endoscopic Draf IIa has been shown to achieve an 86.6% patency rate with an average follow-up of 32 months.[8]

On failure of endoscopic frontal sinusotomy, the traditional gold standard for recalcitrant frontal sinusitis was the frontal sinus obliteration procedure via an external osteoplastic flap. Despite reported success rates ranging from 75% to 93%, frontal sinus obliteration is also associated with issues such as persistent frontal headaches, delayed mucocele formation, and difficulty in monitoring recurrent disease postoperatively.[34–36] As an alternative, the endoscopic modified Lothrop procedure (EMLP) was described in the early 1990s as a purely transnasal technique aimed at restoring

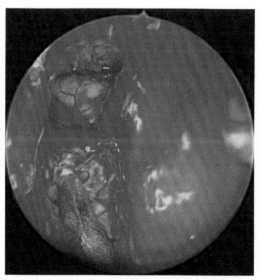

Fig. 2. Seventy-degree endoscopic view of right frontal sinus following a revision Draf IIa dissection.

frontal sinus ventilation and drainage.[37,38] The final goal of this procedure is to create a common outflow tract for both frontal sinuses, and involves the following key steps:

1. Identification of the frontal recess bilaterally
2. Identification of the frontal sinus posterior table (marks the posterior limit of dissection)
3. Partial resection of bilateral anterior middle turbinates (to create room for visualization and instrumentation)
4. Resection of the superior nasal septum (usually 2 × 2 cm in size to permit binostril instrumentation)
5. Drilling out the frontal sinus floor (drill anteriorly through the nasofrontal bone before communicating medially to avoid inadvertent intracranial entry)
6. Drilling out the frontal sinus intersinus septum
7. Final shape of the EMLP should resemble a horse-shoe (**Figs. 3** and **4**).

Since its original description, there have now been multiple studies describing the effectiveness of the EMLP.[39] Adamson and Sindwani[40] recently published a systematic review and meta-analysis on 18 articles that have been published on this procedure since 1990. In a series of almost 400 patients, these investigators found that the overall rate of frontal sinus ostium patency was 95.9% at a mean follow-up of 28.5 months (range, 1–90 months), with 82% of patients reporting symptomatic improvement. Furthermore, the rate of major complications such as cerebrospinal fluid leak, tension pneumocephalus, and posterior table dehiscence was found to be less than 1%. The EMLP clearly appears to be an effective surgical procedure with relatively low morbidity. However, more important questions are where the EMLP fits in the spectrum of frontal sinus procedures and what specific indications should be considered before embarking on this more technically demanding surgery.

In the review by Anderson and Sindwani,[40] the most common indications for EMLP were chronic frontal sinusitis and mucocele formation. However, a more interesting

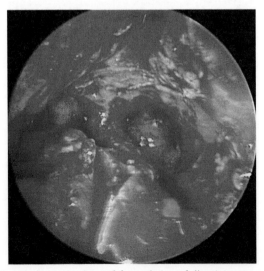

Fig. 3. Intraoperative endoscopic view of frontal sinus following an endoscopic modified Lothrop procedure (EMLP).

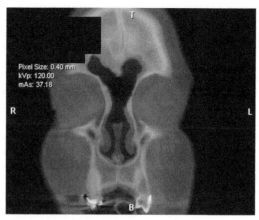

Fig. 4. Postoperative coronal CT following EMLP.

finding is that patients underwent an average of 4.8 sinus procedures prior to EMLP. In this regard, the authors certainly believe that there are specific reasons why an endoscopic Draf IIa procedure would fail, including:

- Stripped mucosa in the frontal recess with resultant neo-osteogenesis (**Fig. 5**)
- Lateralized middle turbinate remnants
- Posttraumatic frontal recess stenosis
- Frontal bone osteomyelitis
- Type 3 or 4 frontal recess cells with narrow anterior-posterior diameter of the frontal recess.

Although this list is not exhaustive, it provides insight into the anatomic and etiologic factors for persistent frontal sinus disease. Thus, with these considerations and in the context of a failed complete Draf IIa dissection, the EMLP should be considered for the maximum endoscopic management of chronic frontal sinusitis. In addition to its high reported success rates, an animal study has shown a nonsignificant trend toward improved frontal sinus mucociliary clearance times following EMLP.[41]

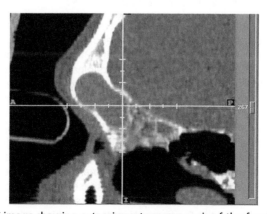

Fig. 5. Sagittal CT image showing extensive osteoneogenesis of the frontal recess.

INTRAOPERATIVE CT FOR MAXIMAL ENDOSCOPIC SINUS SURGERY

As previously described, one of the concepts of maximal ESS techniques includes the complete removal of involved mucosa and bony partitions to facilitate disease resolution and to prevent recurrence. The challenge of employing this technique is that bony partitions are adjacent to the skull base and orbit, a fact that may limit a surgeon's enthusiasm for complete ESS. Image guidance systems have been used for the last 20 years to help in the localization of critical structures, especially in revision surgery and in massive nasal polyposis.[42] However, this technology is based on preoperative CT scans and does not reflect intraoperative changes that have occurred during the dissection. In light of the concerns regarding incomplete bony dissection leading to disease persistence, the use of a low-dose intraoperative CT has been recently described as a technique to evaluate the completeness of surgery.[43–45]

The Xoran xCAT (Xoran Technologies, Ann Arbor, MI, USA) is a low-dose, portable volume CT scanner that can perform a sinus scan in approximately 30 seconds. With an isotropic spatial resolution of 0.4 mm, it can produce images with reliable bony detail to evaluate the paranasal sinuses and skull base. Furthermore, these real-time intraoperative images can be exported to all compatible image-guided surgery (IGS) systems within 5 to 10 minutes.[44] During a cadaveric dissection course, Das and colleagues[43] have shown that intraoperative CT scanning with the xCAT is feasible. When updated scans were loaded into IGS machines, the accuracy improved at both the anterior and posterior skull base during image registration.

Two case series have described the use of intraoperative CT scanning in the clinical setting for evaluation of surgical completeness. Jackman and colleagues[44] evaluated 20 patients with CRS who had an intraoperative CT scan following standard ESS. Six patients (30%) required additional surgery because of various reasons including residual uncinate, incompletely dissected type 3 frontal recess cell, and residual posterior ethmoid partitions. Two patients had mucoceles, which were removed and confirmed on the intraoperative scan. Similarly, Batra and colleagues[45] reported that intraoperative CT resulted in 24% of patients requiring additional surgical intervention in a series of 25 patients with both inflammatory disease and skull base tumors. Ultimately, these early studies have shown that intraoperative CT is a feasible and viable option for ensuring completeness of surgical technique during ESS. Additional prospective evaluation is required to further study whether this technology will lead to lower revision rates and, ultimately, better outcomes for patients.

NASALIZATION: IS IT MAXIMUM SURGERY FOR POLYPS?

In the discussion of maximal ESS techniques, the concept of nasalization should be mentioned. Originally described by Jankowski and colleagues[46] for the treatment of nasal polyposis, this procedure combines radical sphenoethmoidectomy with middle turbinate resection. Although this technique was originally popularized in France, Jankowski's group has published several articles describing its effectiveness in long-term nasal polyp management.[47–49] To date, the best evidence comes from a retrospective case series review comparing nasalization versus standard ESS techniques for diffuse and severe nasal polyposis. Five years after surgical intervention, the nasalization group of 37 patients had improved symptom scores and endoscopic findings compared with the cohort of 36 patients treated with ESS. Perhaps the most significant finding was that nasalization resulted in a markedly lower recurrence rate of 22.7% versus 58.3% in the ESS group.[49] Despite these results, a significant limitation would be the historical nature of the study, a recall rate of less than 80%, and the lack of randomization between the 2 groups. Nonetheless, this work and the impact of a diseased and polypoid middle turbinate on recurrent disease may warrant further investigation.

IMPLICATIONS FOR CLINICAL PRACTICE

This article aims to highlight some of the reasons why maximal techniques in ESS play a role in the management of CRS. By examining the anatomic, etiologic, and postoperative factors that may lead to recalcitrant disease, there is clear evidence to support this surgical philosophy. Although "maximum technique" may not be required for all patients, the procedures presented are a reflection of the severity of inflammatory disease often afflicting our patients and requiring surgical intervention. Ultimately, the goals of ESS will remain the same: to provide an adjunctive role in the long-term management of patients with CRS. Diligent postoperative care and continued medical therapy will be paramount for successful long-term outcomes.

IMPLICATIONS FOR RESEARCH

While there is research to support maximal techniques in ESS, much of the evidence is extrapolated from retrospective reviews or corroborative laboratory studies. This limitation also afflicts surgeons who favor minimal techniques in ESS. Future studies should be designed in a prospective manner directly comparing the 2 different philosophies in CRS management. Until then, the debate regarding extent of surgery in ESS will surely continue. Furthermore, long-term data examining topical medications and intraoperative CT are required to further define their role in inflammatory disease management.

REFERENCES

1. Kennedy DW. Prognostic factors, outcomes and staging in ethmoid sinus surgery. Laryngoscope 1992;102(12 Pt 2 Suppl 57):1–18.
2. Levine HL. Functional endoscopic sinus surgery: evaluation, surgery, and follow-up of 250 patients. Laryngoscope 1990;100(1):79–84.
3. Ramadan HH. Surgical causes of failure in endoscopic sinus surgery. Laryngoscope 1999;109(1):27–9.
4. Gliklich RE, Metson R. Effect of sinus surgery on quality of life. Otolaryngol Head Neck Surg 1997;117(1):12–7.
5. Senior BA, Kennedy DW, Tanabodee J, et al. Long-term results of functional endoscopic sinus surgery. Laryngoscope 1998;108(2):151–7.
6. Bhattacharyya N. Clinical outcomes after revision endoscopic sinus surgery. Arch Otolaryngol Head Neck Surg 2004;130(8):975–8.
7. Musy PY, Kountakis SE. Anatomic findings in patients undergoing revision endoscopic sinus surgery. Am J Otolaryngol 2004;25(6):418–22.
8. Chiu AG, Vaughan WC. Revision endoscopic frontal sinus surgery with surgical navigation. Otolaryngol Head Neck Surg 2004;130(3):312–8.
9. Chiu AG. Osteitis in chronic rhinosinusitis. Otolaryngol Clin North Am 2005;38(6): 1237–42.
10. Lee JT, Kennedy DW, Palmer JN, et al. The incidence of concurrent osteitis in patients with chronic rhinosinusitis: a clinicopathological study. Am J Rhinol 2006;20(3):278–82.
11. Cho SH, Min HJ, Han HX, et al. CT analysis and histopathology of bone remodeling in patients with chronic rhinosinusitis. Otolaryngol Head Neck Surg 2006; 135(3):404–8.

12. Kennedy DW, Senior BA, Gannon FH, et al. Histology and histomorphometry of ethmoid bone in chronic rhinosinusitis. Laryngoscope 1998;108(4 Pt 1):502–7.
13. Cohen M, Kofonow J, Nayak JV, et al. Biofilms in chronic rhinosinusitis: a review. Am J Rhinol Allergy 2009;23(3):255–60.
14. Costerton JW, Stewart PS, Greenberg EP. Bacterial biofilms: a common cause of persistent infections. Science 1999;284(5418):1318–22.
15. Stewart PS, Costerton JW. Antibiotic resistance of bacteria in biofilms. Lancet 2001;358(9276):135–8.
16. Chiu AG, Antunes MB, Palmer JN, et al. Evaluation of the in vivo efficacy of topical tobramycin against *Pseudomonas* sinonasal biofilms. J Antimicrob Chemother 2007;59(6):1130–4.
17. Desrosiers M, Bendouah Z, Barbeau J. Effectiveness of topical antibiotics on *Staphylococcus aureus* biofilm in vitro. Am J Rhinol 2007;21(2):149–53.
18. Uren B, Psaltis A, Wormald P. Nasal lavage with mupirocin for the treatment of surgically recalcitrant chronic rhinosinusitis. Laryngoscope 2008;118(9):1677–80.
19. Ha KR, Psaltis AJ, Butcher AR, et al. In vitro activity of mupirocin on clinical isolates of *Staphylococcus aureus* and its potential implications in chronic rhino-sinusitis. Laryngoscope 2008;118(3):535–40.
20. Desrosiers M, Myntti M, James G. Methods for removing bacterial biofilms: in vitro study using clinical chronic rhinosinusitis specimens. Am J Rhinol 2007;21(5):527–32.
21. Harvey RJ, Goddard JC, Wise SK, et al. Effects of endoscopic sinus surgery and delivery device on cadaver sinus irrigation. Otolaryngol Head Neck Surg 2008;139(1):137–42.
22. Penttilä MA, Rautiainen ME, Pukander JS, et al. Endoscopic versus Caldwell-Luc approach in chronic maxillary sinusitis: comparison of symptoms at one-year follow-up. Rhinology 1994;32(4):161–5.
23. Setliff RC. The hummer: a remedy for apprehension in functional endoscopic sinus surgery. Otolaryngol Clin North Am 1996;29(1):95–104.
24. Catalano PJ, Roffman EJ. Evaluation of middle meatal stenting after minimally invasive sinus techniques (MIST). Otolaryngol Head Neck Surg 2003;128(6):875–81.
25. Kennedy DW, Zinreich SJ, Bolger WE. Disease of the sinuses: diagnosis and endoscopic management. Hamilton (Canada): BC Decker; 2000. p. 197–210.
26. St Martin MB, Hitzman CJ, Wiedmann TS, et al. Deposition of aerosolized parti-cles in the maxillary sinuses before and after endoscopic sinus surgery. Am J Rhi-nol 2007;21(2):196–7.
27. Miller TR, Muntz HR, Gilbert ME, et al. Comparison of topical medication delivery systems after sinus surgery. Laryngoscope 2004;114(2):201–4.
28. Moncada S, Palmer RM, Higgs EA. Nitric oxide: physiology, pathophysiology, and pharmacology. Pharmacol Rev 1991;43(2):109–42.
29. Kirihene RK, Rees G, Wormald P. The influence of the size of the maxillary sinus ostium on the nasal and sinus nitric oxide levels. Am J Rhinol 2002;16(5):261–4.
30. Albu S, Tomescu E. Small and large middle meatus antrostomies in the treat-ment of chronic maxillary sinusitis. Otolaryngol Head Neck Surg 2004;131(4):542–7.
31. Cho D, Hwang PH. Results of endoscopic maxillary mega-antrostomy in recalci-trant maxillary sinusitis. Am J Rhinol 2008;22(6):658–62.
32. Woodworth BA, Parker RO, Schlosser RJ. Modified endoscopic medial maxillec-tomy for chronic maxillary sinusitis. Am J Rhinol 2006;20(3):317–9.

33. Hahn S, Palmer JN, Purkey MT, et al. Indications for external frontal sinus procedures for inflammatory sinus disease. Am J Rhinol Allergy 2009;23(3):342–7.
34. Schaefer SD, Close LG. Endoscopic management of frontal sinus disease. Laryngoscope 1990;100(2 Pt 1):155–60.
35. Seiden AM, Stankiewicz JA. Frontal sinus surgery: the state of the art. Am J Otolaryngol 1998;19(3):183–93.
36. Stankiewicz JA, Wachter B. The endoscopic modified Lothrop procedure for salvage of chronic frontal sinusitis after osteoplastic flap failure. Otolaryngol Head Neck Surg 2003;129(6):678–83.
37. Gross WE, Gross CW, Becker D, et al. Modified transnasal endoscopic Lothrop procedure as an alternative to frontal sinus obliteration. Otolaryngol Head Neck Surg 1995;113(4):427–34.
38. Gross CW, Zachmann GC, Becker DG, et al. Follow-up of University of Virginia experience with the modified Lothrop procedure. Am J Rhinol 1997;11(1):49–54.
39. Scott NA, Wormald P, Close D, et al. Endoscopic modified Lothrop procedure for the treatment of chronic frontal sinusitis: a systematic review. Otolaryngol Head Neck Surg 2003;129(4):427–38.
40. Anderson P, Sindwani R. Safety and efficacy of the endoscopic modified Lothrop procedure: a systematic review and meta-analysis. Laryngoscope 2009;119(9): 1828–33.
41. Rajapaksa SP, Ananda A, Cain T, et al. The effect of the modified endoscopic Lothrop procedure on the mucociliary clearance of the frontal sinus in an animal model. Am J Rhinol 2004;18(3):183–7.
42. Smith TL, Stewart MG, Orlandi RR, et al. Indications for image-guided sinus surgery: the current evidence. Am J Rhinol 2007;21(1):80–3.
43. Das S, Maeso PA, Figueroa RE, et al. The use of portable intraoperative computed tomography scanning for real-time image guidance: a pilot cadaver study. Am J Rhinol 2008;22(2):166–9.
44. Jackman AH, Palmer JN, Chiu AG, et al. Use of intraoperative CT scanning in endoscopic sinus surgery: a preliminary report. Am J Rhinol 2008;22(2):170–4.
45. Batra PS, Kanowitz SJ, Citardi MJ. Clinical utility of intraoperative volume computed tomography scanner for endoscopic sinonasal and skull base procedures. Am J Rhinol 2008;22(5):511–5.
46. Jankowski R, Pigret D, Decroocq F. Comparison of functional results after ethmoidectomy and nasalization for diffuse and severe nasal polyposis. Acta Otolaryngol 1997;117(4):601–8.
47. Jankowski R, Bodino C. Evolution of symptoms associated to nasal polyposis following oral steroid treatment and nasalization of the ethmoid—radical ethmoidectomy is functional surgery for NPS. Rhinology 2003;41(4):211–9.
48. Jankowski R, Bodino C. Olfaction in patients with nasal polyposis: effects of systemic steroids and radical ethmoidectomy with middle turbinate resection (nasalization). Rhinology 2003;41(4):220–30.
49. Jankowski R, Pigret D, Decroocq F, et al. Comparison of radical (nasalisation) and functional ethmoidectomy in patients with severe sinonasal polyposis. A retrospective study. Rev Laryngol Otol Rhinol (Bord) 2006;127(3):131–40.

Surgical Salvage for the Non-Functioning Sinus

Rodney J. Schlosser, MD

KEYWORDS

- Endoscopic sinus surgery • Frontal obliteration
- Caldwell-Luc • Cranialization

FRONTAL SINUS

Dysfunctional frontal sinuses occur most often after failed frontal sinus obliteration (FSO), but can also occur after cranialization performed for inflammatory disease, trauma, or neurosurgical approaches. FSOs are known to have a failure rate of approximately 10%,[1] and many times mucoceles occur years after the attempted obliteration. Although cranialization failure rates are not widely reported, they have been known to fail.[2]

Considerations in the surgical approach for dysfunctional frontal sinuses include the patient's original diagnosis; what substance, if any, was used to obliterate the sinus; and the anatomy of the frontal recess and surrounding skull base and orbit. If the situation permits, restoring ventilation to the sinus through reestablishing the natural frontal sinus outflow tract is desirable. With a neoplastic diagnosis, this technique will result in an aerated sinus that can be followed up endoscopically and radiographically for tumor recurrence.

Obliterated cavities are particularly difficult to assess for recurrence, and this technique is generally not recommended when dealing with neoplasms. The substance used for obliteration also impacts the surgical approach. With fat obliteration, removal of all of the fat is typically not required, and simple restoration of the drainage pathway and removal of any grossly infected fat will result in success (**Fig. 1**). Treatment of FSOs using hydroxyapatite or other alloplastic materials is typically much more difficult. These products often become infected and must be completely removed (**Figs. 2** and **3**). Simple marsupialization of the sinus in these cases will not suffice.

Finally, analyzing the anatomy adjacent to the dysfunctional frontal sinus is critical. Dehiscences into the anterior cranial fossa or orbit are very common. In these cases, removing every bit of mucosa from surrounding dura or periorbita to try to obliterate/ablate the sinus is even more difficult, and every effort should be made to restore some

Financial Disclosures: Consultant: BrainLAB, Olympus, Medtronic. Grant support: Antigen Labs, NeilMed.

Department of Otolaryngology – Head and Neck Surgery, Medical University of South Carolina, 135 Rutledge Avenue, Suite 1130, Charleston, SC 29425, USA

E-mail address: schlossr@musc.edu

Otolaryngol Clin N Am 43 (2010) 591–604

doi:10.1016/j.otc.2010.02.015

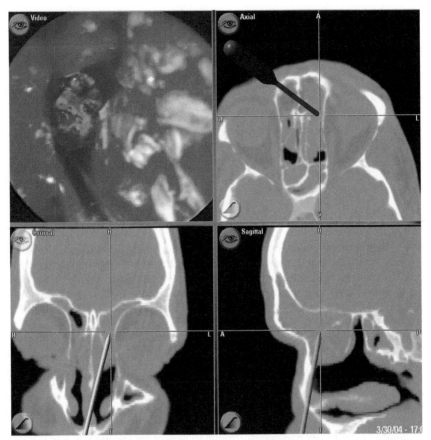

Fig. 1. Triplanar CT imaging in a patient who had undergone osteoplastic flap and oblitera-tion with fat for nasal polyposis. After removal of scar and lateralized middle turbinate, endo-scopic view shows an evacuated mucocele with healthy fat that does not need to be removed.

ventilation pathway into the nasal cavity. Mucoceles with anterior/posterior table dehiscences or orbital dehiscences do very well with simple endoscopic procedures.[3] Additional consideration must be given to the specific location of the pathology, most often a loculated mucocele, on preoperative imaging when planning the surgical approach. Prior radical procedures that strip mucosa and even drill the bony confines of the frontal sinus often result in nonanatomic scarring and multiple loculated pockets (**Fig. 4**). The precise location of these pockets can be difficult to access from below, and simple widening of the native frontal recess may not suffice.

The surgical algorithm to the dysfunctional frontal sinus is much like the approach to primary frontal sinus surgery (**Table 1**). After taking into account the factors described earlier, the simplest approach, and one that is very often successful, is revision endo-scopic frontal sinusotomy. Removal of residual agger nasi or frontal cells and any obstructing synechiae or lateralized middle turbinates often will open the frontal outflow tract (see **Fig. 1**).

In cases of severe osteoneogenesis caused by prior surgery or trauma, a simple frontal sinusotomy may not be possible (**Fig. 5**), and an endoscopic modified Lothrop may be a reasonable alternative. Significant experience in endoscopic frontal sinus

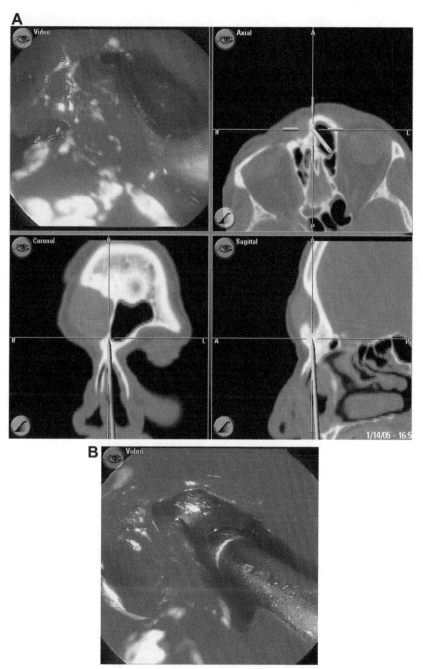

Fig. 2. Triplanar CT shows access to right frontal sinus through endoscopic inner sinus septectomy (*A*). This patient experienced facial trauma and underwent an obliteration and placement of silicone into frontal sinus. After removal of silicone (*B*), the sinus remained patent and the patient is asymptomatic.

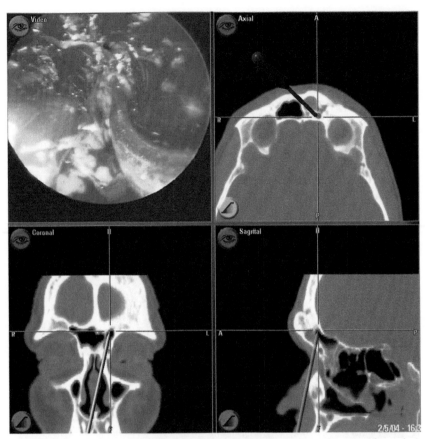

Fig. 3. CT in a patient experiencing chronic headaches after undergoing frontal sinus obliteration with hydroxyapatite. An external approach was needed to remove all hydroxyapatite.

Table 1
Stepwise surgical algorithm for the nonfunctioning frontal sinus

Procedure	Considerations
Endoscopic frontal sinusotomy	Marsupializes sinus, similar to revision endoscopic sinus surgery.
Endoscopic modified Lothrop	Most aggressive endoscopic marsupialization procedure. Needs advanced equipment and experience.
Inner sinus septectomy	Can be performed endoscopically or through a trephine. Results in a safe, ventilated sinus drained through a contralateral frontal recess.
Open approach for marsupialization and sinus preservation	Can be performed through existing scars/wrinkles, brow incision, or coronal incision. May be required for lateral pathology that is inaccessible from below.
Revision obliterative/ablative procedure	Requires major open approach to remove all mucosa from surrounding bone, dura, and periorbita. Significant long-term failure rate.

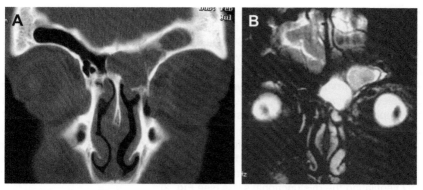

Fig. 4. CT (*A*) and MRI (*B*) show the formation of multiple loculated mucoceles 17 years after a frontal craniotomy.

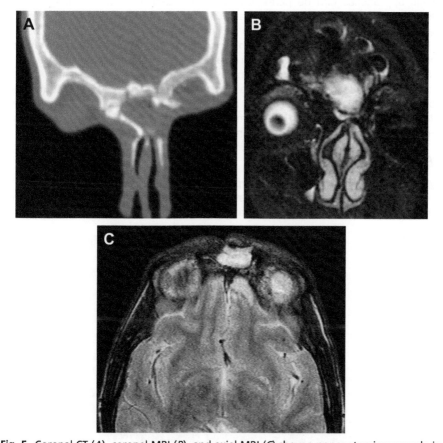

Fig. 5. Coronal CT (*A*), coronal MRI (*B*), and axial MRI (*C*) show a nonanatomic mucocele in a patient who experienced facial trauma. After failing hydroxyapatite reconstruction, he developed a midline mucocele with sinocutaneous fistula, which required an endoscopic Lothrop and external resection of fistula tract to restore drainage into the nasal cavity.

surgery and advanced equipment are needed, because this procedure has a higher complication rate than routine frontal sinus surgery. This stepwise, minimally invasive endoscopic approach to the failed FSO has been described with initial success rates between 81% and 93% with relatively short-term follow-up,[4–6] and most failures can be revised endoscopically with success.

Although the frontal recess can typically be addressed from below, if loculated mucoceles are located laterally and unable to be reached endoscopically, a frontal sinus trephine can be used to marsupializate the mucocele into the native frontal recess. In other cases, removing the inner sinus septum through frontal trephine or endoscopically can provide a route for drainage into the contralateral frontal sinus. Although this route is not anatomic, the inner sinus septectomy is often performed through an area that has not been traumatized by prior surgery, providing a way of safely ventilating the dysfunctional sinus (see **Fig. 2**).

The final option for reventilating the frontal sinus is a formal osteoplastic approach. This approach may be needed in cases of sinocutaneous fistulas, to excise the epithelialized fistula tract, or in conditions not amenable to simple trephine or endoscopic surgery, such as the need to remove alloplastic materials. Even these formal osteoplastic approaches can be performed with the intent to restore drainage of the dysfunctional sinus (**Fig. 6**), and obliteration/ablation is not necessary simply because the approach to the sinus was through an open incision.

The final step in the surgical algorithm for the dysfunctional frontal sinus is a revision obliteration or ablative procedure, such as a Reidel procedure. In most series treating failed obliterations/ablations, more than 80% of patients can be successfully treated with procedures designed to restore ventilation, and fewer than one fifth require revision FSO or ablative operations. Even in these worst-case scenarios, high success rates are reported, although long-term follow-up is required to ensure success, because these radical procedures often take a decade or longer to fail.

MAXILLARY SINUS

Dysfunctional maxillary sinuses are typically the result of failed Caldwell-Luc–type operations performed with the goal of stripping out sinus mucosa believed to be irreversibly diseased. Similar to external approaches to the frontal sinus, these radical

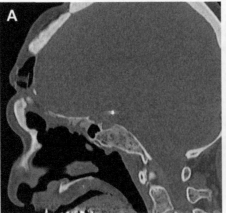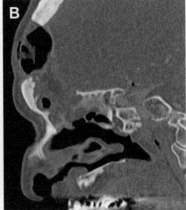

Fig. 6. A mid-brow approach was performed to resect a sinocutaneous fistula and remove the foreign body from prior neurosurgical intervention in this patient (*A, B*). The above and below approach was required to marsupialize this epidural space into the neofrontal sinus.

destructive approaches often result in loculated mucoceles or infected pockets that are difficult to access through standard surgical techniques. In addition, this mucosal stripping leads to reactive, osteitic bone and a contracted sinus with a small lumen (**Fig. 7**).

Similar to preoperative planning for the dysfunctional frontal sinus, planning revision surgery for maxillary pathology must take into account the original diagnosis, the location of subsequent pathology, and involvement of adjacent structures. For patients who had a neoplasm, every effort must be made to restore a functional, ventilated sinus that can be followed up endoscopically and radiographically. In rare situations, a simple revision middle meatal antrostomy may suffice. Similarly, small inferior meatal antrostomies or nasoantral windows are usually insufficient and often close over time. These inferior windows can also result in mucus recirculation around the inferior turbinate remnant (**Fig. 8**).

More commonly, an endoscopic medial maxillectomy (EMM) is needed to obtain an adequate opening for endoscopic visualization, debridement, and topical medications. This approach also provides complete access to the inferior alveolar recess of the maxillary sinus, where loculated pockets from Caldwell-Luc procedures often occur (**Fig. 9**). Care must be taken when performing the EMM to avoid injury to the nasolacrimal duct. The authors also prefer to preserve the anterior one third of the inferior turbinate to avoid atrophic rhinitis,[7,8] an approach that has reported success rates of 95% or higher.

In cases of laterally located pathology in the zygomatic recess of the maxillary sinus, an ipsilateral approach may not provide adequate visualization or access. A transseptal approach will provide the angulation necessary to access this area and marsupialize any pathology into the maxillary sinus proper.[9] Although this approach requires the

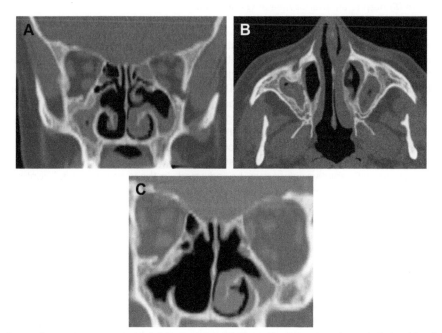

Fig. 7. This patient experienced chronic right-sided maxillary sinusitis after a failed Caldwell-Luc procedure with mucosal stripping resulted in a contracted, osteitic cavity (A, B). An endoscopic medial maxillectomy (C) restored function to this sinus.

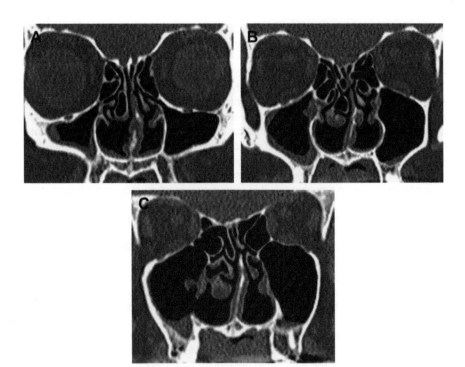

Fig. 8. Simple inferior meatal windows can result in mucus recirculation around the inferior turbinate or its remnant. The uncinate process was left intact (*A*), resulting in mucus recirculation (*B*) despite an inferior meatal window (*C*).

creation of a controlled septal perforation, careful reconstruction with pedicled mucosal flaps can prevent this from resulting in a postoperative perforation. An alternative approach to mucoceles in the inferior and lateral aspects of the maxillary sinus is to perform a canine fossa trephine. This technique has been described[10] most commonly for treating difficult-to-reach polyps, but could also be used for loculated mucoceles. The goal in these cases is, again, to reestablish ventilation and drainage of these pockets into the nasal cavity, rather than ablative mucosal stripping.

When reestablishing an outflow tract from the loculated mucocele into the maxillary sinus proper or directly into the nasal cavity does not seem possible, then revision Caldwell-Luc with ablative intent may be indicated. In these cases, orbital contents typically have herniated into the maxillary sinus and prevent attempts at reventilation (**Fig. 10**). Rather than obliterating with fat or hydroxyapatite in these ablative maxillary sinus procedures, drilling of the surrounding bone to remove mucosal remnants and auto-obliteration and collapse of facial soft tissues into the contracted small defect work well.

SPHENOID SINUS

As with the frontal and maxillary sinuses, radical mucosal stripping procedures are the leading cause of dysfunctional sphenoid sinuses. Although sphenoid obliteration with fat or other materials are not routinely performed for inflammatory disease, some surgeons attempt to remove all mucosa and obliterate with fat in patients with sphenoid cerebrospinal fluid leaks, such as spontaneous leaks or after pituitary surgery.

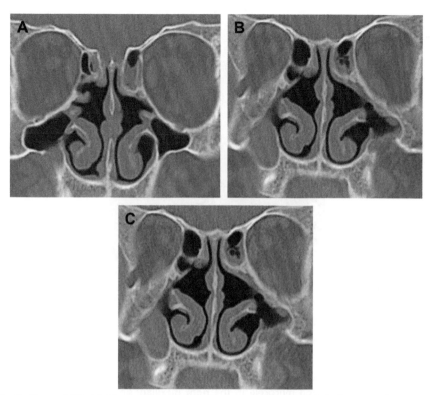

Fig. 9. Coronal CTs (*A–C*) of a failed Caldwell-Luc procedure and inferior meatal antrostomies show the formation of loculated mucoceles in the inferior aspect of the maxillary sinuses. Simple uncinectomies and middle meatal antrostomies (*A*) would only enlarge that portion of the sinus that is already ventilated and not reach the pathology in this case. Bilateral endoscopic medial maxillectomies were successful.

Given the relatively high failure rate of frontal obliteration despite efforts to drill every bit of mucosa out using magnification and open approaches, the sphenoid is difficult to truly obliterate. The risk for injury to surrounding structures makes it unlikely that prior surgeons would drill away the bone except in cases of malignancy. Thus, most attempts to obliterate actually result in a ventilated sphenoid sinus, and any fat placed with obliterative intent actually becomes a biologic packing or dressing that often resorbs. Extreme cases for which cartilage or bone is used to obstruct an obliterated sphenoid may result in iatrogenic mucoceles (**Fig. 11**). Other more common causes of dysfunctional sphenoid sinuses include severe osteitic bone and contracted lumens, which can be caused by iatrogenic mucosal stripping, a fungus ball, or chronic sphenoid sinusitis (**Figs. 12** and **13**).

As with the frontal and maxillary sinuses, imaging of the dysfunctional sphenoid is crucial to surgical planning. MRI is often helpful to determine if opacification is caused by a mucocele, fungus ball, encephalocele, neoplasm, or some other lesion, and can also be useful to determine if loculated pockets exist within the dysfunctional sphenoid. Modern surgical approaches to the sphenoid are typically endoscopic. Unlike the frontal or maxillary sinuses for which obliterative or ablative options exist for extreme cases, no options exist for the sphenoid for reasons cited earlier. Success

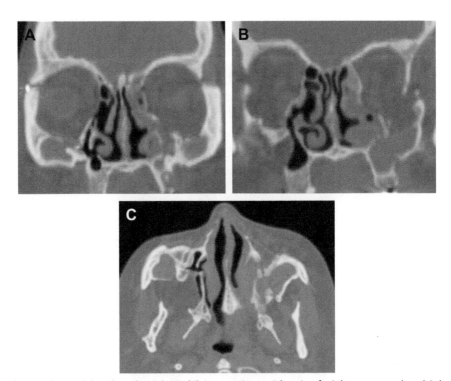

Fig. 10. Coronal (*A*, *B*) and axial CTs (*C*) in a patient with prior facial trauma and multiple surgeries shows a loculated mucocele in the right maxillary sinus. Herniation of orbital contents prevented successful endoscopic marsupialization of this area, and a sublabial approach with drilling away of mucosal remnants and auto-obliteration was successful. An endoscopic medial maxillectomy was performed on the left.

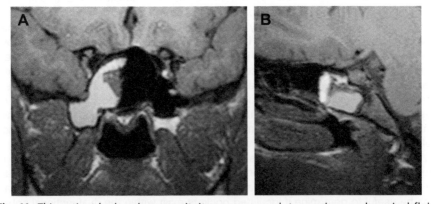

Fig. 11. This patient had undergone pituitary surgery and, to repair a cerebrospinal fluid leak, underwent fat obliteration with cartilage to obstruct the sphenoid outflow. Coronal (*A*) and sagittal (*B*) MRIs show a mucocele in the lateral recess of the sphenoid sinus, where it is extremely difficult to remove all mucosa. Viable fat was still present at surgery.

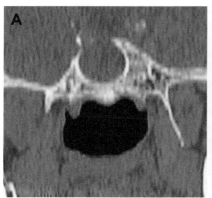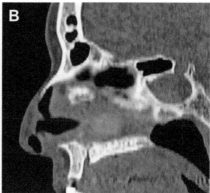

Fig. 12. Coronal (*A*) and sagittal (*B*) CTs in a patient with a fungus ball show the severe osteitic reaction that can occur in these patients.

is inherent on restoring a ventilated sinus with a patent outflow tract. Surgeons typically have two general options for this procedure: unilateral or bilateral approaches.

Unilateral sphenoid sinusotomies can be performed using the transethmoid or direct parasagittal approach, depending on adjacent pathology and surgeon preference. The general underlying principle in either approach is mucosal preservation and maximal sphenoidotomy dimensions. These cases typically have osteitic bone, which has a tendency to scar and contract more than nonosteitic sinuses. Submucosal elevation over the face of the sphenoid will avoid inadvertent entry into the sphenopalatine artery and provide a vascularized flap of nasal mucosa that can be used at the completion of the operation to reline the surgically created sphenoidotomy. After elevating this mucosal flap, the osteitic bone is removed, generally with Kerrison punches, to create as wide a sphenoidotomy as possible. Taking down much of the floor of the sphenoid can often be advantageous in creating a large neoostia. Every effort should also be made to preserve the sphenoid sinus mucosa while resecting this osteitic bone in a submucosal fashion.

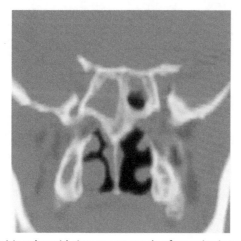

Fig. 13. Severely osteitic sphenoid sinuses can result after stripping mucosa in previously nondiseased areas.

Once the bony opening is enlarged to skull base, orbit, inner sinus septum, and inferiorly as much as possible, the sphenoid sinus mucosa can be incised and any pus, fungal concretions, or other inflammatory mucus within the sinus is removed. The previously elevated nasal mucosal flaps can then be reapproximated to the sphenoid sinus mucosal flap. This approach seems to result in larger postoperative openings, and remucosalization is faster than simply drilling into the sphenoid with large areas of exposed bone.

If unilateral approaches to the dysfunctional sphenoid fail or the unilateral sphenoidotomy does not seem satisfactory, then removal of the inner sinus septum can be helpful. This procedure enlarges the dimensions of the outflow tract and hopefully results in a ventilated sinus.

Similar to removal of the inner sinus septum in the dysfunctional frontal sinus, if the natural outflow tract of the sphenoid scars postoperatively but the inner sinus septectomy remains patent, then the sinus will remain ventilated and safe, even though the outflow tract is nonanatomic through the contralateral sinus. The approach for this surgery is typically similar to that for transseptal pituitary surgery. A large posterior nasal septectomy is performed for access. Bilateral sphenoidotomies are then

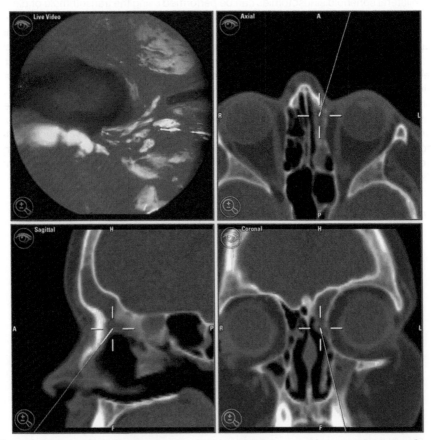

Fig. 14. Prior mucosal stripping has resulted in osteitic bone with mucoceles in nonfunctioning frontal and ethmoid sinuses.

performed so that both sphenoid sinuses, the rostrum, and the planum can be visualized with one view of the endoscope. The inner sinus septum is then removed back to the face of the sella. As with inner sinus septectomy of the frontal sinuses, this site is often untraumatized by prior surgery and less likely to scar and contract than revision surgery through the previously operated area of the native sphenoid os. Care must be taken to perform this inner sinus septectomy with cutting instruments or drills. Twisting and pulling of the inner sinus septum can result in an indirect injury to the internal carotid artery, because the inner sinus septum often inserts onto the carotid.

ETHMOID SINUS

Unlike the dependent sinuses previously described, the ethmoid is a labyrinth of smaller sinuses and is actually less likely to result in a dysfunctional sinus that is isolated from the nasal cavity. Prior surgeries may have stripped mucosa and resulted in osteitic reactive bone. Although formation of obstructed mucoceles is possible in this scenario, it is less common (**Fig. 14**). Given the smaller size of these mucoceles, standard endoscopic approaches with marsupialization into the nasal cavity works well. Similar principles of mucosal preservation do apply. Unlike the larger dependent sinuses, loculations do not often occur and these mucoceles should be opened widely up to skull base and medial orbital wall.

IMPLICATIONS FOR CLINICAL PRACTICE AND RESEARCH

Dysfunctional sinuses occur when mucosa has intentionally or inadvertently been removed. The resulting scar tissue and osteitic reactive bone that separates these sinuses from the nasal cavity makes surgical treatment of these dysfunctional sinuses a challenge. Surgery to restore ventilation either through normal outflow pathways or nonanatomic pathways, such as through inner sinus septectomies or endoscopic medial maxillectomies, should be the initial approach. This technique allows the sinus to regain normal function and has high reported success rates. Revision ablative or obliterative procedures are rarely needed and should be the final option.

REFERENCES

1. Weber R, Draf W, Kratzsch B, et al. Modern concepts of frontal sinus surgery. Laryngoscope 2001;111(1):137–46.
2. Meetze K, Palmer JN, Schlosser RJ. Frontal sinus complications after frontal craniotomy. Laryngoscope 2004;114(5):945–8.
3. Woodworth BA, Neal JG, Palmer JN, et al. Endoscopic management of frontal sinus mucoceles with anterior table erosion. Rhinology 2008;46(3):231–7.
4. Kanowitz SJ, Batra PS, Citardi MJ. Comprehensive management of failed frontal sinus obliteration. Am J Rhinol 2008;22(3):263–70.
5. Chandra RK, Kennedy DW, Palmer JN. Endoscopic management of failed frontal sinus obliteration. Am J Rhinol 2004;18(5):279–84.
6. Hwang PH, Han JK, Bilstrom EJ, et al. Surgical revision of the failed obliterated frontal sinus. Am J Rhinol 2005;19(5):425–9.
7. Woodworth BA, Parker RO, Schlosser RJ. Modified endoscopic medial maxillectomy for chronic maxillary sinusitis. Am J Rhinol 2006;20(3):317–9.
8. Cho DY, Hwang PH. Results of endoscopic maxillary mega-antrostomy in recalcitrant maxillary sinusitis. Am J Rhinol 2008;22(6):658–62.

9. Harvey RJ, Sheehan PO, Debnath NI, et al. Transseptal approach for extended endoscopic resections of the maxilla and infratemporal fossa. Am J Rhinol Allergy 2009;23(4):426–32.

10. Sathananthar S, Nagaonkar S, Paleri V, et al. Canine fossa puncture and clearance of the maxillary sinus for the severely diseased maxillary sinus. Laryngoscope 2005;115(6):1026–9.

Quality of Life Outcomes After Functional Endoscopic Sinus Surgery

Zachary M. Soler, MD, Timothy L. Smith, MD, MPH*

KEYWORDS

- Chronic rhinosinusitis • Quality of life
- Endoscopic sinus surgery • Sinusitis

Clinicians have traditionally focused on objective findings to assess response after a given treatment; however, for many disease processes including chronic rhinosinusitis (CRS), objective measures fail to capture the full burden of disease experienced by the individual patient. The discordance between radiographic findings and patients' symptoms in CRS highlights this dilemma. Numerous studies have shown that the degree of sinonasal inflammation as measured by CT scan or endoscopy fails to correlate with the extent of symptoms experienced by the individual patient.[1] A patient may have debilitating symptoms with only minimal mucosal thickening or vice versa. The lack of agreement between objective assessment and patient-centered assessment is not unique to CRS, but can also be seen in such conditions as obstructive sleep apnea, asthma, and low back pain.[2–5] At present, CRS remains a symptom-based diagnosis (corroborated by objective signs of inflammation) and the extent of symptoms remains the overriding factor motivating patients to seek medical treatment.[6] Given this situation, the study of patient-centered disease impact is critical to understanding outcomes after endoscopic sinus surgery (ESS). To date, a number of rhinologic-specific instruments have been developed to measure quality-of-life (QOL) in patients with rhinologic conditions, including the Chronic Sinusitis Survey (CSS), Rhinosinusitis Disability Index (RSDI), Rhinitis Quality of Life Questionnaire, and most recently the 22-item Sinonasal Outcomes Test (SNOT-22).[7–10] These instruments provide a validated means to objectively quantify a patient's perception of their disease burden both before and after intervention.

Division of Rhinology and Sinus Surgery, Department of Otolaryngology–Head and Neck Surgery, Oregon Sinus Center, Oregon Health and Science University, 3181 South West Sam Jackson Park Road, PV-01, Portland, OR 97239, USA
* Corresponding author.
E-mail address: smithtim@ohsu.edu

Otolaryngol Clin N Am 43 (2010) 605–612
doi:10.1016/j.otc.2010.03.001
0030-6665/10/$ – see front matter © 2010 Elsevier Inc. All rights reserved.

IN GENERAL, QOL IMPROVES AFTER ESS

In general, patient-reported symptoms and QOL improve after ESS. One of the earliest studies was published by Kennedy[11] in 1992, wherein 97% of 120 patients reported improvement in symptoms (85% marked improvement) after ESS with a mean follow-up of 18 months. A follow-up study on the same cohort showed these results to be durable up to 7.8 years after surgery.[12] The development of validated, disease-specific QOL instruments in the mid 1990s added an additional layer of sophistication to ESS outcomes research. A recent literature review identified 45 articles published between 1966 and 2004 dedicated to the question of whether ESS leads to improvements in symptoms or QOL.[13] In that report, all 45 studies demonstrated improvements in CRS-related symptoms and QOL, including 11 prospective studies and 5 that used validated QOL instruments.

Since that time, additional large prospective studies have been published using validated CRS-specific QOL instruments or symptom scales. Ling and Kountakis[14] followed a cohort of 158 patients for 12 months after ESS, reporting statistically significant improvements in patient visual analog scale scores for Rhinosinusitis Task Force symptoms. Major Rhinosinusitis Task Force symptom scores ranged from 4.5 to 5.7 (0–10 point scale) at baseline and improved to 0.3 to 0.9 after ESS, representing a greater than 80% change from baseline. SNOT-22 scores were also shown to improve by 77% after surgery.

Bhattacharyya[15] performed a similar study following 100 patients for an average of 19 months after ESS. RSDI symptoms were examined at preoperative and postoperative time points using Likert scales (0–5 range). After surgery, statistically significant decreases in major (facial pressure, nasal congestion, nasal obstruction, rhinorrhea, and hyposmia) and minor symptoms were noted ($P<.001$ for all). The net change in major symptom score ranged from 1.5 to 2.3 points (0–5 range) with effect sizes noted to be large.

Recent studies have also focused on nonspecific symptoms, such as fatigue and bodily pain. Chester and coworkers[16] performed a systematic review and meta-analysis of available studies looking at the effect of ESS on fatigue, vitality, energy, and malaise. All 28 identified studies described substantial improvement in fatigue following ESS. A similar study by the same author showed improvements in bodily pain scores as recorded by the SF-36 instrument.[17]

One of the most comprehensive studies was published by Smith and colleagues in 2009.[18] This multi-institutional study prospectively followed 302 patients at three medical centers for an average of 17.4 months after ESS. Mean scores improved on the RSDI by 18.9 points (15.8%; $P<.001$) and the CSS by 21.2 points (21.2%; $P<.001$). Among patients with poor baseline QOL, 71.7% experienced clinically significant improvement on the RSDI and 76.1% on the CSS.

The available literature provides a wealth of evidence demonstrating that CRS-specific symptoms and QOL improve after ESS to statistically significant levels; however, a "statistically significant" improvement may not necessarily translate into a clinically relevant change as perceived by the individual patient. One of the burdens of QOL research is to identify what has been called the "minimal clinically important difference" (MCID). The MCID is the minimal change in symptom or QOL after a given intervention that is perceptible and relevant to the individual patient. Establishing an MCID for a particular disease state and QOL instrument can be a difficult task. Until recently, little had been done to specifically define the MCID for CRS symptoms or CRS-specific QOL instruments. Instead, estimates of MCID were extrapolated from other disease states and used by proxy. For example, there has been much interest using visual analog scales for measuring pain in the operative and emergency department setting. Prior studies have shown the MCID for acute pain to be between 0.9 and 1.3 (10-point scale).[19–21] Recent studies reporting scaled symptom scores by Ling and Kountakis,[14] Bhattacharrya,[15] and Smith and coworkers[22] all easily reach this threshold of clinical relevance. Similarly, estimates of MCID exist for general QOL instruments, such as the SF-36, wherein 10 to 12.5 points (100-point scale) represents the minimum change believed to be clinically relevant for such diseases as asthma, chronic obstructive pulmonary disease, and coronary artery disease.[23] Studies by Smith and coworkers[18] and Kennedy[11] evaluating long-term changes in SF-36 scores easily exceed these extrapolated thresholds.

The difficulty of defining an MCID is not unique to rhinologic QOL outcomes research. The most widely accepted solution in other disease states has been to use statistical constructs, such as standard error and standard deviation, to define the MCID. Generally speaking, QOL changes become clinically meaningful when they approximate half of the standard deviation of the baseline QOL value for the given population. This seemingly arbitrary definition of clinical relevance has been validated across many disease-specific and general QOL instruments.[24] Considering the multi-institutional outcomes study by Smith and colleagues,[18] this threshold of clinical significance was exceeded for both the disease-specific (CSS, RSDI) and general QOL improvements after ESS. Recently, attention has been given to defining the MCID for CRS-specific QOL instruments including the Rhinitis Quality of Life Questionnaire and SNOT-22. **Table 1** shows the available published MCID values for CRS-specific QOL instruments.[10,18,25]

Even with the beneficial outcomes seen after ESS, one must not confuse "improvement" with complete symptomatic resolution or "cure." ESS is most typically reserved for patients who are refractory to standard medical treatments. The preponderance of the QOL studies show that these patients experience statistically and clinically significant improvement after ESS, but will likely still be left with some measurable burden of disease. For example, patients in the Bhattacharyya[15] study showed average postoperative symptom scores ranging from 1 to 1.4 (0–5 scale). **Table 2** shows symptom

Table 1
Minimal clinically important difference for chronic rhinosinusitis quality of life survey instruments

QoL Survey Instrument		
Domains	Score Range	MCID
RSDI total	0–120	≥ 10.35
Physical	0–44	≥ 3.80
Functional	0–36	≥ 3.45
Emotional	0–40	≥ 4.20
CSS total	0–100	≥ 9.75
Symptoms	0–100	≥ 13.25
Medications	0–100	≥ 12.60
SNOT-22	0–110	≥ 8.90
RQLQ	0–6	≥ 0.62

Abbreviations: CSS, Chronic Sinusitis Survey; MCID, minimal clinically important difference; QOL, quality of life; RQLQ, Rhinitis Quality of Life Questionnaire; RSDI, Rhinosinusitis Disability Index; SNOT-22, 22-item Sinonasal Outcomes Test.

Table 2
Individual symptom scores before and after endoscopic sinus surgery in a cohort of 152 patients with chronic rhinosinusitis

Symptoms (N = 152)	Range	Preop Mean ± SD	Postop Mean ± SD	P Value
Nasal discharge	0–10	5.49 ± 3.06	3.38 ± 2.75	<0.001
Nasal congestion	0–10	6.52 ± 2.84	3.36 ± 2.79	<0.001
Facial pain	0–10	5.45 ± 2.91	2.34 ± 2.56	<0.001
Decreased olfaction	0–10	5.54 ± 3.58	2.57 ± 3.06	<0.001
Headache	0–10	4.13 ± 3.22	4.01 ± 3.27	0.699
Fatigue	0–10	6.03 ± 3.01	3.24 ± 2.80	<0.001
Toothache	0–10	3.32 ± 3.25	1.17 ± 2.08	<0.001
Sinus congestion	0–10	7.16 ± 2.46	3.37 ± 2.85	<0.001

Abbreviation: SD, standard deviation.
$P<.05$, significant.
Data from Soler ZM, Mace J, Smith TL. Symptom-based presentation of chronic rhinosinusitis and symptom-specific outcomes after endoscopic sinus surgery. Am J Rhinol 2008;22:297–301.

scores from a different cohort both before and after ESS.[22] Similarly, the multi-institutional Smith and coworkers[18] study reported average postoperative RSDI and CSS scores well above the norms for those without CRS.[18] These studies were done at tertiary referral centers and usually include a disproportionate number of patients with severe phenotype and revision surgical status. As such, reported results might not be fully generalizable to all patients undergoing ESS.

VARIOUS CLINICAL FACTORS CAN INFLUENCE QOL

Most patients perceive improvement in symptoms and QOL after ESS. There is variability, however, as to the degree with which any individual patient improves. Much attention has been given to identifying clinical factors that might enable treating physicians to predict a favorable or unfavorable outcome. Studies have looked at demographic factors (age, gender, ethnicity), medical comorbidities (asthma, allergies, aspirin (ASA) triad disease, depression, fibromyalgia, smoking, prior sinus surgery), and phenotypic qualities (polyposis, eosinophils) to identify characteristics that might allow outcome prediction.[18,26–34] The results of these studies can at times seem conflicting given the subtle but important differences in study design and analysis, and the interrelatedness of various factors, which makes confounding difficult to fully eliminate.

Several factors have been shown to worsen baseline sinusitis-specific QOL, including ASA triad disease, depression, fibromyalgia, female gender, and nonwhite ethnicity.[18,27,29,33] Patients with polyps and those of male gender have been shown to have slightly higher baseline QOL than the average CRS patient.[26,33] Asthma, allergies, age, and revision surgical status seem to have little or no affect on baseline QOL.[18,28,31–33] Regardless of their affect on baseline disease-specific QOL, few of the previously mentioned factors seem to influence the degree of improvement afforded by ESS. For example, patients with comorbid depression have worse disease-specific QOL scores at baseline and postoperatively compared with those without depression. They experience the same absolute level of improvement with ESS, however, as those without depression.[27] At any one point in time a depressed patient has worse QOL than a nondepressed patient, but the absolute change in

QOL after ESS is similar to those without depression. Similar results have been seen when closely examining patients with ASA triad disease, fibromyalgia, female gender, and nonwhite ethnicities.[18,29,30,33] One recent study reported that a history of prior sinus surgery predicted less improvement in QOL after ESS.[18] In that study, patients undergoing primary ESS were 2.1 times more likely to improve as patients undergoing revision surgery (95% confidence interval, 1.2–3.4; $P<.006$). No other factor was found to be similarly predictive by multivariate regression analysis.

Patients with nasal polyposis represent a unique clinical subgroup. The presence of nasal polyps naturally leads to worse objective disease severity as defined by imaging and endoscopic grading systems.[15] Except for symptoms of nasal congestion, however, these patients seem to have a lighter burden of disease as measured by patient-centered symptom scores and QOL compared with patients without nasal polyps.[26] Most clinicians have met the archetypal patient with polyps completely filling the nasal cavity yet relatively few complaints. Despite better preoperative QOL scores, patients with polyps tend to improve after ESS to a similar degree as those without polyps.

Recently, the authors reported the impact of mucosal eosinophilia on QOL outcomes in 102 patients with CRS.[34] At the time of ESS, the degree of mucosal eosinophilia was quantified by microscopy. Although all patients demonstrated improvement after ESS, the subgroup of patients with mucosal eosinophilia greater than 10 eosinophils per high-powered field showed less improvement in disease-specific (CSS, RSDI) and general (SF-36) QOL than those without eosinophilia (<10 eosinophils per high-powered field) at an average follow-up of 16 months. Interestingly, patients without polyps but with mucosal eosinophilia performed the worst after ESS and patients without polyps or eosinophilia performed the best. The difference in outcomes between the groups clearly exceeded a threshold one would consider clinically relevant. Without pathologic review, these patients might otherwise be indistinguishable on clinical grounds alone. These findings are not unexpected and serve to support the commonly held clinical belief that patients with eosinophilic inflammation are especially difficult to treat.

IMPORTANT WEAKNESSES EXIST IN CURRENT QOL OUTCOMES STUDIES

Outcomes research for CRS has steadily improved over the last 25 years from short-term, single-institution studies of a retrospective nature to prospective, multi-institution studies using validated disease-specific QOL instruments. Despite these improvements, important weaknesses still exist in the current literature. The lack of a control arm is perhaps the biggest shortcoming of most studies. A control arm serves to minimize the chance that observed improvements simply represent the natural resolution of the disease process. Additionally, a control arm minimizes the placebo affect associated with any given treatment.

Randomized, double-blind, placebo-controlled trials remain the gold standard for many disease processes (level 1 evidence) and serve as the foundation for evidence-based reviews, such as the Cochrane Database. The tenants of a randomized, double-blind, placebo-controlled trials, however, are not easily applied to surgical outcomes because obvious problems with randomization, blinding, and sham surgeries arise. To the authors' knowledge, only two randomized studies have compared medical regimens with ESS for adult patients with CRS.[35,36] Both of these were done outside of the United States and showed no difference in outcomes when comparing ESS with medical treatments of CRS. The *Cochrane Review* of these trials concluded that available evidence does not demonstrate ESS conferring additional benefit over medical treatment alone.[37] The impact of the *Cochrane Review* has been mitigated, however, by the fact that patients were randomized to ESS before receiving maximal medical treatments. The comparison was ESS versus a medical regimen as initial treatment of CRS. This up-front, direct comparison between surgery and medical therapy does not justly model current typical practice patterns. The typical current paradigm is first to treat CRS patients with maximal available medical treatments, which often include antibiotic and anti-inflammatory regimens. Only those who fail these interventions are offered ESS, usually followed by ongoing medical treatments. To best mimic current treatment paradigms, one would begin with a cohort that has failed maximal medical management, and compare further treatment with ESS plus ongoing medical management with a control arm of continued medical management (level 2 evidence). Studies with this construct would represent the strongest evidence likely to be achieved in the United States.

FUTURE OUTCOMES STUDIES SHOULD INCORPORATE HISTOLOGIC, MOLECULAR, AND GENETIC INFORMATION

The initial objective of ESS outcomes research was to assess the effectiveness of ESS as a therapeutic option for CRS in general. Current thinking is that CRS represents a generic diagnosis of which there are many underlying etiologies and phenotypic subtypes. Various classification schemes exist often based on clinical features, such as presence of polyps or mucosal eosinophilia, although little consensus exists. As subtypes of CRS are identified and precisely classified, it will be important to understand variations in outcomes related to available therapies. Perhaps the greatest goal is to develop a comprehensive model of multiple pretreatment factors that predict disease-specific QOL outcomes after treatment. This model would include demographic, clinical, and radiographic measures as previously discussed. The discovery that mucosal eosinophilia predicts QOL outcomes after ESS suggests that further investigation is needed to define the underlying basis and characteristics of the inflammatory infiltrate comprising CRS. Evaluating cellular counts and other histologic parameters of mucosal inflammation represents a fairly crude method of assessment compared with current molecular and genetic methodology. The study of molecular markers of inflammation and their genetic underpinnings remains a nascent research front just now beginning to flourish. Future studies need to incorporate genetic markers and molecular markers of genetic expression into predictive models before a clear, comprehensive picture of outcomes is finally realized.

SUMMARY

An abundance of evidence exists supporting the efficacy of ESS to improve long-term QOL outcomes in patients with CRS. Both CRS-specific and general QOL improve after ESS to levels considered statistically significant and clinically relevant. Variability in individual patient QOL can in part be explained by demographic factors, medical comorbidities, and histologic inflammatory phenotypes.

Continued QOL outcomes research is necessary in both the medical and surgical treatment of CRS. Control arms should be incorporated where possible to minimize confounding and placebo effects. An overarching goal is to develop a comprehensive model of multiple pretreatment factors that predicts QOL outcomes and guides clinical decision making. This model needs to incorporate clinical, histologic, molecular, and genetic information to fully account for individual variability.

REFERENCES

1. Stewart MG, Smith TL. Objective versus subjective outcomes assessment in rhinology. Am J Rhinol 2005;19:529–35.
2. Weaver EM, Kapur V, Yueh B. Polysomnography vs self-reported measures in patients with sleep apnea. Arch Otolaryngol Head Neck Surg 2004;130:453–8.
3. Kemp JP, Cook DA, Incaudo GA, et al. Salmeterol improves quality of life in patients with asthma requiring inhaled corticosteroids. J Allergy Clin Immunol 1998;101:188–95.
4. Fuchs-Clement D, Le Gallais D, Varray A, et al. Factor analysis of quality of life in patients with chronic obstructive pulmonary disease before and after rehabilitation. Am J Phys Med Rehabil 2001;80:113–20.
5. Gronblad M, Hurri H, Kouri JP. Relationships between spine mobility, physical performance tests, pain intensity, and disability assessments in chronic low back pain patients. Scand J Rehabil Med 1997;29:17–24.
6. Rosenfeld RM, Andes D, Bhattacharyya N, et al. Clinical practice guidelines: adult sinusitis. Otolaryngol Head Neck Surg 2007;137(Suppl 3):S1–31.
7. Leopold D, Ferguson BJ, Piccirillo JF. Outcomes assessment. Otolaryngol Head Neck Surg 1997;117(3 Pt 2):S58–68.
8. Gliklich RE, Metson R. Techniques for outcomes research in surgery for chronic sinusitis. Laryngoscope 1995;105:387–90.
9. Benninger MS, Senior BA. The development of the rhinosinusitis disability index. Arch Otolaryngol Head Neck Surg 1997;123:1175–9.
10. Hopkins C, Gillett S, Slack R, et al. Psychometric validity of the 22-item Sinonasal Outcome Test. Clin Otolaryngol 2009;34:447–54.
11. Kennedy DW. Prognostic factors, outcomes, and staging in ethmoid sinus surgery. Laryngoscope 1992;102:1–18.
12. Senior BA, Kennedy DW, Tanabodee J, et al. Long-term results of functional endoscopic sinus surgery. Laryngoscope 1998;108:151–7.
13. Smith TL, Batra PS, Seiden AM, et al. Evidence supporting endoscopic sinus surgery in the management of adult chronic rhinosinusitis: a systematic review. Am J Rhinol 2005;19:537–43.
14. Ling FT, Kountakis SE. Important clinical symptoms in patients undergoing functional endoscopic sinus surgery for chronic rhinosinusitis. Laryngoscope 2007; 117:1090–3.
15. Bhattacharyya N. Symptom outcomes after endoscopic sinus surgery for chronic rhinosinusitis. Arch Otolaryngol Head Neck Surg 2005;130:329–33.
16. Chester AC, Sindwani R, Smith TL, et al. Fatigue improvement following endoscopic sinus surgery: a systematic review and meta-analysis. Laryngoscope 2008;118:730–9.
17. Chester AC, Sindwani R, Smith TL, et al. Systematic review of change in bodily pain after sinus surgery. Otolaryngol Head Neck Surg 2008;139:759–65.
18. Smith TL, Litvack JR, Hwang PW, et al. Determinants of outcomes of sinus surgery: a multi-institutional prospective cohort study. Otolaryngol Head Neck Surg 2010;142:55–63.
19. Powell CV, Kelly AM, Williams A. Determining the minimum clinically significant difference in visual analog pain score for children. Ann Emerg Med 2001;37:28–31.
20. Todd KH, Funk KG, Funk JP, et al. Clinical significance of reported changes in pain severity. Ann Emerg Med 1996;27:485–9.
21. Kelly AM. Does the clinically significant difference in visual analog scale pain scores vary with gender, age, or cause of pain? Acad Emerg Med 1998;5:1086–90.

22. Soler ZM, Mace J, Smith TL. Symptom-based presentation of chronic rhinosinusitis and symptom-specific outcomes after endoscopic sinus surgery. Am J Rhinol 2008;22:297–301.
23. Wyrwick KW, Tierney WM, Babu AN, et al. A comparison of clinically important differences in health-related quality of life for patients with chronic lung disease, asthma, or heart disease. Health Serv Res 2005;40(2):577–92.
24. Norman GR, Sloan JA, Wyrwick KW. Interpretation of changes in health related quality of life: the remarkable universality of half a standard deviation. Med Care 2003;41:582–92.
25. Turner D, Schunemann HJ, Griffith LE, et al. Using the entire cohort in the receiver operating characteristic analysis maximizes precision of the minimal important difference. J Clin Epidemiol 2009;62:374–9.
26. Poetker DM, Mendolia-Loffredo S, Smith TL. Outcomes of endoscopic sinus surgery for chronic rhinosinusitis associated with sinonasal polyposis. Am J Rhinol 2007;21:84–8.
27. Mace J, Yvonne ML, Carlson NE, et al. Effects of depression on quality of life improvement after endoscopic sinus surgery. Laryngoscope 2008;118:528–34.
28. Litvack JR, Griest S, James KE, et al. Endoscopic and quality of life outcomes after revision endoscopic sinus surgery. Laryngoscope 2007;117:2233–8.
29. Soler ZM, Mace J, Smith TL. Fibromyalgia and chronic rhinosinusitis: outcomes after endoscopic sinus surgery. Am J Rhinol 2008;22:427–32.
30. Robinson JL, Griest S, James KE, et al. Impact of aspirin intolerance on outcomes of sinus surgery. Laryngoscope 2007;117:825–30.
31. Colclasure JC, Gross CW, Kountakis SE. Endoscopic sinus surgery in patients older than sixty. Otolaryngol Head Neck Surg 2004;131:946–9.
32. Reh DD, Mace J, Robinson JL, et al. Impact of age on presentation of chronic rhinosinusitis and outcomes after endoscopic sinus surgery. Am J Rhinol 2007; 21:207–13.
33. Smith TL, Mendolia-Loffredo S, Loehrl TA, et al. Predictive factors and outcomes in endoscopic sinus surgery for chronic rhinosinusitis. Laryngoscope 2005;115:1–7.
34. Soler ZM, Sauer DA, Mace J, et al. Impact of mucosal eosinophilia and nasal polyposis on quality of life outcomes after sinus surgery. Otolaryngol Head Neck Surg 2010;142(1):64–71.
35. Ragab SM, Lung VJ, Scadding G. Evaluation of the medical and surgical treatment of chronic rhinosinusitis: a prospective, randomised, controlled trial. Laryngoscope 2004;114:923–30.
36. Hartog B, van Benthem PP, Prins LC, et al. Efficacy of sinus irrigation versus sinus irrigation followed by functional endoscopic sinus surgery. Ann Otol Rhinol Laryngol 1997;106:759–66.
37. Khalil H, Nunez DA. Functional endoscopic sinus surgery for chronic rhinosinusitis. Cochrane Database Syst Rev 2006;3:CD004458. DOI:10.1002/14651858.CD004458.pub2.

Extended Endoscopic Techniques for Sinonasal Resections

Richard J. Harvey, MD[a],*, Richard M. Gallagher, MD[b],
Raymond Sacks, MD[c]

KEYWORDS

- Endoscopic • Skull base • Tumor • Sinonasal
- Angiofibroma • Juvenile nasopharyngeal angiofibroma
- Inverted papilloma • Osteoma

Endoscopic resections of benign neoplastic disease of the anterior skull base and paranasal sinuses is now widely practiced.[1] Selected malignancies can also be successfully managed by an endoscopic approach.[2,3] However, the approach should never dictate the surgery performed. Anatomic location and areas involved by a pathologic condition should always be the determining factor. Similarly, pathology such as inverted papilloma, should never imply a particular surgery (endoscopic medial maxillectomy or lateral rhinotomy). Although endoscopic resection has replaced many open approaches at our institutions, the authors still use a combination of techniques to remove extensive disease.

The endoscopic surgeon performing extended procedures should be equally comfortable performing a similar open procedure. Endoscopic surgery should not imply conservative surgery. If a pathologic lesion is considered irresectable via an open approach then it is axiomatic that this is true for the endoscopic option. There are a variety of open approaches that can be applied and they have been well described,[4,5] however, they have a limited role in the management of benign disease. The midface degloving approach is perhaps 1 open approach that is still sometimes used to manage lesions for which an endoscopic approach may not suffice.

[a] Rhinology and Skull Base Surgery, Department of Otolaryngology/Skull Base Surgery, St Vincent's Hospital, 354 Victoria Street, Darlinghurst, Sydney, New South Wales 2010, Australia
[b] Rhinology and Skull Base, Department of Otolaryngology/Skull Base Surgery, St Vincent's Hospital, Suite 1002b, 438 Victoria Street, Darlinghurst, Sydney, New South Wales 2010, Australia
[c] Department of Otolaryngology/Head & Neck Surgery, Concord General Hospital, 354 Victoria Street, Concord, Sydney, New South Wales 2010, Australia
* Corresponding author.
E-mail address: richard@sydneyentclinic.com

Otolaryngol Clin N Am 43 (2010) 613–638
doi:10.1016/j.otc.2010.02.016

The authors believe the foundations of successful extended endoscopic surgery, whether for accessing a lateral frontal mucocele or removing malignant disease, relies on 5 important concepts: preoperative planning (surgery and equipment required), obtaining appropriate surgical access, micro- and macrovascular control; reconstruction of nasolacrimal physiology; and postoperative care of the large endoscopic cavity (**Table 1**).

PREOPERATIVE PLANNING

The philosophy of complete endoscopic resection can be retained without the need for traditional en bloc surgery. The limits of the area to be resected and bone removed can often be defined before surgery begins. An attempt should be made to define the surgical margins preoperatively. This ensures that a surgical plan is adhered to and will enhance total removal. The authors believe there needs to be a shift away from the patho-etiology focus of traditional teachings and emphasize the need to resect anatomic zones or regions, therefore tailoring surgery to the exact extent of disease and preserving normal structures. This is not pathology-specific surgery but site-specific surgery. The ability to gain good visualization and access to the anatomic region of the lesion is essential. Particularly in malignant disease, being able to accurately map resection margins is vital for intra- and postoperative decision making (**Fig. 1**). Further resection of positive frozen section margins can be inaccurate if many (>10) biopsies are taken. Postoperatively, accurate surgical mapping aids radiation oncologists in defining treatment fields and assists focused endoscopic surveillance.

ENDOSCOPIC SURGICAL ACCESS

There are 4 areas notorious for recurrence and present challenging access[1]:

1. Anterolateral maxilla
2. Frontal sinus
3. Supraorbital ethmoid cell
4. Floor of a well-pneumatized maxillary sinus.

Table 1 Foundations of extended endoscopic surgery	
Preoperative planning	Ensure that imaging, skill, equipment, and a predefined surgical plan are created
Surgical access	Accessing anterolateral disease of the maxilla and within the frontal sinus requires unconventional or combination techniques
Anatomic orientation	Preoperatively defining a structured approach to identify fixed anatomic landmarks
Vascular control	Microvascular management: preoperative reduction of associated inflammatory changes, anesthetic techniques, and intraoperative vasoconstriction Macrovascular control with a structured approach to the ethmoidal, sphenopalatine, internal maxillary, and carotid artery
Reconstruction	Ensuring a functional lacrimal system, the formation of a final cavity that will allow relatively normal nasal physiology Reconstruction of dura or periorbita
Postoperative management of the large cavity	Controlling adhesions, crusting, bacterial colonization and facilitating mucosalization

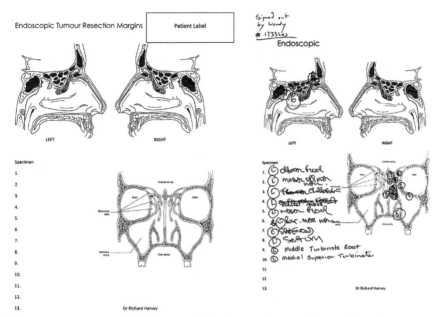

Fig. 1. Systematic systems to ensure pathologic resection margins greatly aid communication between nursing staff, the pathology and radiation oncology teams. Blank template on the left and an operative example from surgery on the right.

Many staging systems have been developed for benign pathologic conditions commonly managed endoscopically. Examples by Cannady and colleagues,[6] Jameson and Kountakis,[7] Krouse,[8] and Woodworth and colleagues[9] all touch on important aspects in the groupings of their patients. However, unlike malignant staging, it is fundamentally the completeness of surgical resection of the tumor that dictates the final outcome for benign disease. These staging systems reflect surgical complexity of access rather than intrinsic disease factors such as nodal or metastatic spread. Synchronous and metachronous malignant disease may occur but the effect of these events on outcome is unlikely to be reflected in these staging systems. Potentially, the difficult or higher-stage tumors are simply those lesions associated with more difficult access.

Predefining regions or zones that require endoscopic access and resection has become an important process in our institution (**Table 2**). The limits of tissue removal may too easily align with surgeon comfort rather than anatomic boundaries defined by the presurgical clinical and radiological examination. The principles of en bloc resection, from its oncologic foundations in managing malignant disease, are often followed by some surgeons to ensure that the appropriate margins have been reached. With careful planning and preoperative evaluation of radiology, it is possible to define the zone of resection likely to be required. **Table 2** outlines our current surgical approach to endoscopic resection.

Accessing Anterolateral Disease

Five zones were developed and are used at the Medical University of South Carolina (MUSC) Rhinology and Skull Base and St Vincent's Rhinology and Skull Base Divisions when planning surgical access in endoscopic tumor removal (**Fig. 2A; Table 3**).

Table 2
Surgical access planning

Anatomic Site	Pathology Involves	Surgical Access Consideration
Anterolateral maxilla and infratemporal fossa	Zone 2/3	Appropriate angled instruments need to be available; 40° burrs and debriders are not angled enough for zone 3; 60–75° instruments are usually required
	Zone 3 or 4	Ancillary techniques required such as maxillary trephine, maxillotomy, or trans-septal access
	Zone 5	An open approach may be better
Frontal sinus	Medial quarter of orbital roof	Unilateral access with a Draf 2a or 2b
	Medial half of orbital roof or lateral posterior and anterior walls	Draf 3 Possible trephine
	Orbital roof lateral to midpoint	External trephine or osteoplastic flap required
	Frontal recess	Draf 2b or 3 required as reconstruction of the recess with exposed bone requires greater intervention
Supraorbital ethmoid	Anterior ethmoidal artery	A dehiscent anterior ethmoidal artery may be obscured on imaging because of a nearby pathologic lesion; control is required in approach
	Orbitocranial cleft	The potential for dural or periorbital injury needs to be balanced with pathology and risk of recurrence
Maxillary floor	Dental roots	Damage to roots likely or pathology may be of odontogenic nature with tooth extraction or endodontics required
	Low maxilla relative to nasal floor	Angled instruments or ancillary access, such as maxillary trephination or modified medial maxillectomy required

Zone 1: tumor is limited to

- Septum
- Turbinates
- Middle meatus
- Ethmoid
- Frontal
- Sphenoid sinuses
- Medial orbital wall.

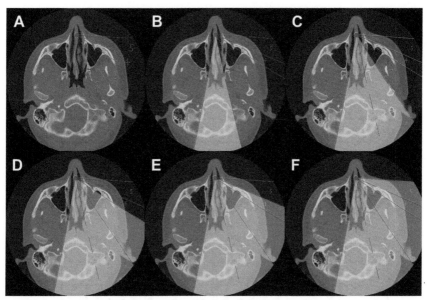

Fig. 2. MUSC zones: the MUSC endoscopic resection zones (*A*). Zones 1 to 5 demonstrate increasing anterior and lateral disease (*B–F*). 1, nasal cavity; 2, medial to infraorbital nerve (ION); 3, lateral to ION and up to the zygomatic recess of the maxilla; 4, the anterior maxillary sinus wall; 5, premaxillary tissue. (*From* Harvey RJ, Sheahan PO, Schlosser RJ. Surgical management of benign sinonasal masses. Otolaryngol Clin North Am 2009;42(2):353–75; with permission.)

Surgery may include turbinectomies, septectomy, middle meatal antrostomy (MMA), frontal, sphenoid, ethmoid surgery. Basic endoscopic sinus surgery instrumentation is required (see **Fig. 2**B).

Zone 2: tumor extends to involve

- Maxillary sinus medial to the inferior orbital nerve (ION)
- Limited posterior wall or
- Maxillary floor.

MMA or modified endoscopic medial maxillectomy[10,11] (MMM) is needed for tumor surveillance. Sinus surgery to include MMA ± MMM and sphenopalatine artery management and some angled instrumentation is needed (see **Fig. 2**C).

Zone 3: tumor involves

- Maxilla lateral to ION and up to the zygomatic recess
- Nasolacrimal duct or medial buttress may need resection.

Surgery may require dacrocystorhinostomy (DCR), possible trans-septal approach, trephine, total medial maxillectomy (TMM)[12] or maxillotomy,[13] medial buttress removal. Traditional open approaches are described for tumors in this location (sublabial Caldwell-Luc type approach, open lateral rhinotomy, and midface degloving). Angled instrumentation is mandatory for ipsilateral surgery (see **Fig. 2**D).

Zone 4: Tumor involves

- Anterior maxillary wall without extension into premaxillary soft tissue.

Table 3
Surgical resection zones

MUSC Zone	Anatomic Region	Surgery Techniques	Instrumentation
Zone 1	Tumor limited to septum, turbinates, middle meatus, ethmoid, frontal, sphenoid sinuses, medial orbital wall (inverted papilloma, hemangioma, chondroma)	Surgery includes turbinectomy and septectomy	Basic endoscopic sinus surgery instrumentation
Zone 2	Tumor extends to involve maxillary sinus medial to the inferior orbital nerve (ION), limited posterior wall or maxillary floor (inverted papilloma, juvenile nasopharyngeal angiofibroma)	Middle meatal antrostomy, frontal recess surgery (Draf 1–3, trephine, or osteoplastic), sphenoid, ethmoid surgery. Some sinus surgery to include sphenopalatine artery management or modified endoscopic medial maxillectomy needed for tumor surveillance	Angled instrumentation and bipolar diathermy/endoscopic clip applicators. Maxillary trephination may be used. Rongeurs or chisel required for bone removal
Zone 3	Tumor involves nasolacrimal duct, medial buttress, or maxilla lateral to ION and up to the zygomatic recess (inverted papilloma, juvenile nasopharyngeal angiofibroma)	Requires dacrocystorhinostomy, possible trans-septal approach, possible endoscopic Denker maxillotomy, or open approach (sublabial Caldwell-Luc type approach)	Angled instrumentation has limitations in access. Standard endoscopic sinus surgery instruments via trans-septal approach or maxillary trephine may be required
Zone 4	Tumor involves anterior maxillary wall with minimal extension into premaxillary soft tissue	Surgery requires trans-septal approach, endoscopic Denker maxillotomy or premaxillary endoscopic sinus surgery approach. Sublabial open type approach Open lateral rhinotomy/midface degloving	Endoscopic sinus surgery instruments via trans-septal approach or maxillary trephine may be required Angled ipsilateral endoscopic instruments of little utility
Zone 5	Tumor involves premaxillary tissue or skin	Surgery requires open approach	Open surgical instrumentation

Surgery requires trans-septal dissection with direct drilling to the anterior maxillary wall (mucosal side) or 1 of the previously described external approaches (see **Fig. 2**E).

Zone 5: tumor involves premaxillary tissue and/or skin.

Surgery requires open approach (see **Fig. 2**F).

Modified medial maxillectomy

This technique is widely used to manage access to the maxilla, infratemporal fossa, maxillary artery, and maxillary sinus floor. It is technically the same as that described as a salvage procedure for chronic maxillary sinusitis (**Fig. 3**).[10,11] A modified medial maxillectomy also ensures dependent drainage for a final cavity that may not have normal mucocillary function. In additional, it provides excellent access for postoperative care and surveillance.

Trans-septal Access

Our current technique involves the creation of a large posterior based septal flap in the contralateral nasal cavity.[14] This mucoperichondrial/periosteal flap is pedicled posteriorly on the septal branch of the sphenopalatine artery. The anterior incision commences at the hemitransfixion, or mucosquamous junction (**Fig. 4**C). The lateral incision starts well lateral on the nasal floor near the inferior meatus (see **Fig. 4**A). Foreshortening of the flap after elevation occurs and additional width is important for adequate reconstruction. The superomedial incision is made high, under the nasal dorsum (see **Fig. 4**B). The flap is then raised back to the middle turbinate and reflected between septum and middle turbinate to prevent injury during the subsequent tumor removal (see **Fig. 4**D). The ipsilateral mucosa over this area is raised as an inverted-U flap with a random blood supply based inferiorly from the nasal floor (see **Fig. 4**E). Beginning at the head of the inferior turbinate, a window of septal cartilage is removed posteriorly (see **Fig. 4**F). An area of 1.5×2 cm is removed to allows the endoscope and instrument to work comfortably through the septum. This approach is ideal for zone 3 or 4 pathologic conditions.

Maxillary Trephination

The development of specialized instrument sets for maxillary trephination (**Fig. 5**) has greatly assisted the ease with which an additional port for endoscope or instrument can be deployed. Robinson and colleagues[15–17] have help to redefine the landmarks for the placement of these trephines. The safest entry point for a canine fossa puncture was where a vertical line drawn through the midpupillary line was bisected by a horizontal line drawn through the floor of the pyriform aperture. The placement of the trephine can assist access to the maxillary floor, retraction for infratemporal tumors, and early access for maxillary artery ligation and control. This is an excellent adjunct to lateral infratemporal fossa or lateral maxillary lesion. However, for those pathologic conditions involving the anterior wall itself, the trephine does not improve surgical access and will come through tumor in its approach.

Maxillotomy

Endoscopic maxillotomy or endoscopic Denker maxillotomy has been described and can provide similar access to the trans-septal approach.[13] This procedure involves the removal of the medial buttress via osteotomies (**Fig. 6**). A premaxillary plane is raised and the entire medial buttress is removed. The lacrimal apparatus is disrupted as with a total medial maxillectomy. However, the additional bone removal disrupts the

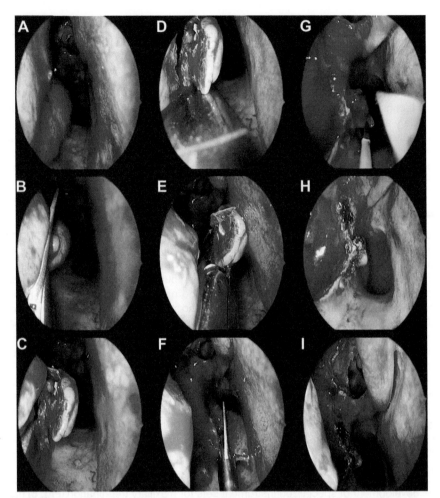

Fig. 3. The modified medial maxillectomy. Although originally designed as a salvage procedure for recalcitrant inflammatory maxillary sinusitis, modified medial maxillectomy is a quick and simple procedure to enhance access to the maxillary sinus floor, roof, and infratemporal fossa. The stepwise approach: (*A*) simple antrostomy, (*B*) excision of turbinate up to natural os, (*C*) down Kerrison Rongeur divided the medial maxillary wall from os to floor, (*D*) osteotome runs low on floor to posterior maxillary sinus wall, (*E*) grasping forceps push the segment posteriorly and perpendicular to the nasal cavity, (*F*) scissors remove the segment close to the vertical palatine bone (*G, H*) bipolar diathermy of the posterior turbinate remnant, (*I*) finished right cavity dramatically improving access to the maxillary sinus, orbital floor, and infratemporal fossa via the posterior wall.

anterior superior alveolar nerve, potentially transecting the canine root and may lead to loss of lateral support of the alar cartilage to the piriform aperture. When performed via a direct nasal or endoscopic route, the resulting alar retraction and collapse is never as severe compared with similar lateral rhinotomy approaches but can still occur. The authors prefer the trans-septal approach for most lateral pathologic conditions but maxillotomy is a good option if the medial buttress bone is directly involved in pathology.

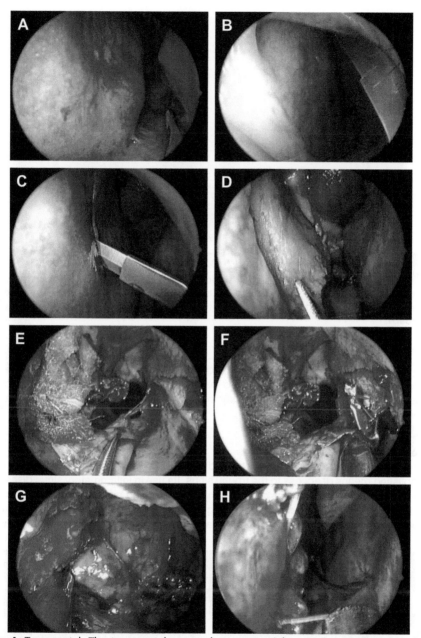

Fig. 4. Trans-septal. The trans-septal approach to access right anterior maxillary inverted papilloma: (*A*) lateral incision in the left nasal floor, (*B*) high left septal incision under dorsum, (*C*) anterior incision almost at the mucosquamous junction, (*D*) large left septal flap reflected between septum and middle turbinate; the septal cartilage is on view, (*E*) a right mucosal flap based inferiorly, (*F*) a 1.5 × 2.0 cm window of septum being removed, starting at the head of the inferior turbinate, (*G*) access through the septum to the right anterior maxilla, (*H*) the left nasal cavity after closure. (*From* Harvey RJ, Sheehan PO, Debnath NI, et al. Transseptal approach for extended endoscopic resections of the maxilla and infratemporal fossa. Am J Rhinol Allergy 2009;23(4):426–32; with permission.)

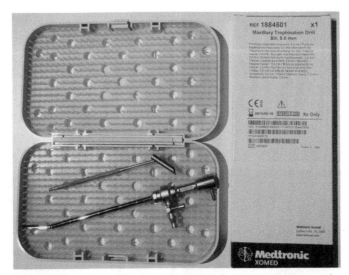

Fig. 5. Specialized maxillary trephine kits allow an additional instrument for retraction, endoscopic camera access, or the ability to address the internal maxillary artery before tumor debulking when the nasal cavity is filled with pathology not allowing a simple approach.

Frontal Sinus

The coronal incision/osteoplastic flap and browline incision/frontal trephine are 2 important open adjuncts that are used to manage frontal sinus extension. Trans-facial incisions are rarely used. Blepharoplasty incision or orbital crease approaches have been described recently.[18,19]

Lateral frontal sinus and trephination

The modified endoscopic Lothrop procedure (MELP, Draf 3, frontal drillout) is an established means of access to the frontal sinus. Its use in inflammatory sinus disease and as access for treatment of cerebrospinal fluid leak and benign neoplasms is well documented.[20,21] In the treatment of benign lesions, particularly inverted papilloma, drilling of bone at the site of attachment rather than the use of scraping techniques

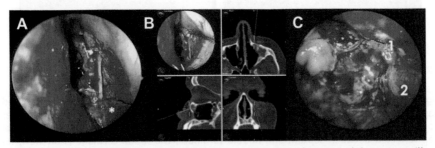

Fig. 6. Endoscopic maxillotomy is an alternative to trans-septal surgery. (A) A premaxillary plan is elevated anterior to the left maxilla and osteotome used to remove the lateral buttress of the pyriform aperture through to the maxillary sinus. (B) Image-guided surgery pictures to assist orientation to the area being excised. (C) The final left maxillary cavity (1, zygomatic recess; 2, buccal fat covered with periosteum).

may reduce the risk of recurrence.[1,22] Therefore, to adequately treat these lesions, access is required such that an angled drill can be used under vision with bone contact.

The ability to contact the bone under vision with the head of a 70° diamond burr defines good access.[23] Post Draf 3, lateral endoscopic access to the anterior and posterior walls of the frontal sinus is excellent for 95% of anatomy (Timperley D and Harvey RJ, unpublished data, 2010). Access to the orbital roof was limited (10.3 ± 4.6 mm from medial orbital wall). Access to the orbital roof is reliable in the medial orbital quarter only. For a frontal sinus pneumatized beyond the midorbital point, only 10% of lateral orbital roofs were contacted. For lesions between these points, the anterior-posterior distance between the olfactory fossa and the outer periostium of the nasofrontal beak may help to define which lesions are amenable to endoscopic access. Access correlated with this distance between the olfactory fossa and outer periostium of the nasofrontal beak (r = 0.6, $P<.01$) (Timperley D and Harvey RJ, unpublished data, 2010).

Disease of the frontal sinus is often not accessible for a total resection via a transnasal only approach[9] even when a Draf 3 has been performed. Other adjunctive procedures may be necessary. The frontal trephine[24] and osteoplastic flap form the basis of achieving additional access. Understanding the need for these in the preoperative assessment is key. They are easy to perform but the need for them should be defined preoperatively and not discovered as unexpectedly necessary during the surgery. Use of magnetic resonance imaging and computed tomography (CT) help in this assessment.

Frontal trephine is an excellent adjunct for lesions lateral to the midorbital point.[25,26] The formation of a small 1- to 2-cm incision and bone window allows dissection instrument and endoscope to facilitate dissection (**Fig. 7**). Frontal trephine can also be used to allow an above and below visualization and dissection technique. The midorbital exit point for the supraorbital neurovascular pedicle and awareness of the supratrochlear nerve bundles is important to ensure safe dissection.[27]

Frontal recess

Access is not the only concern. Reconstruction of the frontal recess may be necessary if the pathologic lesion has been removed from within the frontal sinus. A combination of maximal widening of the frontal recess (Draf 2a, b or 3),[28] mucosal preservation, and possible sialastic sheet stenting for 7 to 21 days postoperatively may be appropriate in this circumstance. In addition, inadvertent frontal recess obstruction may occur if the surgery is performed adjacent to frontal recess. A Draf 2a[28] is routinely performed for most endoscopic resections. This ensures correct localization of the frontal recess, posterior table, and aids postoperative care.

Supraorbital Ethmoid Cell

The supraorbital ethmoid (SOE) cell presents a unique surgical problem for the treating rhinologist. Any anterior approach (open or endoscopic) will have great difficulty in removing disease from the increasingly narrow orbitocranial cleft of the SOE, formed between the orbit roof and anterior cranial fossa, as dissection proceeds posterior. Instrumentation may simply not fit into this cleft. Even with removal of orbital bone (the medial wall and roof) and ethmoid roof, the cleft of dura and periorbita is still restrictive (**Fig. 8**). Only a subcranial or frontal craniotomy approach allows elevation of the anterior cranial fossa dura and removal of the superior bone; the disease in this cleft can then be addressed. Identification of disease in this area preoperatively

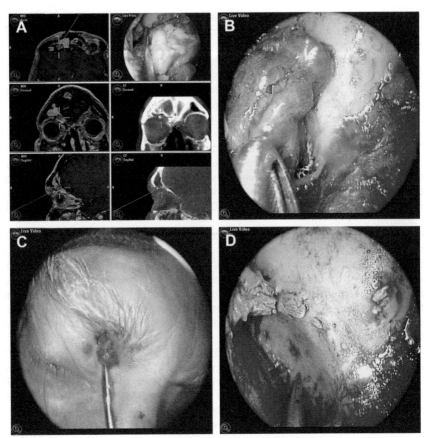

Fig. 7. A mucopyocele presenting 9 years after an attempted obliteration. (*A*) The image-guided pictures of the right frontal/supraorbital mucopyocele. (*B*) Trans-trephine endoscopic dissection and mobilization of the mass. (*C*) The mass being removed via a frontal trephine. (*D*) The final cavity demonstrating the postexcision space between posterior frontal sinus bone and the orbital roof (periorbita only).

is important to balance the approach-related morbidity and need for completeness of resection.

Dental Roots

The adult maxillary sinus pneumatizes below the nasal floor in most adults. The bone between dental roots and sinus mucosa is on average only 2 mm for the second premolar tooth. Significant morbidity can arise from aggressive drilling in this area. Identifying the maxillary dental relationship is important for preoperative counseling. A modified medial maxillectomy (see **Fig. 3**) facilitates access, postoperative care, and follow-up for pathologic conditions in the maxillary sinus floor.

ORIENTATION USING FIXED ANATOMIC LANDMARKS

Easy disorientation can occur during open or endoscopic surgery within the complex anatomy of the skull base. However, the anatomy for endoscopic surgeons has its

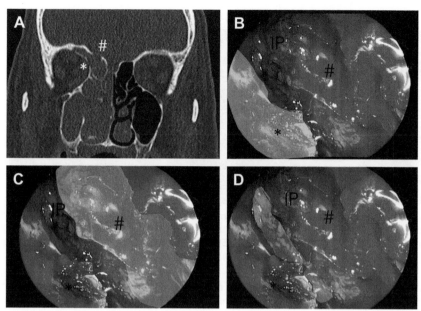

Fig. 8. SOE cell problem in tumor resection. The SOE cell forms a narrow cleft between orbit (*) and anterior cranial fossa (#). The inverted papilloma (IP) can be seen in this cleft. The CT scan (A) is for reference. The orbital wall (B), anterior cranial fossa (C) and SOE (D) arrangement makes resection and especially drilling challenging in these cases. (*From* Harvey RJ, Sheahan PO, Schlosser RJ. Surgical management of benign sinonasal masses. Otolaryngol Clin North Am 2009;42(2):353–75; with permission.)

foundations in functional endoscopic techniques.[29] Uncinectomy and removal of the bulla have little meaning to those removing large bulky pathologic lesions from the paranasal sinus system. Large tumors, such as inverted papilloma or malignancy, may have significantly distorted or destroyed these functional anatomic features. Although it is important to include the natural ostia into any final endoscopic resection cavity, the steps to gain orientation for tumor resection differ from surgery for inflammatory disease. Where landmarks have been removed or altered by a pathologic lesion, the use of fixed anatomic landmarks is required.

Discovering fixed anatomy allows safe dissection and completeness of removal. The nasal floor, posterior choana, eustachian tube opening, skull base, sella, and orbital wall are the fixed anatomic features that we seek out during endoscopic surgery. Finding traditional anatomic landmarks around the periphery of a tumor will always be the mainstay of endoscopic orientation. Similarly, the contralateral paranasal sinus anatomy can be used to find key landmarks, such as the sphenoid roof, for small lesions. However, for bulky tumors that span nearly orbit to orbit, these techniques may not be practical. Discovery of the maxillary sinus leads to location of the orbital floor (maxillary sinus roof) and finding the sphenoid sinus allows identification of the skull base (sphenoid sinus roof). However, significant tumor bulk can sit between these 2 key landmarks and prevent quick progress (**Fig. 9**). Image-guided surgery can greatly enhance our confidence and orientation in this situation.[30] But image-guided surgery is an accessory not always available, accurate, or reliable.

During endoscopic surgery, we follow a structured approach to the identification of fixed landmarks to allow quick and easy orientation in relation to the skull base.

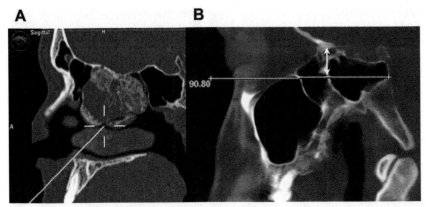

Fig. 9. Finding normal anatomy and fixed anatomic landmarks, such as the sphenoid roof, is important to ensure surgery progresses quickly and safely. The maxillary sinus roof (or orbital floor) intersects at approximately 50% the height of the sphenoid anterior wall (A, B).

A stepwise approach is followed: floor of nose and inferior turbinate, posterior choana and eustachian tube orifice, maxillary sinus roof (orbital floor) and posterior wall, and then the medial orbital wall. The next group of landmarks are in the posterior skull base, superior turbinate (defining the lateral boundary of the olfactory cleft), skull base (sphenoid roof to posterior frontal table), and a clear view of the orbital axis (optic nerve to lamina papyracea) (**Fig. 10**). The superior turbinate serves as a key landmark in endoscopic sinus surgery.[31,32] However, when the superior turbinate is not available, previously resected or replaced by a pathologic lesion, transitioning from the anterior group to the posterior group of landmarks can be challenging. Superior dissection can potentially damage the olfactory fossa or posterior ethmoid roof. The use of the orbital floor and orbital axis as a fixed landmark is of great value in skull base surgery.[33] "Stay below or at the level of the orbital floor as dissection proceeds posteriorly and one will avoid the skull base" (see **Fig. 9**). When bulky disease fills the operative area, it can assist debulking of tumor and further posterior discovery of a safe entry to the sphenoid, thus allowing identification of the skull base.

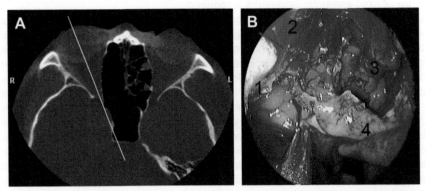

Fig. 10. Defining the right orbital axis. The ability to see or localize the entire length of the axis is essential to orientation in the skull base. Orbital morbidity is significantly low if the surgeon is able to complete this task (A, B).

Using the nasal floor as a reference, the parallel line extending from the maxillary sinus roof (orbital floor) allows safe entry to the sphenoid sinus. This rule allows a safe route of entry into the sphenoid when all other anatomic features have been distorted. Once the sphenoid roof is located, the remainder of the skull base can be identified by working from posterior to anterior.

The medial orbital floor was also noted to approximate to 40% of the sphenoid height. There was approximately 14 mm and no less than 10 mm between this landmark and carotid, optic nerve, ethmoid roof, and anterior ethmoidal artery.[34] From radiological study, there seems to be a mean vertical distance of 11.0 ± 2.9 mm to sphenoid roof, correlating to a maxillary roof line intersecting the anterior sphenoid face at $52 \pm 13\%$ of its height,[35] and direct distance of at least 10 mm from the orbital floor[34] to critical anatomy. This distance encompasses the bite size of many commonly used surgical instruments. Orlandi and colleagues[32] acknowledged that perforation of the basal lamella at the level of the maxillary sinus roof is a safe maneuver in proceeding to posterior ethmoidectomy. Defining the highest maxillary sinus roof point allows easier identification of the transition to the medial orbital wall. The authors' alternative guides to the skull base, medial orbital wall, and sphenoid sinus are described in **Table 4**.

VASCULAR CONTROL FOR EXTENDED PROCEDURES

Vascular control is arguably the most common reason for incomplete resection, and not just for endoscopic cases. Endoscopic resection of benign and malignant tumors of the nasal fossae, paranasal sinuses, anterior skull base, and beyond requires good access and a dry surgical field. Poor hemostasis can lead to imprecise removal of tumor, increased difficulty in recognizing the most important anatomic landmarks and identifying the sinus outflow pathways. Poor hemostasis enhances the risks of

Table 4	
Commonly used characteristics or guides for finding fixed anatomy in endoscopic surgery	
Endoscopic Anatomy	**Identifying Feature**
Skull base	Different color (white)
	No evidence of translucency (ie, air cell seen through it)
	Follow the back wall of the frontal sinus posterior
	Follow the sphenoid roof anterior
	Partitions become broad based on the skull base
	Palpate behind partitions before removing them to identify level of roof
Orbital wall	Balloting the eye will cause movement if lamina papyracea has been removed
	Manipulation of the medial wall creates mass movement (Cohen's sign)
	In similar parasaggital plane as natural ostium of maxillary sinus
	Define the junction of roof to vertical medial wall
	Color change (yellow or off-white)
Sphenoid sinus	Ostium medial and posterior to superior turbinate
	Ostium located 12–15 mm superior to posterior choana arch
	Locate the contralateral sphenoid and remove the intersinus septum
	Follow the septum posterior and find the ostium or face in the submucoperiosteal layer
	Removal of the medial and inferior partition of the most posterior ethmoid cell (Bolger's box)
	Enter the sphenoid face at or below the level of the orbital floor

intraoperative complications and postoperative scarring. Most importantly, it leads to an incomplete operation. It is therefore important that surgeons who perform endoscopic tumor resections have a complete understanding of the anatomy and in particular the vascular supply to the nose and paranasal sinuses. The concept of controlling microvasculature in addition to larger artery/arteriolar structures (macrovascular) is an important process to ensure a workable operative field for prolonged endoscopic surgery. A structured approach to the management of both capillary bed and major blood vessels results in complete and thorough tumor resection.[36] Monopolar cautery, as a result of possible current dispersion, should not be used within the sphenoidal sinus, on the skull base, or intracranially. Bipolar cautery with endoscopic forceps is preferred or Ligge clip applicator.

Microvascular Control

Preoperative management of associated infective or inflammatory surrounding mucosa is important. It is common preoperative practice at our institution to give systemic glucocorticosteroids to reduce the obstructive mucosal changes associated with large tumors. This greatly improves the operative field and we believe enhances the return of normal mucosal function. The choice of anesthetic is important. Total intravenous anesthesia with remifentanil and propofol is associated with better mucosal hemostasis.[37,38] Cotton pledgets containing adrenaline 1:1000 are placed in the nasal cavity over the areas of surgical access for 10 minutes before the surgical procedure. The middle turbinate, lateral nasal wall, and septum are infiltrated with 1% naropin with adrenaline 1:100,000. Warm water irrigation has been advocated for hemostasis in nasal mucosa[39,40] and frequent saline irrigation is used to control the intraoperative field.[41] Reverse Trendelenburg of the operative table to 10 to 30° has a profound effect by decreasing regional mucosal blood flow by 38%[42] and reduces dural venous pressure.[43–45]

Macrovascular Control

The blood supply of the nose and paranasal sinuses is from the external (sphenopalatine artery) and internal (anterior and posterior ethmoid arteries) carotid systems.

The sphenopalatine artery is the terminal branch of the maxillary artery and provides 90% of the blood supply to the nose and sinuses. It is therefore the key artery that needs to be controlled when resecting tumors. This requires an understanding of the variable branching of the sphenopalatine artery and of the anatomy of the pterygopalatine fossa allowing competent sphenopalatine artery ligation.[46] The size of tumor may require dissection of the posterior wall of the maxillary antrum to expose the maxillary artery and enable more lateral vascular control (**Fig. 11**). A modified medial maxillectomy is usually required for access (see **Fig. 3**).[10,11] In known vascular tumors, such as juvenile nasopharyngeal angiofibromas, this can be achieved preoperatively by angiography and embolization.

The anterior and posterior ethmoid arteries are more difficult arteries to approach and identify. The ethmoid arteries are usually within the bone of the ethmoid roof and only 20% can be simply clipped.[47] The key to identifying the arteries is to dissect the lamina papyracea to the level of the frontoethmoidal suture line (**Fig. 12**) and then to gradually dissect posteriorly elevating the periorbita.[48,49] The anterior ethmoidal artery can be seen passing medially into the roof of the ethmoid (see **Fig. 12**). Once mobilized, ligation can then be performed. Further dissection posteriorly will identify the posterior ethmoid artery (about 10–15 mm posterior) much closer to the orbital apex.[50,51] Alternative approaches are either via a mini-Lynch incision[52] (**Fig. 13**) or

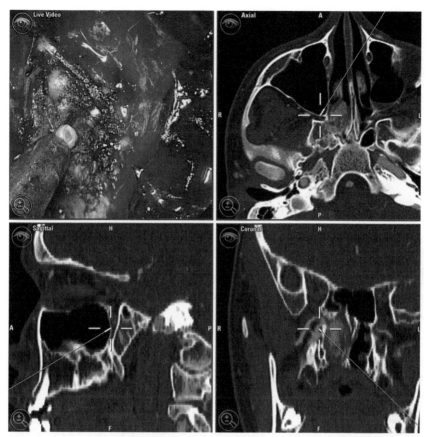

Fig. 11. Ligation of the right internal maxillary artery via removal of the right posterior maxillary sinus wall before resection. Controlled devascularization of a large pathologic lesion dramatically improves the endoscopic surgical field.

transcaruncular incision and dissection within the orbit with the use of the endoscope to identify the arteries. The authors favor a complete endoscopic trans-nasal approach, which has always proved to be successful.

The management of vessels related to the cavernous carotid artery and pituitary gland is more difficult. The inferior hypophyseal arteries are the most likely point of bleeding during sellar and pituitary surgery, and it is possible during methodical dissection to identify these arteries and to ligate as required. A recurrent superior hypophyseal artery may lie within the vasculature of the pituitary stalk and injury can result in optic nerve, pituitary, or hypothalamic injury.[53,54]

Special mention should be given to the management of injury to the cavernous carotid artery during dissection. The internal carotid artery is a robust structure and small bleeding points directly on the artery can be managed potentially with bipolar diathermy, suturing, or even a muscle patch, although the risk of subsequent false aneurysm is high (**Fig. 14**). Significant injury to the artery is potentially catastrophic and requires immediate packing of the operative site, cessation of surgery, stabilization of the patient, angiography, and the consideration of coiling.

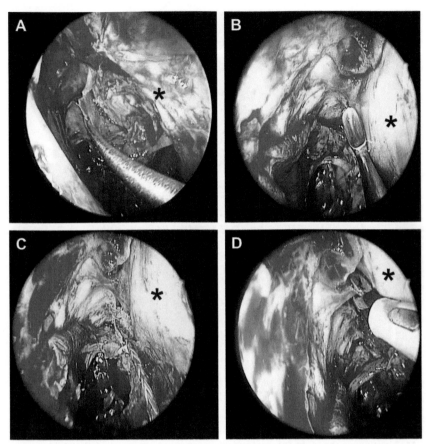

Fig. 12. Ligation of the left anterior ethmoidal artery. (*A*) Removal of the medial orbital wall (*periorbita). (*B*) Removal of the bony anterior ethmoidal artery canal with curette or diamond drill. (*C*) Mobilization of a long segment. (*D*) This allows clips or bipolar forceps to control the vessel.

In summary, complete tumor resection requires good vascular control. The only way to achieve this is for the surgical team to have a structured approach to how they are going to manage the vascular supply to the tumor and paranasal sinuses. Typically the tumor may need to be resected until the sphenopalatine artery can be identified at which point it should be immediately controlled, which will reduce most of the blood supply to the tumor. If required, dissection can be continued laterally into the pterygopalatine fossa and beyond to control the maxillary artery. Superiorly, when the lamina can be appropriately dissected, the anterior and posterior ethmoidal arteries should be ligated. This enables tumor resection in a relatively bloodless field.

RECONSTRUCTION

Attention should be paid to restoring nasal physiology as part of any endoscopic resection. Although this may seem pedantic after several hours of tumor removal, a working cavity results in return of function and a more satisfied patient in the

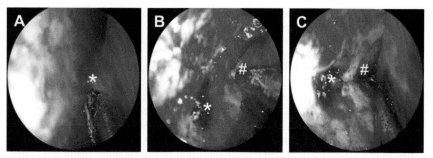

Fig. 13. Endoscopic orbital ligation of the anterior ethmoidal artery. (*A*) A 1- to 1.5-cm external incision with subperiosteal dissection to the anterior ethmoidal artery orbital exit point (*). (*B*) Further 10- to 14-mm dissection reveals the posterior ethmoidal artery exit point (#). (*C*) Final view with both arteries controlled before removal of a large juvenile nasopharyngeal angiofibroma.

long-term. Connecting natural drainage pathways with the surgical cavity prevents mucus recirculation. Avoidance of large sump formation, particularly in the maxillary sinus ensures dependent drainage and easy access to saline irrigation to those areas in which mucocillary function may not fully return. Dural reconstruction can be successfully made[30] with free grafts or pedicled flaps[2,55] and is not discussed here.

Managing the Nasolacrimal System

The management of the lacrimal system creates distinct problems and concerns for the endoscopic surgeon involved in the treatment of neoplastic sinonasal disease. The lower nasolacrimal duct should simply be removed and reconstructed when disease is adjacent or involves this area. Working around this structure simply decreases visualization and increases the risk of positive margins. Consideration for

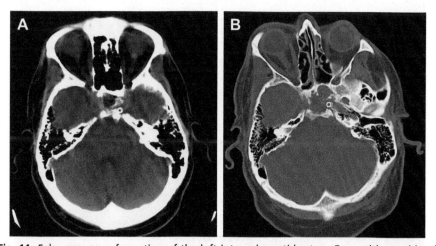

Fig. 14. False aneurysm formation of the left internal carotid artery. Even with good local control, internal carotid artery injury (from an outside center attempt at sublabial hypophysectomy) can result in subsequent false aneurysm. Indiscriminant packing should be avoided in this situation if possible. (*A*) Soft tissue and (*B*) bone window CT images with a previously placed stent that did not prevent false aneurysm formation.

reconstruction is made when resection of the lacrimal system during surgical approach occurs or from tumor involvement.

Need for resection of lacrimal system during surgical approach

In patients with tumors in zone 3 and 4, it is often necessary to resect the nasolacrimal duct for the purpose of access and vision. The duct should never be retained and compromise the access and the dissection to avoid postoperative epiphora. There are reliable reconstructive techniques with greater than 95% lacrimal patency should the lower lacrimal system need to be removed.[56–58] If the nasolacrimal duct is divided sharply, then reconstruction with marsupialization of the retained distal duct with or without stenting will suffice (**Fig. 15**). Endoscopic DCR can be used to provide a robust and reliable patency but is rarely warranted.

Involvement of the lacrimal system by tumor

The surgical approach to the resection of the lacrimal system is dependent on the extent of the involvement of the lacrimal system by the tumor.

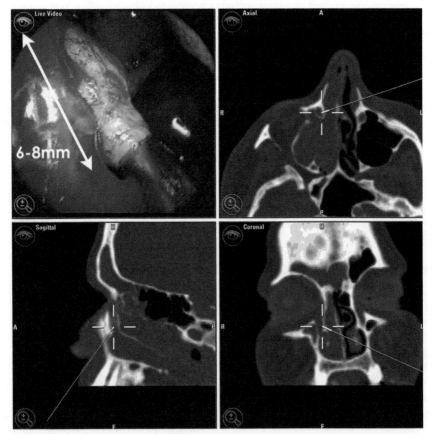

Fig. 15. Image-guided surgery pictures from a right medial maxillectomy. The membranous right nasolacrimal duct is exposed for 6 to 8 mm in its distal portion and marsupialized to the nasal cavity rather than a formal DCR.

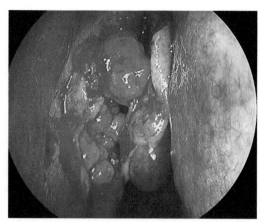

Fig. 16. Inverted papilloma within the right lacrimal sac requires partial or subtotal sac removal. Reconstruction needs to be appropriate for the degree of sac loss.

1. Tumor involves nasolacrimal duct. The nasolacrimal duct can be completely resected along with the tumor and typically no formal reconstruction is required. After the surgical margin is defined, the remaining duct can be simply marsupialized. Should the remaining duct be less than 5 mm then a formal DCR is preferred.
2. Tumor involves the lacrimal sac. A formal endoscopic DCR with wide bone removal should be performed for access. The medial sac wall can be safely sacrificed and DCR completed using standard techniques. Occasionally the lateral sac mucosa needs to be resected and reconstruction can be achieved by the placement of a free mucosal graft (**Fig. 16**). A 3-mm punch biopsy cutter is used on a Blakesley forcep to preserve the common canniculus opening and mucosa. The remaining lateral sac is removed. A central perforation of the graft is created with the same 3-mm punch biopsy instrument. The graft is placed to provide near complete mucosal apposition preserving the common canniculus. Stenting is used and a Gelfoam donut dressing is used to secure the graft (**Fig. 17**).
3. Tumor involves the common canalliculus. The entire sac and common canalliculus need to be resected and reconstruction is required by the insertion of a glass Jones tube through the medial canthus (**Fig. 18**). This is best performed by an ocular plastic surgeon and an endoscopic surgeon.

POSTOPERATIVE MANAGEMENT

Leaving a large endoscopic cavity without good postoperative control usually results in a wound bed covered with large crusting (a combination of dry blood and mucus) and superficial bacterial colonization. High-volume positive-pressure squeeze bottle irrigations are used from the first postoperative day. The authors find that this improves patient comfort, breathing, and counterintuitively reduces bleeding.[39–41] Antibiotics are given for 14 days postoperatively as there is exposed bone and foreign material in the cavity.

Packing has a limited role. Extensive tight ribbon gauze is generally not necessary and is uncomfortable for the patient.[59] Sialastic sheeting is used routinely to cover the anterior septum, particularly for trans-septal approaches.[14] Prolonged endoscopic surgery is associated with significant excoriation and mucosal abrasion to anterior septum even with careful technique. Heavy fibrinous exudate can occur and can cause nasal obstruction, adhesion, and discomfort if not managed; 0.4-mm silastic

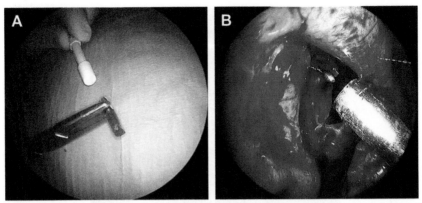

Fig. 17. Cutting out the common cannuliculus with a circular biopsy punch (*A*) from the right lacrimal sac (*B*).

sheeting secured with a through and through prolene suture assists with this problem. Exposed bone is covered with Gelfoam or SurgiFlo (Johnson & Johnson Medical) **(Fig. 19)**. A gloved Merocel dressing is placed as a middle meatal spacer or in the new cavity created, less for hemostasis and more for preventing extensive crusting. The dressing is secured with a trans-septal prolene suture. The gloved Merocel spacer is removed on day 7. This generally provides a moist environment with a soft clot that can easily be suctioned in the outpatient clinic. Pain management has evolved in the past few years in our experience. Combination acetaminophen and opiates are used initially. The extensive bone exposure often results in a secondary pain phenomenon around postoperative days 5 to 10, similar to that experienced by tonsillectomy patients undergoing secondary healing. Nonsteroidal anti-inflammatory drugs greatly help to reduce this phenomenon.

IMPLICATIONS FOR RESEARCH

Further research is required on optimal wound healing for large resection cavities created by the extended surgery. Long-term follow-up of sinonasal function greatly assists in defining the role for extended endoscopic resection. Health cost and economic studies are required to demonstrate a cost advantage to managing patients via an endoscopic approach. This type of surgery often involves long operating time but substantial savings in postoperative care, recovery, and inpatient stay.

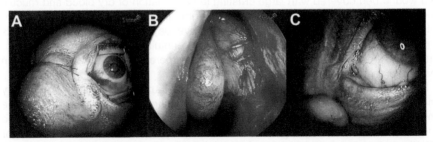

Fig. 18. Jones tubes. Exposure of the left medial canthus (*A*). The glass Jones tube in situ (*B*) and the final external position (*C*).

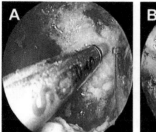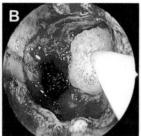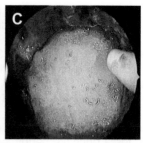

Fig. 19. A trans-septal approach to a left maxillary inverted papilloma. (*A*) The attachment site in the left zygomatic recess is drilled directly. (*B, C*) The large bone exposed cavity is covered with Surgiflo to encourage granulation and prevent heavy crusting. High-volume saline irrigations always accompany this postoperative care.

IMPLICATIONS FOR CLINICAL PRACTICE

Endoscopic techniques developed from managing inflammatory sinus disease have little relevance in large tumor resections. The focus for these cases should be on appropriate surgical access, early vascular control, and complete excision. Our greater understanding of sinonasal physiology and endoscopic evaluation should allow the creation of a functional cavity even after large resections. A postresection nasal cavity with extensive adhesions, chronic mucosal inflammation, and mucus recirculation should be a relic of days when surgery was performed under a headlight.

REFERENCES

1. Harvey RJ, Sheahan PO, Schlosser RJ. Surgical management of benign sinonasal masses. Otolaryngol Clin North Am 2009;42(2):353–75.
2. Harvey RJ, Stamm AC, Vellutini E, et al. Closure of large skull base defects after endoscopic trans-nasal craniotomy. J Neurosurg 2009;111(2):371–9.
3. Lund V, Howard DJ, Wei WI. Endoscopic resection of malignant tumors of the nose and sinuses. Am J Rhinol 2007;21(1):89–94.
4. Danesi G, Panciera DT, Harvey RJ, et al. Juvenile nasopharyngeal angiofibroma: evaluation and surgical management of advanced disease. Otolaryngol Head Neck Surg 2008;138(5):581–6.
5. Weissler MC, Montgomery WW, Turner PA, et al. Inverted papilloma. Ann Otol Rhinol Laryngol 1986;95(3 Pt 1):215–21.
6. Cannady SB, Batra PS, Sautter NB, et al. New staging system for sinonasal inverted papilloma in the endoscopic era. Laryngoscope 2007;117(7):1283–7.
7. Jameson MJ, Kountakis SE. Endoscopic management of extensive inverted papilloma. Am J Rhinol 2005;19(5):446–51.
8. Krouse JH. Endoscopic treatment of inverted papilloma: safety and efficacy. Am J Otolaryngol 2001;22(2):87–99.
9. Woodworth BA, Bhargave GA, Palmer JN, et al. Clinical outcomes of endoscopic and endoscopic-assisted resection of inverted papillomas: a 15-year experience. Am J Rhinol 2007;21(5):591–600 [erratum appears in Am J Rhinol 2008;22(1):97].
10. Cho DY, Hwang PH. Results of endoscopic maxillary mega-antrostomy in recalcitrant maxillary sinusitis. Am J Rhinol 2008;22(6):658–62.
11. Woodworth BA, Parker RO, Schlosser RJ. Modified endoscopic medial maxillectomy for chronic maxillary sinusitis. Am J Rhinol 2006;20(3):317–9.

12. Wormald PJ, Ooi E, van Hasselt CA, et al. Endoscopic removal of sinonasal inverted papilloma including endoscopic medial maxillectomy. Laryngoscope 2003;113(5):867–73.

13. James D, Crockard HA. Surgical access to the base of skull and upper cervical spine by extended maxillotomy. Neurosurgery 1991;29(3):411–6.

14. Harvey RJ, Sheehan PO, Debnath NI, et al. Transseptal approach for extended endoscopic resections of the maxilla and infratemporal fossa. Am J Rhinol Allergy 2009;23(4):426–32.

15. Robinson SR, Baird R, Le T, et al. The incidence of complications after canine fossa puncture performed during endoscopic sinus surgery. Am J Rhinol 2005; 19(2):203–6.

16. Robinson S, Wormald PJ. Patterns of innervation of the anterior maxilla: a cadaver study with relevance to canine fossa puncture of the maxillary sinus. Laryngoscope 2005;115(10):1785–8.

17. Robinson S, Patel N, Wormald PJ. Endoscopic management of benign tumors extending into the infratemporal fossa: a two-surgeon transnasal approach. Laryngoscope 2005;115(10):1818–22.

18. Knipe TA, Gandhi PD, Fleming JC, et al. Transblepharoplasty approach to sequestered disease of the lateral frontal sinus with ophthalmologic manifestations. Am J Rhinol 2007;21(1):100–4.

19. Seiberling K, Floreani S, Robinson S, et al. Endoscopic management of frontal sinus osteomas revisited. Am J Rhinol Allergy 2009;23(3):331–6.

20. Chen C, Selva D, Wormald PJ. Endoscopic modified Lothrop procedure: an alternative for frontal osteoma excision. Rhinology 2004;42(4):239–43.

21. Yoon BN, Batra PS, Citardi MJ, et al. Frontal sinus inverted papilloma: surgical strategy based on the site of attachment. Am J Rhinol Allergy 2009;23: 337–41.

22. Chiu AG, Jackman AH, Antunes MB, et al. Radiographic and histologic analysis of the bone underlying inverted papillomas. Laryngoscope 2006;116(9): 1617–20.

23. Chandra RK, Schlosser R, Kennedy DW. Use of the 70-degree diamond burr in the management of complicated frontal sinus disease. Laryngoscope 2004; 114(2):188–92.

24. Zacharek MA, Fong KJ, Hwang PH. Image-guided frontal trephination: a minimally invasive approach for hard-to-reach frontal sinus disease. Otolaryngol Head Neck Surg 2006;135(4):518–22.

25. Batra PS, Citardi MJ, Lanza DC. Combined endoscopic trephination and endoscopic frontal sinusotomy for management of complex frontal sinus pathology. Am J Rhinol 2005;19(5):435–41.

26. Chiu AG, Vaughan WC. Management of the lateral frontal sinus lesion and the supraorbital cell mucocele. Am J Rhinol 2004;18(2):83–6.

27. Seiberling K, Jardeleza C, Wormald PJ. Minitrephination of the frontal sinus: indications and uses in today's era of sinus surgery. Am J Rhinol Allergy 2009;23: 229–31.

28. Weber R, Draf W, Kratzsch B, et al. Modern concepts of frontal sinus surgery. Laryngoscope 2001;111(1):137–46.

29. Stammberger HR, Kennedy DW. Paranasal sinuses: anatomic terminology and nomenclature. The Anatomic Terminology Group. Ann Otol Rhinol Laryngol Suppl 1995;167:7–16.

30. Harvey RJ, Smith JE, Wise SK, et al. Intracranial complications before and after endoscopic skull base reconstruction. Am J Rhinol 2008;22(5):516–21.

31. Bolger WE, Keyes AS, Lanza DC. Use of the superior meatus and superior turbinate in the endoscopic approach to the sphenoid sinus. Otolaryngol Head Neck Surg 1999;120(3):308–13.

32. Orlandi RR, Lanza DC, Bolger WE, et al. The forgotten turbinate: the role of the superior turbinate in endoscopic sinus surgery. Am J Rhinol 1999;13(4): 251–9.

33. Stamm AC, Nogueira JF Jr, Harvey RJ. Revision endoscopic skull base surgery. In: Kountakis SE, Jacobs J, Gosepath J, editors, Revision sinus surgery, vol. 1. Heidelberg (Germany): Springer; 2008. p. 289–300.

34. Casiano RR. A stepwise surgical technique using the medial orbital floor as the key landmark in performing endoscopic sinus surgery. Laryngoscope 2001; 111(6):964–74.

35. Harvey RJ, Shelton BS, Timperley D, et al. Using fixed anatomical landmarks in endoscopic skull base surgery. Am J Rhinol Allergy 2010. [Epub ahead of print].

36. Harvey RJ, Gallagher RM. Endoscopic vascular control of the anterior skull base. Presented at Annual Scientific Conference. Melbourne, Australia, March 25, 2006.

37. Eberhart LH, Folz BJ, Wulf H, et al. Intravenous anesthesia provides optimal surgical conditions during microscopic and endoscopic sinus surgery. Laryngoscope 2003;113(8):1369–73.

38. Wormald PJ, van Renen G, Perks J, et al. The effect of the total intravenous anesthesia compared with inhalational anesthesia on the surgical field during endoscopic sinus surgery. Am J Rhinol 2005;19(5):514–20.

39. Stangerup SE, Thomsen HK. Histological changes in the nasal mucosa after hot-water irrigation. An animal experimental study. Rhinology 1996;34(1):14–7.

40. Stangerup SE, Dommerby H, Lau T, et al. Hot-water irrigation as a treatment of posterior epistaxis. Rhinology 1996;34(1):18–20.

41. Kassam A, Snyderman CH, Carrau RL, et al. Endoneurosurgical hemostasis techniques: lessons learned from 400 cases. Neurosurg 2005;19(1):E7.

42. Gurr P, Callanan V, Baldwin D. Laser-Doppler blood flowmetry measurement of nasal mucosa blood flow after injection of the greater palatine canal. J Laryngol Otol 1996;110(2):124–8.

43. Iwabuchi T, Sobata E, Suzuki M, et al. Dural sinus pressure as related to neurosurgical positions. Neurosurgery 1983;12(2):203–7.

44. Tankisi A, Cold GE. Optimal reverse Trendelenburg position in patients undergoing craniotomy for cerebral tumors. J Neurosurg 2007;106(2):239–44.

45. Haure P, Cold GE, Hansen TM, et al. The ICP-lowering effect of 10 degrees reverse Trendelenburg position during craniotomy is stable during a 10-minute period. J Neurosurg Anesthesiol 2003;15(4):297–301.

46. Simmen DB, Raghavan U, Briner HR, et al. The anatomy of the sphenopalatine artery for the endoscopic sinus surgeon. Am J Rhinol 2006;20(5):502–5.

47. Floreani SR, Nair SB, Switajewski MC, et al. Endoscopic anterior ethmoidal artery ligation: a cadaver study. Laryngoscope 2006;116(7):1263–7.

48. Camp AA, Dutton JM, Caldarelli DD. Endoscopic transnasal transethmoid ligation of the anterior ethmoid artery. Am J Rhinol Allergy 2009;23(2):200–2.

49. Pletcher SD, Metson R. Endoscopic ligation of the anterior ethmoid artery. Laryngoscope 2007;117(2):378–81.

50. Simmen D, Raghavan U, Briner HR, et al. The surgeon's view of the anterior ethmoid artery. Clin Otolaryngol 2006;31(3):187–91.

51. Han JK, Becker SS, Bomeli SR, et al. Endoscopic localization of the anterior and posterior ethmoid arteries. Ann Otol Rhinol Laryngol 2008;117(12):931–5.

52. Woolford TJ, Jones NS. Endoscopic ligation of anterior ethmoidal artery in treatment of epistaxis. J Laryngol Otol 2000;114(11):858–60.
53. van Overbeeke J, Sekhar L. Microanatomy of the blood supply to the optic nerve. Orbit 2003;22(2):81–8.
54. Krisht AF, Barrow DL, Barnett DW, et al. The microsurgical anatomy of the superior hypophyseal artery. Neurosurgery 1994;35(5):899–903 [discussion: 903].
55. Harvey RJ, Sheahan PO, Schlosser RJ. Inferior turbinate pedicle flap for endoscopic skull base defect repair. Am J Rhinol Allergy 2009;23(5):522–6.
56. Wormald PJ. Powered endoscopic dacryocystorhinostomy. Otolaryngol Clin North Am 2006;39(3):539–49.
57. Mann BS, Wormald PJ, Mann BS, et al. Endoscopic assessment of the dacryocystorhinostomy ostium after endoscopic surgery. Laryngoscope 2006;116(7):1172–4.
58. Tsirbas A, Davis G, Wormald PJ, et al. Revision dacryocystorhinostomy: a comparison of endoscopic and external techniques. Am J Rhinol 2005;19(3):322–5.
59. von Schoenberg M, Robinson P, Ryan R. Nasal packing after routine nasal surgery–is it justified? J Laryngol Otol 1993;107(10):902–5.

Evolution of Endoscopic Skull Base Surgery, Current Concepts, and Future Perspectives

João Flávio Nogueira, MD[a],*, Aldo Stamm, MD, PhD[b],
Eduardo Vellutini, MD[c]

KEYWORDS

• Endoscopic skull base surgery • Endoscopic techniques
• Expanded endonasal approaches • Neurosurgery

Endoscopic techniques have influenced almost all of the surgical specialties. From open procedures to minimally invasive approaches, the endoscope, and its ability to reach areas within the human body, has gained popularity among specialists, creating a revolution in some fields. Two of the fields in which endoscopes provided a true revolution are otolaryngology and neurosurgery.[1,2]

Endoscopic skull base (ESB) surgery is now a rapid growing field for otolaryngologists and neurosurgeons. Of course, to perform safe and effective ESB procedures, a multidisciplinary team is paramount and this team should include an anesthesiologist, endocrinologist, pathologist, radiologist, intensive care unit specialists, and specialized paramedical staff.[1–3]

The current limits for endoscope-assisted skull base procedures are constantly changing. In the past decades we moved from endoscopic closure of cerebrospinal fluid (CSF) leaks, to a myriad of lesions extending from the cribriform plate to the craniocervical junction and laterally to the infratemporal fossa and petrous apex. These recent advances are termed "expanded endonasal approaches" (EEA) and they provide access to the anterior, middle, and posterior cranial fossae.[1–5]

However, all of these advances were dependent on several technical and technological components, which included high endoscopic anatomic knowledge, advanced endoscopic surgical techniques and skills, crystal clear endoscopes and cameras, CT

[a] ENT Institute of Fortaleza, Fortaleza, Brazil
[b] São Paulo ENT Center – Hospital Professor Edmundo Vasconcelos, São Paulo, Brazil
[c] DFV Neuro, São Paulo, Brazil
* Corresponding author. Rua Dr José Furtado, 1500 Fortaleza, Ceará 60822-300, Brazil.
E-mail address: joaoflavioce@hotmail.com

Otolaryngol Clin N Am 43 (2010) 639–652
doi:10.1016/j.otc.2010.02.017
0030-6665/10/$ – see front matter © 2010 Elsevier Inc. All rights reserved.

and MRI, specially designed instruments, powered instrumentation, and more recently, image guidance systems. However, even with all the evolution in this field, complications still occur.[1–3]

OBJECTIVES

In this content the authors discuss some important factors for the evolution of ESB surgery and EEA, highlighting historical landmarks but also addressing the current concepts, complications, and the future of this promising field for clinical research and surgical techniques and technology.

BRIEF HISTORY

Although the history of skull base surgery is intrinsically linked with the evolution of pituitary surgery, the history of ESB surgery starts with the capability to close small dural defects through the nose.[6]

With the evolution of endoscopic sino-nasal procedures for inflammatory diseases since the 1980s, purely endoscopic approaches for the evaluation and treatment of CSF rhinorrhea were also developed.[6,7] These endoscopic approaches allowed the complete closure of CSF leaks through a minimally invasive perspective, but with safety and good results.[8] The use of free grafts and other types of materials allowed surgeons to close small defects, traumatic, spontaneous, and iatrogenic CSF leaks from the 1990s to 2000s.

However, the paucity of good closure results with large (>2 cm) dural defects was still a limiting factor for the EEA. Problems, such as infections, meningitis, and ventriculitis, were serious complications.[9–11] Also, the location of the pathology relative to important neural and vascular structures was another important limiting factor, but for many tumors the endonasal corridor provided the most direct access with the least manipulation of neural and vascular structures.[1,9–11]

This important anatomic consideration drove surgeons to other ESB applications, such as pituitary adenomas.[9–11] Since the 1990s, several surgeons published reports with good results that popularized the use of endoscopes in this area.[1,10,11] The functional and endocrinologic results were better when compared with open microscopic approaches, but tumors with suprasellar or lateral (into cavernous sinus) invasion were still a challenge, mainly because of a lack of specialized instruments and an inability to control vascular lesions and to close large dural defects with assistance of endoscopes.[1,10,11]

The works of several important authors allowed the evolution regarding these limiting factors. The limitations in technology and instrumentation were overcome. However, the real revolution occurred in 2004 when doctors from Argentina designed and used pediculated nasoseptal flaps for the closure of big CSF defects.[2,12–14] At first the doctors were discredited, but the good results obtained with those pediculated, robust, reconstructive tissues forced the endoscopic surgeons to use it.

Although this evolution (ie, the ability to safely remove large tumors endoscopically) did not change the philosophy of tumor removal, it closed the large, created dural defects with good success rates, which was the last limiting factor for the EEA. Since 2006 several other types of pediculated flaps were designed and developed, such as inferior and medium turbinates flaps, pericranial flaps, and palatal flaps, among others.[2,14–17] Along with the flaps, several endoscopic approaches were described and the authors are going to discuss them.

CURRENT CONCEPTS

Several endoscopic approaches, following the endonasal corridor, exist according to the size and location of the tumor. However, in some cases of large tumors, combined procedures may still be required.[1–3]

The choice of a surgical approach depends on patient comorbidities, tumor characteristics (location, proximity to important neurovascular structures), and the skills and comfort level of the surgeons. If nerves or vessels need to be mobilized to reach the tumor, then an alternative microscopic approach should be considered. Relative contraindications to an endonasal approach include tumor involvement of superficial tissues, the need for vascular reconstruction, and the duration of surgery.[1,2]

Potential current advantages of ESB surgery include the lack of external incision, decreased trauma to normal soft tissue and bone, improved visualization, increased access, improved outcomes, fewer complications, rapid recovery, decreased hospitalization, and cost.[1,2,10] Disadvantages include unfamiliar anatomy, physiologic sinonasal alterations with potential postoperative complications, a long learning curve, and still some technological limitations.[1]

The current concepts of EEA rely on endoscopes to provide a better field of image with angulated views when compared with microscopes. However, because we use rigid instruments, this capability is only achieved if the endoscopes reach the surgical field.

The nose and paranasal sinuses have several important anatomic landmarks and potential natural barriers to the skull base, such as the nasal septum, turbinates, and sphenoid rostrum, among others.

To access important skull base structures through the nose you have to create a pathway for instruments and the surgeons. The current concept of a multidisciplinary team is important and EEA should always be done with the presence of two or more surgeons.[1,2]

The current ESB pathways from anterior to posterior are transfrontal, transcribriform, transplanum, trans-sellar, transclival, and transodontoid/craniocervical junction (**Fig. 1**). Also, there are the ESB lateral approaches, which include all orbital, transpterygoid, and infratemporal accesses.[1] Each one of these approaches has its own applications, important landmarks, and pitfalls. A brief discussion of these approaches follows.

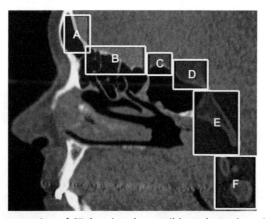

Fig. 1. Sagittal reconstruction of CT showing the possible endonasal surgical accesses to the skull base. (A) transfrontal, (B) transcribriform, (C) transplanum, (D) trans-sellar, (E) transclival, (F) transodontoid/craniocervical junction.

The transfrontal approach provides access to the floor and posterior wall of the frontal sinus. Examples of lesions found in this area include inflammatory sinus disease, erosive mucocoeles, and frontal osteomas, among others.[1] The transfrontal approach is the anterior limit of an endonasal craniofacial resection for malignant sinonasal neoplasms and for these approaches a Draf III procedure and complete ethmoidectomy is common practice. To close defects in this area, a nasal septal flap can be used, although the use of free grafts is also successful according to the size of the dural defect.

The trans-cribriform access extends from the crista galli to the planum sphenoidal and across the roof of the ethmoid sinuses (fovea ethmoidalis) to the orbital roof. This module is most often used for sino-nasal malignancies and esthesioneuroblastomas and olfactory groove meningiomas.

Often, a Draf III procedure and complete ethmoidectomy is necessary. Sometimes, in cases of malignances, a nasal septal flap cannot be used because the surgeon may suspect compromised margins. In these cases, to close the dural defect, a turbinate, palatal, or even pericranium flap may be used (**Figs. 2** and **3**).

The transplanum module provides access to suprasellar lesions, such as pituitary tumors with extra-sellar extension, meningiomas, and craniopharyngiomas. It is limited anteriorly by the posterior ethmoidal artery and posteriorly by the optic canals.

To allow good transplanum access, a complete ethmoidectomy, wide opening of the sphenoid sinus, and occasionally middle turbinate removal, are performed. An example of a meningioma requiring a transplanum approach is depicted in **Figs. 4** and **5**. The use of a nasal septal flap, pediculated at the sphenopalatine artery, is possible for the closure of the dural-created defects. Sometimes, according to the size of the defect, two nasal septal flaps are required.

The trans-sellar access is the current standard approach for pituitary lesions but may be combined with other approaches for tumors with extra-sellar or lateral extension. It is limited laterally by the cavernous internal carotid artery (ICA), superiorly by the optic canal, and inferiorly by the clivus.

Several techniques regarding this approach are described.[18] From trans-nasal direct to binostril, removing the posterior part of the nasal septum, middle turbinates, or preserving these structures, the best technique is the one most comfortable for the surgeons and the team. Of course, the size and invasion of the lesion are important factors when choosing the appropriate access. The sino-nasal postoperative complications are another important factor.

The key to a successful trans-sellar approach is the exposition. Some tips to perform this approach are

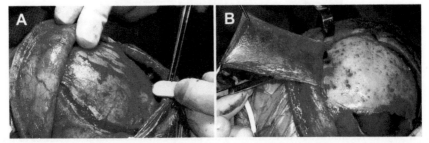

Fig. 2. Pericranium flap. (*A*) Harvesting the flap in a traditional fashion. (*B*) Size of the flap and frontal sinus anterior wall created defect to cross the flap into the nasal cavity.

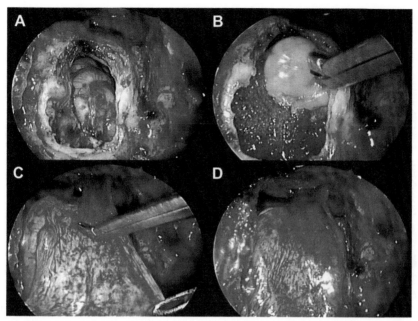

Fig. 3. Endoscopic view, with a 45-degree, 4 mm endoscope of the surgical site. (*A*) After a Draf III procedure and well exposition of the tumor and its margins, resection with clear margins (frozen sections) and resulting large anterior fossa skull base defect. (*B*) Layered reconstruction with absorbable material, fat and fascia lata. (*C*) Pericranium flap rotation, under endoscopic view, into the nasal cavity. Special care was taken to avoid torsion of the flap (*D*) pericranium flap final aspect. Note the frontal sinus maintained lateral drainage pathway.

- Wide opening of the sphenoid sinus, visualizing ICA and optic canals
- Wide exposition of sellar dura and quadrangular incision, differently from most authors that preconize cruciate incisions. The quadrangular or rectangular incision is made with a #11 blade having the following limits

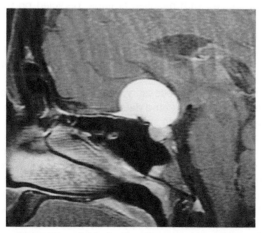

Fig. 4. Sagittal view of MRI, T1-weighted, of a planum sphenoidal meningioma.

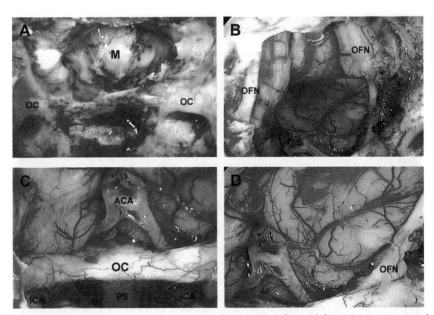

Fig. 5. Endoscopic surgical view of resection of a planum sphenoidal meningioma, transplanum approach. (*A*) Endoscopic view (0 degree, 4 mm) of the aspect of the tumor. (*B*) Endoscopic view (45 degree, 4 mm) of surgical field. (*C*) Endoscopic view (0 degree, 4 mm) of important anatomic landmarks. (*D*) Endoscopic view (45 degree, 4 mm) of the final aspect of the surgical field. ACA, anterior communicating artery; ICA, internal carotid artery; M, meningioma; OC, optic canal; OC, optic chiasma (for **Fig. 5**C); OFN, olfactory nerve; PS, pituitary stalk.

> Lateral: medial to ICAs and cavernous sinus
> Superior: inferior to the superior intercavernous sinus
> Inferior: superior to the inferior intercavernous sinus (**Fig. 6**).

The dura is removed without the need of creating a flap. Also, trans-sellar approaches may be closed with nasoseptal flaps, pedicled on the sphenopalatine artery.

The transclival approach is indicated for clival bone lesions, such as chordomas, chondrosarcomas, and meningiomas. It is a challenging access because it requires several advanced endoscopic skills and specially designed long instruments, such as drills.[2]

Also, a wide sphenoidotomy is necessary. Sometimes a complete bilateral ethmoidectomy is also performed. The created defects can be closed with the assistance of nasal-septal flaps pediculated at the sphenopalatine artery (**Fig. 7**).

The transodontoid/craniocervical junction approach provides access to the upper cervical spine (C1 and C2) and foramen magnum.[19] It is indicated for several lesions, including rheumatoid degeneration of the upper cervical spine, malignant tumors, basilar invagination of the spine, and compression of the brainstem. Long handpiece drills are also paramount for this surgery. It is important to remember that removal of the ring of C1 and odontoid decompresses the brainstem anteriorly but still requires stabilization of the spine posteriorly. This approach is limited laterally by the parapharyngeal ICA and the vertebral arteries (**Fig. 8**).

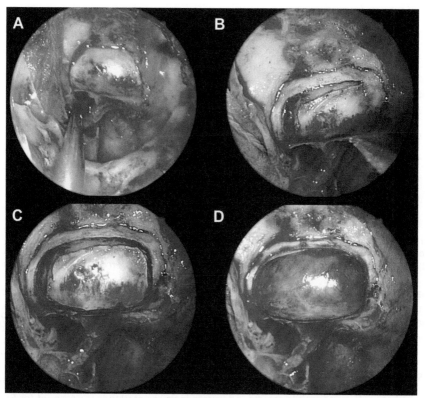

Fig. 6. (*A*) Exposure of sellar dura. (*B*) Incisions for a quadrangular or rectangular area in sellar dura. (*C*) Incision complete. (*D*) Exposure of the pituitary tumor.

The transorbital approach is used for intraconal lesions that are inferior and medial to the optic nerve, such as hemangiomas and schwannomas. Access is between the inferior and medial rectus muscles with preservation of extraocular muscle function (**Fig. 9**).

The transpterygoid/infratemporal fossa approach allows full access to the lateral recess of the sphenoid sinus. Meningiomas, malignant tumors, and schwannomas may require this approach. Further laterally, tumors of the infratemporal fossa

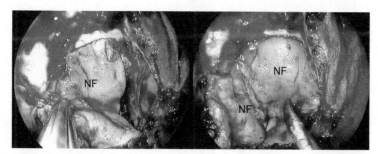

Fig. 7. Endoscopic view (0 degree, 4 mm) of reconstruction after a transclival approach. The closure of the defect is done with nasal septal pediculated flaps (NF) from both sides of the nasal septum.

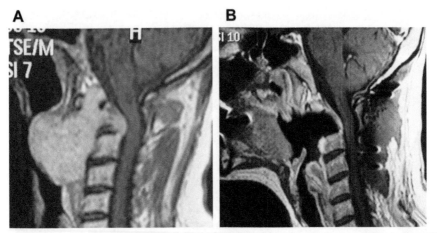

Fig. 8. Giant cell carcinoma of the cervical spine. (*A*) Preoperative, T1-weighted MRI showing infiltration of the C1 and C2 vertebra bodies. Note the compression of the medulla. (*B*) Postoperative, T1-weighted MRI showing the complete resection of C1 and C2 vertebrae.

(mandibular nerve [V3] schwannoma) may be approached. This approach requires a medial maxillectomy for full access to the posterolateral wall of the maxillary sinus. The lateral pterygoid plate is a useful landmark for locating foramen ovale, where V3 tumors are located.[1,20]

INSTRUMENTATION

To achieve safe and feasible results, adequate instrumentation is paramount for ESB surgery. Its absence may be considered a formal absolute contraindication for ESB procedures. These instruments include[2]

- High-quality cameras and endoscopes
- Long handpiece drills with diamond burs
- Powered instrumentation

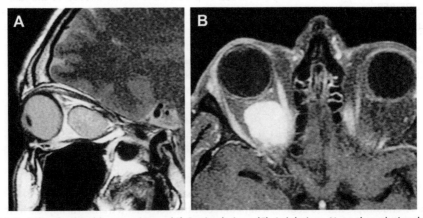

Fig. 9. MRI of orbital hemangioma. (*A*) Sagittal view. (*B*) Axial view. Note the relationship between the tumor and orbital muscles and nerve.

- Specialized hand dissection instruments
- Long bipolar forceps
- Image guidance system, although not paramount, it may assist in revisionary cases with disturbed anatomy.

COMPLICATIONS

The most important innovation in ESB surgery for the prevention of complications has been the introduction of multidisciplinary teams.[1,2] The potential benefits of team surgery include improved visualization, increased operative efficiency, improved decision making and problem solving, and modulation of individual enthusiasm. This multidisciplinary approach concept is important in modern ESB. The team approach is still a novel concept in medicine. Although the multidisciplinary team has evolved only in the last few decades, survival and complication rates have decreased since the introduction of this approach.[2]

The team concept assumes critical importance when complications occur. There are several technological challenges in performing EEA. Strategies for minimizing intraoperative blood loss are paramount and may include preoperative embolization when feasible.[1]

Other complications, such as infectious, endocrinologic, and neurologic, should also be managed with a team effort. Infectious complications are rare with ESB surgery. This rarity is attributed to minimal bacterial colonization of the nasal cavity and sinuses, use of prophylactic perioperative antibiotics, and skull base reconstruction with vascularized flaps. Non-vascularized materials, such as bone cement or titanium plates, can also be used but they may increase the risk for infection.[1,2,10]

Postoperative CSF leaks are managed clinically with a lumbar drainage catheter or aggressively with endoscopic surgical repair. In almost all cases, the repair can be augmented with a small fascial or fat graft or with repositioning of the mucosal flap.[1]

However, one of the most important complications is ICA injury. An experienced team of surgeons can maintain visualization, even with profuse bleeding, and gain control with bipolar electrocautery, application of hemostatic materials, and local packing.[1,2,10,11] Indiscriminate packing should be avoided but if necessary, aneurysm clamps can be placed across an injured ICA. Once intraoperative control is achieved, angiography is performed with possible sacrifice of the vessel.

FUTURE PERSPECTIVES AND IMPLICATIONS

One of the primary restrictions of ESB surgery was the lack of binocular or stereoscopic vision. Used to microscopes, especially some neurosurgeons were not encouraged to perform endoscopic procedures since monocular endoscopes and monitors create a two-dimensional (2D) image that impairs depth perception, hand- eye coordination, and the ability to estimate size.[21,22]

This lack of stereoscopic vision has contributed to the steep learning curve in the field of ESB surgery and the authors think that the next obvious step in the evolution of ESB surgery will be the development of high-definition stereoendoscopes that produce a three-dimensional (3D) image. Although such stereoendoscopes exist, their use in ESB surgery has been limited because of the larger diameter and poor resolution of earlier generations.[21]

There are several reports showing the use of purely stereoendoscopes in several medical areas; however, there are few works in ESB surgery.[21] Also, there is equipment that can convert 2D into 3D images. Its use has been limited to few institutions, because it requires special polarized glasses and eye accommodation by the surgeon.

We used a 2D to 3D converter in some ESB procedures and it really increased the depth perception; however, the quality of images were still not good (**Fig. 10**). The implications of this potential technology are the development of stereoscopic ESB surgery techniques and training programs.

Several studies show that EEA decreases the postoperative discomfort and hospitalization time and enables a quick recovery in patients operated in comparison with the conventional microscopic technique.[2,10]

However, perioperative and especially postoperative sinonasal complications, such as infection, bleeding, crusting, nasal synechias, nasal septum perforations, nasal obstruction, among others, are common.[2]

Unfortunately, at present, to access the various areas of the skull base, we rely on rigid, straight instruments. Because of these instrumental limitations we still have to remove important structures, such as the nasal septum, turbinates, and others, to properly visualize the surgical field.

The authors think that a forthcoming technological development of ESB surgery is the introduction of flexible endoscopes and instruments to perform more minimally invasive procedures, allowing fewer traumas to the nose and paranasal sinuses, minimizing such postoperative sino-nasal problems.

This already happens in other surgical areas, such as laparoscopic surgery, in which a flexible tool allows surgeries such as cholecystectomy, without the need of external openings, completely through oral, gastric or vaginal cavities. Natural orifice transluminal endoscopic surgeries (NOTES) have gained special attention[23] recently. Although it is still potentially inappropriate to use these instruments (**Fig. 11**) in the nose, mainly because of their diameter, with advances in technology these instruments tend to become smaller, providing the potential applicability in endoscopic sino-nasal inflammatory diseases and ESB procedures.

Another future technology is the use of virtual augmented reality (AR) combined with image guidance systems in ESB surgery (**Fig. 12**). Although AR technology provides

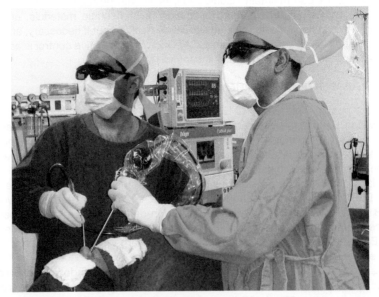

Fig. 10. Stereoscopic 3D endoscopic skull base surgery. The surgeons must wear special polarized glasses to obtain depth perception.

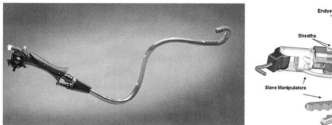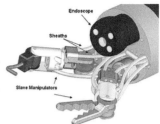

Fig. 11. NOTES equipment. Note illustration of instrument with an endoscopic lens and arms with different instruments. (*Courtesy of* Karl Storz Company.)

more information by linking real image data with virtual image data, it is still a novel field of investigation in ESB surgery.[24,25] However, some authors have reported the clinical use of AR navigation systems to provide information on virtual objects superimposed on real images during surgery.[25] Those systems were perceived as an improved navigational experience because the augmented see-through effect allowed direct understanding of the surgical anatomy beyond the visible surface and direct guidance toward surgical targets.

The implications of AR in ESB surgery are many, such as to locate, through a virtual-reality environment, the lesion and its limits, along with important adjacent structures.

Robotic skull base surgery (**Fig. 13**) is also a future perspective and some cadaveric studies have been performed to use robots in ESB surgery.[26,27] The application of robotic technology to surgery has rapidly expanded over the last years. The main advantage that these systems can offer is the ability to perform bimanual surgery in confined cavities with instrumentation that exceeds the capabilities of the human hand, providing the surgeon with a 3D view of the surgical field. Significant advances in surgical robotics have been made; however, a true role for robotic-based applications in skull base surgery has not been completely defined. Because of the large diameters of the surgical robotic arms, most of the studies for robotic skull base applications are done through transantral accesses to the pituitary gland and the optic chiasm.[26,27]

Several other novel approaches may be developed to allow the use of robotic technology for two surgeons to perform endoscopic manipulation of the pituitary gland and surrounding structures. These approaches and the robot itself may expand the indications of minimally invasive approaches to the central skull base, the pituitary fossa, and in the near future, areas of current limitation.

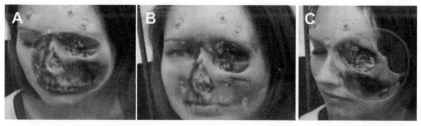

Fig. 12. Augmented-reality example. (*A*) Augmented-reality projected image of CT 3D reconstruction scan into patients face. (*B*) The projected image is dynamic. If the patient moves, the corresponding part of the examination will move according to the patient. (*C*) Note lateral view.

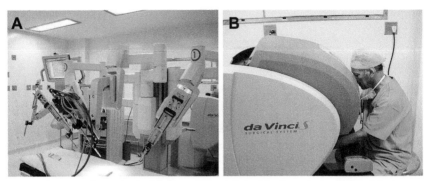

Fig. 13. Robotic endoscopic skull base surgery. (*A*) Da Vinci surgical system with the ports. (*B*) Control unit.

All of these future perspectives may completely change skull base surgery in a clinical perspective, because it may introduce other procedures that enhance diagnostic capabilities, and in a surgical perspective, because it introduces other surgical instruments, technologies, and equipment that may require different skills for surgeons.

SUMMARY

Endoscopic skull base surgery is a constantly growing and changing medical field. Some of the major obstacles to ESB surgery, including endoscopic anatomic knowledge and skills to treat vascular and dural defects, are being managed effectively; however, the techniques, technology, and equipments will continue to evolve. The limits of ESB have not been realized and the future is promising with all of these advances.

IMPLICATIONS FOR CLINICAL PRACTICE

The clinical implications of these advances and future perspectives in techniques and technologies include the possibility of treating lesions in areas of difficult access within the skull base, brain, or even cervical spine, with less morbidity for patients. Endoscopic approaches should be considered in the surgical options for many pathologies of the ventral skull base.

IMPLICATIONS FOR RESEARCH

The implications for research are the continuous development of newer instruments and products to allow these procedures. Augmented reality, three-dimensional endoscopes, and robotic surgery are likely to lead to an advance. Additionally, a better understanding of the nasal physiology, especially after the resection of tumors using this access route, is still required.

REFERENCES

1. Snyderman CH, Pant H, Carrau RL, et al. What are the limits of endoscopic sinus surgery?: the expanded endonasal approach to the skull base. Keio J Med 2009; 58(3):152–60.
2. Harvey RJ, Nogueira JF, Schlosser RJ, et al. Closure of large skull base defects after endoscopic transnasal craniotomy. Clinical article. J Neurosurg 2009; 111(2):371–9.

3. Stamm AC, Vellutini E, Harvey RJ, et al. Endoscopic transnasal craniotomy and the resection of craniopharyngioma. Laryngoscope 2008;118(7):1142–8.
4. Kassam A, Snyderman CH, Mintz A, et al. Expanded endonasal approach: the rostrocaudal axis. Part I. Crista galli to the sella turcica. Neurosurg Focus 2005; 19:E3.
5. Kassam A, Snyderman CH, Mintz A, et al. Expanded endonasal approach: the rostrocaudal axis. Part II. Posterior clinoids to the foramen magnum. Neurosurg Focus 2005;19:E4.
6. Gandhi CD, Christiano LD, Eloy JA, et al. The historical evolution of transsphenoidal surgery: facilitation by technological advances. Neurosurg Focus 2009;27(3):E8.
7. Kennedy DW. Technical innovations and the evolution of endoscopic sinus surgery. Ann Otol Rhinol Laryngol Suppl 2006;196:3–12.
8. Banks CA, Palmer JN, Chiu AG, et al. Endoscopic closure of CSF rhinorrhea: 193 cases over 21 years. Otolaryngol Head Neck Surg 2009;140(6):826–33.
9. Prevedello DM, Doglietto F, Jane JA Jr, et al. History of endoscopic skull base surgery: its evolution and current reality. J Neurosurg 2007;107(1):206–13.
10. Doglietto F, Prevedello DM, Jane JA Jr, et al. Brief history of endoscopic transsphenoidal surgery–from Philipp Bozzini to the First World Congress of Endoscopic Skull Base Surgery. Neurosurg Focus 2005;19(6):E3.
11. Lee SC, Senior BA. Endoscopic skull base surgery. Clin Exp Otorhinolaryngol 2008;1(2):53–62.
12. Hadad G, Bassagasteguy L, Carrau RL, et al. A novel reconstructive technique after endoscopic expanded endonasal approaches: vascular pedicle nasoseptal flap. Laryngoscope 2006;116(10):1882–6.
13. El-Sayed IH, Roediger FC, Goldberg AN, et al. Endoscopic reconstruction of skull base defects with the nasal septal flap. Skull Base 2008;18(6):385–94.
14. Harvey RJ, Sheahan PO, Schlosser RJ. Inferior turbinate pedicle flap for endoscopic skull base defect repair. Am J Rhinol Allergy 2009;23(5):522–6.
15. Prevedello DM, Barges-Coll J, Fernandez-Miranda JC, et al. Middle turbinate flap for skull base reconstruction: cadaveric feasibility study. Laryngoscope 2009; 119(11):2094–8.
16. Zanation AM, Snyderman CH, Carrau RL, et al. Minimally invasive endoscopic pericranial flap: a new method for endonasal skull base reconstruction. Laryngoscope 2009;119(1):13–8.
17. Oliver CL, Hackman TG, Carrau RL, et al. Palatal flap modifications allow pedicled reconstruction of the skull base. Laryngoscope 2008;118(12):2102–6.
18. Stamm AC, Pignatari S, Vellutini E, et al. A novel approach allowing binostril work to the sphenoid sinus. Otolaryngol Head Neck Surg 2008;138(4):531–2.
19. Cavallo LM, Cappabianca P, Messina A, et al. The extended endoscopic endonasal approach to the clivus and craniovertebral junction: anatomical study. Childs Nerv Syst 2007;23(6):665–71.
20. Harvey RJ, Sheehan PO, Debnath NI, et al. Transseptal approach for extended endoscopic resections of the maxilla and infratemporal fossa. Am J Rhinol Allergy 2009;23(4):426–32.
21. Tabaee A, Anand VK, Fraser JF, et al. Three-dimensional endoscopic pituitary surgery. Neurosurgery 2009;64(5 Suppl 2):288–93.
22. Brown SM, Tabaee A, Singh A, et al. Three-dimensional endoscopic sinus surgery: feasibility and technical aspects. Otolaryngol Head Neck Surg 2008; 138(3):400–2.
23. Babatin MA. NOTES: evolving trends in endoscopic surgery. Saudi J Gastroenterol 2007;13(4):207–10.

24. Ukimura O, Gill IS. Image-fusion, augmented reality, and predictive surgical navigation. Urol Clin North Am 2009;36(2):115–23.
25. Thoranaghatte RU, Giraldez JG, Zheng G. Landmark based augmented reality endoscope system for sinus and skull-base surgeries. Conf Proc IEEE Eng Med Biol Soc 2008;2008:74–7.
26. O'Malley BW Jr, Weinstein GS. Robotic anterior and midline skull base surgery: preclinical investigations. Int J Radiat Oncol Biol Phys 2007;69(Suppl 2):S125–8.
27. Kupferman M, Demonte F, Holsinger FC, et al. Transantral robotic access to the pituitary gland. Otolaryngol Head Neck Surg 2009;141(3):413–5.

Evolving Materials and Techniques for Endoscopic Sinus Surgery

Frank W. Virgin, MD[a], Benjamin S. Bleier, MD[b],
Bradford A. Woodworth, MD[a,c],*

KEYWORDS

- Endoscopic sinus surgery • Skull base surgery
- Cerebrospinal fluid leak • Coblator • Hydrodebrider
- Hemostasis • Robotic surgery • Nasoseptal flap
- Nasal septal flap • Intracranial hypertension
- Laser tissue welding

HEMOSTATIC AGENTS

Hemostasis, both during and after endoscopic procedures, is critical for successful outcomes.[1,2] Intraoperative bleeding, especially in the setting of highly vascular sinonasal tumors and polyposis, remains a common pitfall in performing endoscopic sinus and skull base surgery. Although endoscopic bipolar forceps, suction cautery, and newer technologies, such as radiofrequency coblation, are indispensible for producing intraoperative hemostasis, various topical agents are also effective in controlling diffuse bleeding and, in some cases, also provide postoperative benefits.

Traditionally, nasal packing has been used in postoperative care but can have significant drawbacks. Packing can result in pain, rhinorrhea, infection, disturbance

Disclosures: Frank W. Virgin, MD has no financial disclosures or conflicts of interest. Bradford A. Woodworth, MD is a consultant for ArthroCare ENT and Gyrus ENT, and serves on the Speaker's Bureau for GlaxoSmithKline. Benjamin S. Bleir, MD is a co-inventor on LTW solder (09/18/09), Solder Formulation, and use in Tissue Welding U.S. Pat. Non-Provisional Filing (Docket V4914, PCT/US2009/057419, University of Pennsylvania).
[a] Division of Otolaryngology-Head and Neck Surgery, Department of Surgery, University of Alabama at Birmingham, BDB 563, 1530 3rd Avenue South, Birmingham, AL 35294, USA
[b] Division of Rhinology, Department of Otolaryngology-Head and Neck Surgery, Medical University of South Carolina, Charleston, SC 29425, USA
[c] Gregory Fleming James Cystic Fibrosis Research Center, University of Alabama at Birmingham, 790 McCallum Building, 1918 University Boulevard, Birmingham, AL 35294, USA
* Corresponding author. Division of Otolaryngology-Head and Neck Surgery, Department of Surgery, University of Alabama at Birmingham, BDB 563, 1530 3rd Avenue South, Birmingham, AL 35294.
E-mail address: bwoodwo@hotmail.com

Otolaryngol Clin N Am 43 (2010) 653–672
doi:10.1016/j.otc.2010.02.018
0030-6665/10/$ – see front matter © 2010 Elsevier Inc. All rights reserved.
oto.theclinics.com

of nasal breathing, sensation of intranasal and periorbital pressure, alar necrosis, sleep apnea, and epistaxis on removal.[3–7] Patients undergoing endoscopic sinus surgery, have reported packing and removal of packing to be the most uncomfortable portion of the perioperative experience.[6,8] Topical materials that have absorbable properties or aid with hemostasis have become increasingly popular to help improve patient comfort, obviate the need for removal, and assist with healing (**Table 1**). However, an ideal material has not been developed.

Topical Epinephrine

Epinephrine has been used as a hemostatic agent in surgical procedures for many years. It is inexpensive and easily applied to the surgical field, and has excellent hemostatic properties. However, it has the potential to cause severe complications, such as tachycardia, hypotension, hypertension, and cardiac arrhythmias.[9–11] Hypertension and tachycardia historically are the most commonly observed complications, especially combined with the use of volatile anesthetics such as halothane.[12] However, the combination of topical or injected epinephrine with newer anesthetics, either intravenous (eg, propofol) or volatile (eg, enflurane), has significantly reduced the occurrence of serious side effects.[13] Recently, use of topical epinephrine in endoscopic sinus and skull base surgery has experienced resurgence.

Despite obvious advantages, few studies have evaluated epinephrine's effects on blood loss, systemic levels from topical application, and the ideal concentration for topical use. In 2009, Sarmento Junior and colleagues[14] evaluated varying concentrations of topical adrenaline, including 1:2000, 1:10,000, and 1:50,000. The results of their prospective study showed that the 1:2000 group had a statistically significant decrease in blood loss (objective and subjective measures) and shorter operative

Table 1
Available absorbable hemostatic agents

Name/Trade Name	Composition	Hemostasis	Middle Meatus Stent	Scar Tissue Potential
FloSeal	Bovine gelatin particles + thrombin	Excellent	Fair	High
Surgiflo	Porcine gelatin	Good	Fair	Moderate
Merogel	Hyaluronic acid ester	Fair	Good	Low-high
Seprapack	Composite of hyaluron and carboxymethyl cellulose	Fair	Good	Low
Topical adrenaline	NA	Excellent	Poor	Low
Tranexamic acid (Cyklokapron)	NA	Fair	Poor	Low
Epsilon-aminocaproic acid (Amicar)	NA	Poor	Poor	Low
Microporous polysaccharide hemospheres	Purified potato starch	Good	Fair	Low

times. Plasma levels of epinephrine increased in all categories, but more sharply in the 1:2000. Although a trend was seen toward increasing blood pressure in the 1:2000 and 1:10,000 groups, this rise was slow and no adverse events were reported. The authors concluded that 1:2000 epinephrine provided superior hemostasis with minimal risk.

In another recent study, Cohen-Kerem and colleagues[15] evaluated the use of epinephrine/Lidocaine injection versus saline during endoscopic sinus surgery. They measured plasma epinephrine concentrations and surprisingly found that the saline injection group had higher levels 15 minutes after injection. Subjectively, the surgical field had more bleeding in the saline injected group, but the objective findings showed no statistical difference.

The authors' practice routinely uses epinephrine-soaked cotton pledgets to aid with hemostasis. Their preferred concentration is 1:1000, which has provided excellent hemostasis with limited side effects. Prospective trials of large cohorts evaluating ideal concentration and incidence of adverse events are warranted.

Other Topical Hemostatic Agents

In addition to topical epinephrine, numerous absorbable substances have been introduced to aid hemostasis in sinus and skull base surgery. Within the confines of the sinus and nasal cavities, ideal hemostatic agents must have several specific qualities. They must provide hemostasis, conform to an irregular wound bed, and enable healing of the traumatized mucosa without additional detriment to the epithelium. Traditional nasal packing has been substituted largely by absorbable materials designed to improve patient comfort and outcomes. Although many promising agents exist, none have become standard therapy.

Merogel (Medtronic-Xomed, Jacksonville, FL, USA) is a hyaluronic acid ester derivative. It has been used in functional endoscopic sinus surgery as a hemostatic agent and a middle meatal spacer. It was one of the first absorbable materials introduced and has become somewhat of a standard against which newer materials are compared.

In a prospective single-blind randomized control study in 2006, Wormald and colleagues[16] compared nasal cavities packed with Merogel versus no packing. They concluded that the Merogel nasal pack has no significant beneficial or detrimental effect in terms of synechia, edema, or infection when placed in the middle meatus after endoscopic sinus surgery. Recently, Berlucchi and colleagues[17] compared Merogel with traditional nasal packing and showed that Merogel was associated with an improved appearance during nasal endoscopy, fewer adhesions, and improved patient comfort. Merogel has clearly been shown to have no adverse effects on nasal mucosa when used after endoscopic sinus surgery; however, its benefits in terms of long-term outcomes are less apparent.

Sepragel (Genzyme Biosurgery, Cambridge, MA, USA) is a hylan B gel (cross-linked hyaluronic acid molecule) that can be injected into the nasal cavity after endoscopic sinus surgery. Good evidence of its hemostatic properties is not available, but it has been used as a resorbable packing to improve outcomes after endoscopic sinus surgery.

In a trial evaluating postoperative changes after ethmoidectomy with and without the application of Sepragel, Kimmelman and colleagues[18] showed that Sepragel application was associated with a decrease in middle meatal stenosis and synechiae formation, and improved appearance of the nasal mucosa. However, their patient sample size was small and no further studies have shown a clear benefit.

FloSeal (Baxter Healthcare Corporation, Fremont, CA, USA) is a paste of bovine gelatin particles combined with thrombin that can be injected into the sinus cavities. Multiple studies have shown the ability of FloSeal to create hemostasis. Reported bleeding cessation times range from 2.0 to 16.4 minutes.[19–21] When compared with Merogel, which is a nonabsorbable, highly porous, polyvinyl acetal sponge, intraoperative hemostasis was obtained within 3 minutes in both groups.[19]

In addition to its hemostatic properties, evidence shows that postoperative packing with FloSeal does not result in significant patient discomfort.[21] However, concern has been raised regarding increased formation of middle meatal adhesions. When severe, these can cause obstruction of sinus outflow tracts and require revision surgery.

In an initial series in 2003 and a follow-up in 2005 comparing FloSeal with thrombin-soaked gelfoam, Chandra and colleagues[22,23] found a significantly higher number of adhesions in the FloSeal group. Furthermore, in a retrospective analysis of patients who underwent middle turbinate medialization with or without the application of FloSeal, Shrime and colleagues[24] showed that FloSeal was associated with a statistically significant increase in the number of adhesions formed. Thus, solid evidence indicates that FloSeal aids in both intraoperative and postoperative hemostasis, but application of this product increases the risk for adhesion formation.

Surgiflo hemostatic matrix (Ethicon, Inc, West Sommerville, NJ, USA) is a sterile, absorbable porcine gelatin that is combined with Thrombin-JMI (King Pharmaceuticals, Inc, Bristol, TN, USA). The combination of the two materials results in a material that is injectable and conforms to an irregular wound bed. In 2009, Woodworth and colleagues[25] reported on a multicenter, prospective study evaluating success of achieving hemostasis within 10 minutes of Surgiflo application. The study population included patients undergoing primary or revision endoscopic sinus surgery. Bleeding was controlled within 10 minutes in 96.7% of cases and the mean total time to hemostasis was 61 seconds. At 30-day follow up, no evidence of synechiae, adhesions, or infections was seen. Surgiflo is an agent that seems to have very good hemostatic properties; however randomized, controlled trials with long-term follow-up are indicated.

Antifibrinolytics have been in widespread medical use since the 1970s.[26] Epsilon-aminocaproic acid (EACA; Amicar, Lederle Parenterals, Inc, Caroline, Puerto Rico, USA) and tranexamic acid (TA; Cyklokapron, Pfizer, Puurs, Belgium)[27] are pharmaceuticals that competitively bind to lysine-binding sites on plasminogen, preventing the binding of plasminogen to fibrin, its subsequent activation, and the transformation to plasmin. This action prevents fibrinolysis and stabilization of blood clots.[27]

In a study evaluating the hemostatic effects of EACA and TA during endoscopic sinus surgery, Athanasiadis and colleagues[28] applied both agents topically and documented bleeding using standardized videoendoscopy and grading scales. The administration of TA resulted in improved surgical field bleeding at 2, 4, 6, and 8 minutes. However, no significant improvements in surgical field bleeding were seen with EACA. No adverse events were reported with the use of either substance. The results of this limited experience warrant further trials to better determine the effects of TA in endoscopic sinus surgery.

Seprapak (Genzyme, Cambridge, MA, USA) contains a combination of hyaluronic acid and carboxymethyl cellulose. It is packaged as a solid wafer that is inserted into the middle meatus and converted into a gel with saline irrigation. A multicenter, randomized, controlled trial[29] compared Seprapak with no packing in a series of 53 patients undergoing surgery for chronic rhinosinusitis. The primary outcome measure was formation of adhesions. The results of this study showed no long-term difference in formation of adhesions between the groups. However, fewer adhesions at 2 weeks were seen in the Seprapak group, suggesting that packing with Seprapak may reduce the amount of postoperative debridement needed after endoscopic sinus surgery.

Microporous polysaccharide hemospheres (MPH; Medafor, Inc, Minneapolis, MN, USA) are particles produced from purified potato starch that act as a molecular sieve to quickly extract fluids from blood. This osmotic action causes the microporous particles to swell and concentrate serum proteins, platelets, and other formed elements on their surfaces, thereby generating scaffolding for fibrin clot formation. Additionally, MPH is fully resorbed and enzymatically cleared from the wound site within 24 to 48 hours.

In 2008, Antisdel and colleagues[30] published their evaluation of MPH versus FloSeal in the nasal mucosa of New Zealand white rabbits. In this study, the sinus and nasal mucosa was stripped and one side was treated with either FloSeal or MPH, and the other side served as an untreated control. After 2 weeks, animals were euthanized and the surgical site was examined grossly and histologically. The MPH-treated group showed no evidence of remaining substance, and histologically the mucosa resembled that of the untreated mucosa. In contrast, regenerating mucosa treated with FloSeal showed extensive loss of cilia, inflammation, and fibrosis. Residual FloSeal particles were present in the sinus cavity and grossly incorporated within healing mucosa. The results of this study introduced an exciting new material for potential use in endoscopic sinus surgery. Prospective, randomized trials are required to evaluate effects in a human population.

SURGICAL INSTRUMENTS

Arguably, improvements in instrumentation have had the greatest impact on the expansion of endoscopic procedures. Advances in optics and instrumentation have improved surgical outcomes in endoscopic sinus and nasal surgery for inflammatory disease and have allowed endoscopic applications for anterior skull base tumor removal. However, there is continually room for improvement and innovation in endoscopic surgical instrumentation. This article discusses several recent instruments that have evolving applications in endoscopic surgery of the sinus and nasal cavities.

Coblation

Radiofrequency coblation technology (the Coblator; ArthroCare ENT, Austin, TX, USA) was first introduced for use in otolaryngology for tonsil and turbinate surgery. This device uses a bipolar radiofrequency-based plasma process. Radiofrequency energy excites electrolytes in a conductive medium, such as saline, creating precisely focused plasma. The energized particles in the plasma have sufficient energy to break molecular bonds, excising or dissolving tissue at a relatively low temperature, thereby preserving the integrity of surrounding tissue.[31] In contrast to electrocautery, which operates at temperatures of 400°C to 600°C, the Coblator operates at between 40°C and 70°C.[32] Working at lower temperatures, the Coblator causes less collateral damage to surrounding tissues, and thus represents a potentially useful instrument within the confines of the sinus and nasal cavities.

The Coblator has shown clinical effectiveness in removing soft tissue within the sinus and nasal cavities, including adenoids, nasopharyngeal angiofibromas, sinonasal polyposis, and turbinate reduction.[33–36] Recently, Eloy and colleagues[37] investigated blood loss in endoscopic sinus surgery for nasal polyposis using traditional techniques compared with coblation. They found that coblation-assisted nasal polypectomy was associated with a statistically significant lower estimated blood loss and blood loss per minute when compared with the traditional microdebrider removal.

Although nasal polyps have been removed using endoscopy since the inception of endoscopic sinus surgery, sinonasal and anterior skull base neoplasms have traditionally been removed through open surgical approaches, such as a lateral rhinotomy and craniofacial resection. As expertise in using endoscopy to treat inflammatory disease has increased, a natural progression has occurred toward applying these techniques for removing sinonasal and skull base neoplasms.

One of the largest impediments to endoscopic removal of skull base neoplasms has been poor visualization secondary to inadequate control of intraoperative bleeding. Unfortunately, many sinonasal and skull base neoplasms have a robust vascular supply. Debulking these tumors facilitates visualization of tumor attachment sites and increases working space within the sinus cavities. In the past, the microdebrider has been an extremely effective instrument for debulking these tumors, but profuse bleeding is common. The characteristics of the Coblator allow removal of soft tissue and coagulation simultaneously, thus making it an ideal instrument for tumor debulking.

In the authors' experience, the Coblator has become an invaluable tool for tumor debulking in the sinus and nasal cavities. In a review of 23 patients who underwent endoscopic removal of sinonasal or skull base tumors, the coblation device was used in 10 patients (**Fig. 1**) and the microdebrider in the remaining cases (**Fig. 2**). Various data points were collected, including complications and blood loss. Additionally, full operative videoendoscopy was available for all cases and intraoperative bleeding scored using the 11-point Wormald Surgical Field Grading Scale. Findings showed that the Coblator was associated with significantly lower blood loss (350 vs 1000 mL; $P = .00001$), estimated blood loss divided by operative time (66 vs 166 mL/h; $P = .0001$), and Wormald grade (3.3 vs 6.4; $P = .0001$).[38]

In addition to tumor debulking and removal, the Coblator is an excellent tool for reducing and removing encephaloceles. A prospective evaluation of Coblator-assisted endoscopic removal of 13 encephaloceles in 11 patients compared with 7 encephaloceles reduced with traditional bipolar cautery showed that duration of removal was significantly lower in the Coblator group (21.5 vs 65.1 min; $P = .013$), with similar hemostatic properties.[39] Additionally, the authors are now using the Coblator to raise nasoseptal and turbinate flaps for skull base reconstruction.

The limitations of the Coblator are largely caused by the size of the wand and the saline delivery system. The function of the Coblator depends on the presence of a conductive medium. Often when using the device in the sinus and nasal cavities, especially the anterior skull base, the device must be held vertically. This positioning reduces the presence of the conductive medium and causes a reduction in the effectiveness of the device. In most instances this can be overcome by increasing the irrigation delivered. The size of the wand has not been an impediment for debulking

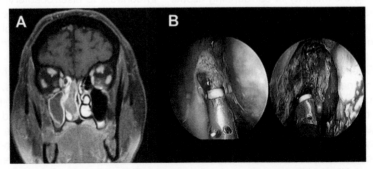

Fig. 1. (*A*) Coronal contrasted MRI showing a malignant melanoma of the skull base. (*B*) The same tumor after debulking using the Coblator.

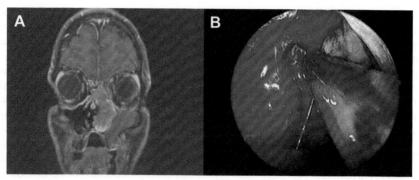

Fig. 2. (*A*) Coronal T1-weighted MRI shows a large esthesioneuroblastoma. (*B*) The bloody field generated by tumor debulking with the microdebrider.

tumors or nasal polyposis, but as the indications in the sinuses increase, designs will require even more specificity for endoscopic sinus procedures.

Hydrodebrider

Despite significant advances in surgical technology and technique, chronic rhinosinusitis remains difficult to control. Multiple studies have shown the presence of bacterial biofilms in patients with this condition.[40–43] Prevailing theories believe that the protection conferred to bacteria from encasing themselves in a self-produced exopolymeric matrix, called a biofilm, provides them with a method of evading host defenses and facilitates their successful colonization of the sinus and nasal cavities. The protection of the matrix results in strong antimicrobial resistance to conventional medical and surgical treatments.[44]

Methods for eliminating biofilms have become an active area of investigation. Chiu and colleagues[45] evaluated 1% baby shampoo irrigations in vitro and in a prospective clinical trial. Baby shampoo is a chemical surfactant that could theoretically reduce the surface tension of thick inspissated mucus, thereby facilitating its clearance, but also potentially break up biofilms from the detergent action. In vitro, 1% baby shampoo prevented the formation of new *Pseudomonas aeruginosa* biofilms, but did not eliminate preformed biofilms. Clinically, most patients noted an improvement in their symptoms. Other substances investigated include mupirocin, citric acid combined with a zwitterionic surfactant (CAZS), and gallium nitrate. All investigations have met with limited success.[44] In 2004, a comprehensive consensus document from five professional otorhinolaryngology societies (The American Academy of Allergy, Asthma and Immunology; the American Academy of Otolaryngic Allergy; the American Academy of Otolaryngology-Head and Neck Surgery; the American College of Allergy, Asthma and Immunology; and the American Rhinologic Society) suggested that elimination of biofilms in patients with chronic rhinosinusitis may require mechanical removal.[46]

In 2007, Desrosiers and colleagues[47] investigated several therapeutics for biofilm removal and their delivery under pressure. CAZS delivered under pressure resulted in the greatest clearance of biofilms in this model. Medtronic subsequently released the Hydrodebrider system as a method for mechanical removal of biofilms and other debris from the sinus and nasal cavities. The Hydrodebrider consists of an endoscopic suction irrigator with 270° articulation designed to apply irrigation under pressure during endoscopic sinus surgery.

Although initial in vitro studies were encouraging, benefit has not been established in clinical trials because an adequate chemical surfactant safe for human use has not been identified. Additionally, little evidence shows the device's long-term therapeutic benefit for chronic rhinosinusitis. However, the Hydrodebrider is currently being used to clear fungal mucin in individuals with allergic fungal rhinosinusitis and during revision surgery in patients with cystic fibrosis for removing purulent debris. Fungal debris or thick inspissated secretions can be eliminated with minimal trauma to the underlying sinonasal mucosa. Continuing investigations of chemical surfactants and the long-term benefits of this system are warranted.

Ultrasonic Aspirator

The ultrasonic aspirator has been used in neurosurgical procedures for the emulsification and removal of cerebellopontine angle tumors, such as acoustic neuromas. The device has also been used for intracranial lesions, such as gliomas, metastatic brain tumors, and meningiomas.[48,49] Intraoral procedures such as tongue reduction and tumor resection are also described.[48–51] The ultrasonic aspirator performs tissue dissection through the ultrahigh frequency movement of the handpiece tip, removing soft tissue and bone through varying the frequency and power.[52,53]

In 2007, Samy and colleagues[52,53] reported on using the ultrasonic aspirator to decompress the facial nerve in cadaveric models. Because the instrument does not rotate like a standard otologic burr, it is less likely to cause tissue damage to surrounding nerve or dura. Although the tissue removal properties could make its use desirable in the sinus and nasal cavities, applicability has been difficult secondary to instrument design.

In 2003, Yamasaki and colleagues[54] reported on a new handpiece designed by Sonopet (M and M Co, Ltd, Tokyo, Japan). The new design was used successfully in transsphenoidal surgery. Despite their initial reports, this device has not become a standard instrument in transsphenoidal surgery. Because it is able to remove various tissue types, including bone, the ultrasonic aspirator deserves further investigation in endoscopic sinus and skull base surgery.

SURGICAL MANAGEMENT

Techniques in endoscopic sinus surgery have changed in many ways since the inception of nasal endoscopy in the late 1970s and early 1980s. A broad range of procedures are now available, such as minimally invasive sinus techniques with or without balloon sinuplasty, functional endoscopic sinus surgery, and nasalization. The breadth and controversies of these are covered in other articles. This article discusses the cutting-edge methods for the endoscopic management of cerebrospinal fluid leaks.

Endoscopic repair of cerebrospinal fluid leaks has been a well-accepted technique over the past 20 years and has become the gold standard, with success rates greater than 90% quoted in numerous patient series.[55–60] Cerebrospinal fluid leaks have multiple causes, but most are broadly classified into traumatic (including accidental and iatrogenic), tumor, spontaneous, and congenital origins. As experience with endoscopic repair of cerebrospinal fluid leaks has increased, it has become clear that the cause of the leak greatly affects successful outcomes.

Management of Elevated Intracranial Pressure

In the subset of patients who have been defined as having spontaneous cerebrospinal fluid leaks, the success rate of endoscopic repair has ranged from 25% to 87%, far below the rates associated with other types of leaks.[61–65] Prior studies have shown that the spontaneous origin most often represents a variant of benign intracranial hypertension (BIH), according to modified Dandy criteria.[66] Clinical, radiographic, and intracranial pressure (ICP) data for the most rigid diagnosis of BIH show that more than 70% of patients with spontaneous leaks meet the diagnosis for BIH. Additionally, prior studies have shown direct evidence of elevated ICP in most patients with spontaneous cerebrospinal fluid leaks, either through obtaining an opening pressure during lumbar tap or monitoring of lumbar cerebrospinal fluid pressure in the postoperative period.[64,66,67]

Management of increased ICP is now known to be crucial for obtaining successful outcomes when repairing spontaneous cerebrospinal fluid leaks endoscopically. Schlosser and colleagues[64] outlined a method for postoperative monitoring and management of elevated ICP in 2004. Lumbar drains are typically placed in all patients with a diagnosis of spontaneous cerebrospinal fluid leaks before repair. The catheter is left in place and postoperatively allowed to drain at a rate of 5 to 10 mL/h. On the second postoperative day the drain is stopped and 3 to 4 hours is allowed to pass to allow cerebrospinal fluid to accumulate.

At this point, the ICP is measured. If the ICP is elevated, then medical treatment in the form of acetazolamide is recommended. If ICPs are significantly elevated (>30–35 cm H_2O), or response to the diuretic is inadequate (<10 cm H_2O), then neurosurgical consultation is sought for consideration of ventriculoperitoneal shunting. In patients with a good diuretic response, the lumbar drain is removed and the patients are started on an oral diuretic.

Woodworth and colleagues[68] reported on their experience with repair of spontaneous cerebrospinal fluid leaks in 2007. Through addressing the elevated pressures at repair using the protocol outlined in the prior study, they were able to achieve a success rate of 89% with first repair and 95% long-term, which approaches the success rate for cerebrospinal fluid leaks of other origins.[68]

Through addressing the elevated ICP in spontaneous CSF leaks, rates of control are similar to those for other causes. Although follow-up data in these studies are as long as 3 years, long-term results are unclear, especially in patients managed with medical treatment alone. Additionally, noninvasive methods of ICP monitoring should be developed for long-term follow-up, which could be applicable to anyone with intracranial hypertension.

Locating Skull Base Defect Site

Endoscopic identification of a cerebrospinal fluid leak is critical in obtaining successful closure. This task can be obvious in the setting of a skull base tumor resection and resultant defect, or can be very challenging in the setting of spontaneous cerebrospinal fluid leaks with the potential to have multiple sites of leakage.

In addition to identifying the leak, methods that show successful closure can also be very useful. Many techniques for identifying the site of leak have been discussed in the literature. One recent method uses high-resolution computerized tomography (HRCT) and intraoperative image guidance systems.[69] The other is the use of intrathecal fluorescein, which has become a time tested strategy that not only allows for the identification of the cerebrospinal fluid leak but also provides intraoperative confirmation of leak repair.

Fluorescein imparts its fluorescent properties to cerebrospinal fluid after intrathecal injection and facilitates identification of skull base defects.[70–75] Although generally considered safe, seizures, radicular symptoms, transient paraparesis or hemiparesis, and myelopathy have been reported.[71,72,76,77] Furthermore, the use of fluorescein for this purpose is not approved by the U.S. Food and Drug Administration, and therefore obtaining informed consent is recommended.

Multiple series have reported extensive experience with intrathecal fluorescein with a very acceptable safety profile.[68,70–74,78,79] A mixture of 0.1 mL of 10% fluorescein diluted in 10 mL of the patient's cerebrospinal fluid or sterile saline (concentrations well below those associated with complications) injected slowly over 10 to 15 minutes has been used for 2 decades with excellent safety (**Fig. 3**), with only one known minor complication reported (a heart arrhythmia that stopped after 24 hours).[65,80] This injection enables accurate identification of cerebrospinal fluid leaks and allows visual confirmation of intraoperative leak cessation after repair.

Laser Tissue Welding

Laser tissue welding (LTW) is a novel technique that uses a biologic solder to produce endoscopic tissue bonds capable of withstanding pressures up to four times those of normal human ICP. Previously described liquid solders have several drawbacks, including gravitational sedimentation, rapid dilution, and the inability to bridge tissue gaps. A new class of polysaccharide-based soldering gels is under investigation that may overcome these obstacles and improve the clinical effectiveness of this technology.

Because transnasal endoscopic surgery has expanded to involve the resection of anterior skull base and intracranial lesions, novel techniques must be developed to reconstruct the resultant defects that may be complicated by postoperative cerebrospinal fluid leaks. LTW has been investigated as an innovative method of skull base repair that is capable of producing tissue bonds that withstand burst pressures exceeding those of human ICP.[81]

The concept of using laser energy to adhere tissue edges was first introduced in 1966 by Yahr and Strully.[82] These bonds relied on the direct transfer of thermal energy from the laser source to the extracellular matrix and were therefore associated with significant local tissue destruction.

Biologic solder materials coupled with wavelength-specific chromophores were introduced in response to these disappointing early results. These materials concentrate the thermal energy within the solder itself, thereby preserving the surrounding

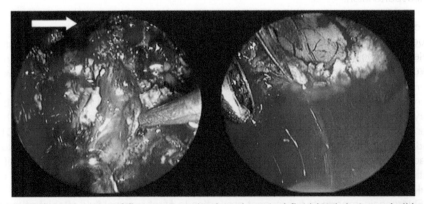

Fig. 3. Endoscopic views of fluorescein-stained cerebrospinal fluid (CSF) during a skull base resection. The right frontal sinus posterior table is illustrated with the arrow to allow for orientation (*left*). The green staining of pooled CSF at the posterior limit of the resection below the planum sphenoidale is shown (*right*).

tissue and resulting in a tissue bond with higher burst strengths than wounds sealed with laser energy alone.[83] The chromophore also has a secondary benefit of providing an objective gauge of the adequacy of the lasing through a predictable color change.[84]

The most extensively studied biologic solder has been an albumin, hyaluronic acid, and indocyanine green solution that maximally absorbs laser energy delivered by an 808-nm diode laser.[85–87] This combination was used in the first human study by Kirsch and colleagues,[84] who reported significantly higher leak threshold pressures in solder-reinforced ureteral incisions than in suture alone (94.2 ± 24.2 mm Hg vs 20.0 ± 2.9 mm Hg; $P<.001$). The bonds produced by this laser/solder platform were also studied previously in rabbit sinonasal mucosa, which showed that when using a bridging graft in a dry bed, LTW can produce welds with burst strengths far exceeding human ICP.[81]

Despite these promising results, clinical investigations have been impeded by several significant drawbacks of the hyaluronic acid solder formulation. As a solution, the solder is subject to gravitational displacement and is rapidly diluted by bleeding or irrigation that are both commonly encountered in active surgical fields.

Another disadvantage is the inability to bridge small gaps at the wound edge. After lasing, a thin denatured albumin matrix remains that lacks the internal stability to maintain the weld integrity without underlying tissue for support. Clinically, areas for which complete tissue apposition is difficult to achieve become potential points of failure with this traditional solder formulation.

These disadvantages have catalyzed investigations into a novel polysaccharide-based solder that may be able to produce superior tissue welds while overcoming the significant problems associated with the hyaluronic acid–based solution. These solders are capable of forming polymeric gels that resist dilution and have considerable intrinsic stability, allowing them to bridge gaps at the wound edge. Furthermore, these gels enable maximal concentration of the chromophore through a pH-dependent precipitation reaction, thereby enhancing the overall lasing efficiency. This new class of biologic soldering gels may overcome the drawbacks of traditional liquid solders and are currently the basis of further investigations.

The ability to produce instant transnasal tissue bonds capable of withstanding pulsatile hydrostatic intracranial pressures has enormous implications in the field of endoscopic anterior skull base surgery. This technology has the potential to obviate the need for lumbar drain placement, dramatically reduce hospital stay, and expand the current boundaries of transnasal endoscopic skull base resections. A novel class of polysaccharide-based soldering gels that may be able to produce these repairs while obviating the limitations of previously described liquid solder formulations is currently under investigation (**Fig. 4**).

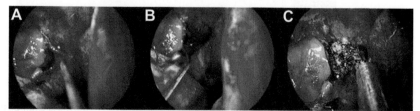

Fig. 4. Endoscopic laser tissue welding of the right maxillary sinus. (*A*) Region of mucosal disruption in posterior fontanelle. (*B*) Application of liquid albumin based solder. (*C*) Application of laser energy resulting in a stable lased coagulum.

Nasal Septal Flaps and Bone Grafts

Skull base defects created by tumor resection, trauma, or spontaneous defects require closure using various techniques. In addition to the size of the defect, other factors that affect successful closure include location of the defect and the presence of elevated ICPs. Various grafting materials have been used in the past with enormous success, including autologous tissue transfer in the form of fascia and fat grafts and various synthetic materials.[88–90] Because of larger defects derived from endoscopic skull base resections and the current understanding of elevated ICPs in patients experiencing spontaneous cerebrospinal fluid leaks, the need for vascularized tissue and more rigid material for grafting to withstand higher ICPs has become apparent. Pedicled nasoseptal flaps and cranial or septal bone grafts have partially filled this void.

In 2006, Hadad and colleagues[91] introduced the pedicled nasoseptal flap based on the septal branch of the sphenopalatine artery. Since its introduction, several authors have published on the successful use of this flap to repair skull base defects of various origins (traumatic, spontaneous, and posttumor resection).[91–95] In these reports, skull base repairs were largely limited to the middle and posterior portions of the anterior skull base.

In their study on the use of the nasoseptal flap in pediatric patients, Shah and colleagues[95] reported data suggesting that this flap was limited by the size of the septum and that its use should be avoided in children younger than 10 years because of the paucity of tissue for rotation available in this group.

The authors' group prospectively collected data on using the pedicled nasoseptal flap for repairing skull base defects involving the frontal sinus (Woodworth BA, unpublished data, 2010). In this study, 12 patients (average age, 49 years) underwent nasoseptal flap reconstruction for spontaneous cerebrospinal fluid leaks (n = 6), tumor resection (n = 5), and traumatic cerebrospinal fluid leaks (n = 1). Average defect size (length vs width) was 21 × 15 mm and average length involving the posterior table was 12.5 mm (6–30 mm). Average follow-up was 30 weeks (2–48 weeks). Satisfactory coverage was obtained in 11 of 12 patients. The one patient who had insufficient overlay of the frontal sinus portion of the defect had decreased flap length from a prior septal perforation. The authors' experience showed that this pedicled flap is useful for repairing even the most anteriorly based defects (3 cm) in the appropriately selected patient (**Fig. 5**).

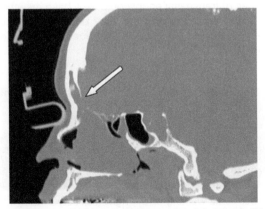

Fig. 5. Sagittal computed tomography scan showing a frontal sinus skull base defect successfully repaired using a pedicled nasal septal flap.

Patients with large defects and those with cerebrospinal fluid leaks in the setting of elevated ICP require special attention and often more rigid grafting materials. In 2003, Bolger and McLaughlin[96] described their experience with the use of cranial bone grafts, finding that the cranial bone stock provided an excellent material that could be easily molded and placed. In 20 patients, all grafts were successfully incorporated into the repair and all defect repairs were intact at follow-up. Other investigators also have had excellent success with septal bone grafts.[80] The use of vascularized tissue and bone grafts has improved the ability to repair even the most challenging defects.

INTRAOPERATIVE COMPUTED TOMOGRAPHY AND IMAGE GUIDANCE SYSTEM

Surgical navigation initially became available in the 1980s. Early intraoperative CT imaging was performed using a CT-dependent frame that served as fiducial markers for the computer during neurosurgical procedures.[97] However, this technique was abandoned because of the impractical nature of using large CT scanners in the operating room and the large doses of radiation required for image acquisition. Images acquired preoperatively and applied to stereotactic navigation systems intraoperatively has become the standard in sinus and skull base surgery. The current systems provide excellent detail of anatomic variations and anatomic changes after prior surgical procedures. However, one drawback of these systems is that the images are obtained preoperatively and the navigation system gives no real-time information during the surgical procedure.

The xCAT (Xoran Technologies, Ann Arbor, MI, USA) is a compact, portable volume CT scanner that can provide 0.4-mm thick images of the paranasal sinuses in less than 3 minutes. When coupled with existing surgical navigation systems, the xCAT can provide real-time surgical updates. This system uses cone beam technology, which reduces the amount of radiation exposure. The effective radiation dose is as low as 0.25 mSv, whereas the radiation dose from a standard CT is on average 10 times higher.[98] The xCAT has been used in both sinus and skull base surgery for real-time updates of image guidance systems.[99,100]

Revision sinus surgery, especially revision surgery for frontal sinus disease, can be very challenging. Additionally, large anterior skull base tumors, both benign and malignant, are being addressed using endoscopic techniques. Real-time intraoperative CT provides the surgeon with verification of surgical completeness and could prove to be an invaluable tool in endoscopic sinus and skull base surgery.

ROBOTIC SKULL BASE SURGERY

Over the past decade a generalized trend has been seen toward more minimally invasive surgical approaches in all surgical specialties. Robotic-assisted surgery has continued to grow in multiple specialties, including urology, cardiac surgery, gynecology, and, most recently, minimally invasive head and neck.[101–104] Several series have shown the effectiveness of transoral robotic surgery in the management of oral cavity, oropharynx, and supraglottic lesions.[102,105] The benefits of the robot include three-dimensional visualization and the ability to use two-handed techniques through small openings. In the setting of head and neck surgery, this has allowed resection of tumors that previously required highly morbid approaches.

Although treatment of skull base pathology using endoscopic techniques is minimally invasive, several limitations have been encountered. Endoscopes, although greatly improved since their first introduction, only provide a two-dimensional visual field. Additionally, endoscopic resection of skull base tumors requires surgeons to use one hand to control the endoscope and the other for instrumentation.

If robotic technology could be applied to surgery of the skull base, this would improve visualization and enable two-handed techniques. Several centers have performed early feasibility studies on the use of robotic surgery on the skull base. In 2007, O'Malley and colleagues[106] performed a feasibility study on the use of transoral robotic surgery for the parapharyngeal space and infratemporal fossa. They were able to transfer their technique from a preclinical cadaver model to a human subject. However, their experience in cadaver and canine models has shown that access to the midline and anterior skull base was not possible through a purely transoral approach. Through modifying their technique and placing trocars transcervically, they were able to gain access to these areas and successfully perform a series of procedures.[107]

Hanna and colleagues[108] developed a different approach that allowed them to access to the anterior and mid-line skull base and perform two-handed watertight dural closure. In their cadaver experiments, they used bilateral Caldwell-Luc antrostomies, traditional maxillary antrostomies, and a septectomy to gain access to the skull base. These preclinical feasibility studies have established that the skull base is accessible using robotic technology. The applicability of this technology will grow as smaller robotic instruments are developed.

IMPLICATIONS FOR RESEARCH

Endoscopic sinus surgery has expanded and evolved as a result of the advances in materials, technology, and techniques over the past 10 to 20 years; however, further research is still needed. Hemostatic agents are widely used in sinus surgery, but each agent has benefits and limitations requiring continued evaluation in large-scale randomized trials. Comparing hemostatic properties and the long-term effects of these agents is necessary to establish the best formulations to use in patient care.

New technologies in surgical instrumentation, such as the Coblator and ultrasonic aspirator, have the potential to expand the indications for endoscopic surgery. Surgeon and industry collaborations are necessary to advance current equipment designs and explore novel technology aimed at solving these limitations. Although the Hydrodebrider shows promise, future investigations and designs of efficacious surfactants that are safe for human use are required to help reduce the presence of mucosal biofilms in chronic rhinosinusitis. In the future, robotic surgery could revolutionize the field of endoscopic sinus and skull base surgery to allow surgeries to be performed with extreme precision, fewer complications, and improved outcomes. However, robotic surgery for these indications is still in its infancy and requires further feasibility studies, development of miniaturized instrumentation, and eventually extensive human trials. Unlike robotics, intraoperative CT scanning, although available, is currently limited by additional cost and lack of widespread applicability.

Management of intracranial hypertension in individuals with spontaneous cerebrospinal fluid leaks has improved successful repair rates. However, the optimal long-term monitoring and management of these patients remains unclear. Laser tissue welding technology promises to improve wound strength and improve the ability to repair cerebrospinal fluid leaks. Clinical trials are required to evaluate the short- and long-term effectiveness of tissue welding and further delineate the limitations of this technique.

IMPLICATIONS FOR CLINICAL PRACTICE

Endoscopic sinus and skull base surgery is a field rife with technological progress. Although hemostasis within the confines of the sinus and nasal cavities has continued to be a limitation of endoscopic procedures, topical epinephrine and other novel topical hemostatic agents have shown promise in decreasing intraoperative bleeding and, thus, improving surgical field visualization. Innovations in instrumentation have allowed increased expertise in endoscopic sinus and skull base surgical procedures. The Coblator provides excellent hemostatic properties and tissue removal. The Hydrodebrider currently is effective in managing chronic sinusitis in patients with cystic fibrosis and in treating allergic fungal sinusitis. Progress with bone grafts, pedicled vascularized flaps, and, potentially, laser tissue welding has improved the success in repairing large and anteriorly based skull base defects. Additionally, understanding of the role increased ICP plays in the successful repair of cerebrospinal fluid leaks has enabled most to be closed using endoscopic techniques. Finally, robotic surgery is an exciting new frontier that will likely expand minimally invasive treatment of benign and malignant disease of the sinuses and anterior skull base in the near future.

REFERENCES

1. Kennedy DW. Technical innovations and the evolution of endoscopic sinus surgery. Ann Otol Rhinol Laryngol Suppl 2006;196:3–12.
2. Senior BA, Kennedy DW, Tanabodee J, et al. Long-term results of functional endoscopic sinus surgery. Laryngoscope 1998;108(2):151–7.
3. Civelek B, Kargi AE, Sensoz O, et al. Rare complication of nasal packing: alar region necrosis. Otolaryngol Head Neck Surg 2000;123(5):656–7.
4. Johannessen N, Jensen PF, Kristensen S, et al. Nasal packing and nocturnal oxygen desaturation. Acta Otolaryngol Suppl 1992;492:6–8.
5. Vaiman M, Eviatar E, Shlamkovich N, et al. Use of fibrin glue as a hemostatic in endoscopic sinus surgery. Ann Otol Rhinol Laryngol 2005;114(3):237–41.
6. von Schoenberg M, Robinson P, Ryan R. Nasal packing after routine nasal surgery–is it justified? J Laryngol Otol 1993;107(10):902–5.
7. Weber R, Hochapfel F, Draf W. Packing and stents in endonasal surgery. Rhinology 2000;38(2):49–62.
8. Kao NL. Endoscopic sinus. Arch Otolaryngol Head Neck Surg 1995;121(7):814–5.
9. Anderhuber W, Walch C, Nemeth E, et al. Plasma adrenaline concentrations during functional endoscopic sinus surgery. Laryngoscope 1999;109(2 Pt 1):204–7.
10. van Hasselt CA, Low JM, Waldron J, et al. Plasma catecholamine levels following topical application versus infiltration of adrenaline for nasal surgery. Anaesth Intensive Care 1992;20(3):332–6.
11. Yang JJ, Wang QP, Wang TY, et al. Marked hypotension induced by adrenaline contained in local anesthetic. Laryngoscope 2005;115(2):348–52.
12. O'Malley TP, Postma GN, Holtel M, et al. Effect of local epinephrine on cutaneous bloodflow in the human neck. Laryngoscope 1995;105(2):140–3.
13. John G, Low JM, Tan PE, et al. Plasma catecholamine levels during functional endoscopic sinus surgery. Clin Otolaryngol Allied Sci 1995;20(3):213–5.
14. Sarmento KM Jr, Tomita S, Kos AO. Topical use of adrenaline in different concentrations for endoscopic sinus surgery. Braz J Otorhinolaryngol 2009;75(2):280–9.
15. Cohen-Kerem R, Brown S, Villasenor LV, et al. Epinephrine/Lidocaine injection vs. saline during endoscopic sinus surgery. Laryngoscope 2008;118(7):1275–81.

16. Wormald PJ, Boustred RN, Le T, et al. A prospective single-blind randomized controlled study of use of hyaluronic acid nasal packs in patients after endoscopic sinus surgery. Am J Rhinol 2006;20(1):7–10.

17. Berlucchi M, Castelnuovo P, Vincenzi A, et al. Endoscopic outcomes of resorbable nasal packing after functional endoscopic sinus surgery: a multicenter prospective randomized controlled study. Eur Arch Otorhinolaryngol 2009; 266(6):839–45.

18. Kimmelman CP, Edelstein DR, Cheng HJ. Sepragel sinus (hylan B) as a postsurgical dressing for endoscopic sinus surgery. Otolaryngol Head Neck Surg 2001; 125(6):603–8.

19. Baumann A, Caversaccio M. Hemostasis in endoscopic sinus surgery using a specific gelatin-thrombin based agent (FloSeal). Rhinology 2003;41(4):244–9.

20. Gall RM, Witterick IJ, Shargill NS, et al. Control of bleeding in endoscopic sinus surgery: use of a novel gelatin-based hemostatic agent. J Otolaryngol 2002; 31(5):271–4.

21. Jameson M, Gross CW, Kountakis SE. FloSeal use in endoscopic sinus surgery: effect on postoperative bleeding and synechiae formation. Am J Otol 2006; 27(2):86–90.

22. Chandra RK, Conley DB, Haines GK 3rd, et al. Long-term effects of FloSeal packing after endoscopic sinus surgery. Am J Rhinol 2005;19(3):240–3.

23. Chandra RK, Conley DB, Kern RC. The effect of FloSeal on mucosal healing after endoscopic sinus surgery: a comparison with thrombin-soaked gelatin foam. Am J Rhinol 2003;17(1):51–5.

24. Shrime MG, Tabaee A, Hsu AK, et al. Synechia formation after endoscopic sinus surgery and middle turbinate medialization with and without FloSeal. Am J Rhinol 2007;21(2):174–9.

25. Woodworth BA, Chandra RK, LeBenger JD, et al. A gelatin-thrombin matrix for hemostasis after endoscopic sinus surgery. Am J Otol 2009;30(1):49–53.

26. Wellington K, Wagstaff AJ. Tranexamic acid: a review of its use in the management of menorrhagia. Drugs 2003;63(13):1417–33.

27. Mannucci PM. Hemostatic drugs. N Engl J Med 1998;339(4):245–53.

28. Athanasiadis T, Beule AG, Wormald PJ. Effects of topical antifibrinolytics in endoscopic sinus surgery: a pilot randomized controlled trial. Am J Rhinol 2007;21(6):737–42.

29. Woodworth BA, Chandra RK, Hoy MJ, et al. The Seprapak dressing after endoscopic sinus surgery: a randomized, controlled trial. ORL J Otorhinolaryngol Relat Spec, in press.

30. Antisdel JL, Janney CG, Long JP, et al. Hemostatic agent microporous polysaccharide hemospheres (MPH) does not affect healing or intact sinus mucosa. Laryngoscope 2008;118(7):1265–9.

31. Chinpairoj S, Feldman MD, Saunders JC, et al. A comparison of monopolar electrosurgery to a new multipolar electrosurgical system in a rat model. Laryngoscope 2001;111(2):213–7.

32. Palmer JM. Bipolar radiofrequency for adenoidectomy. Otolaryngol Head Neck Surg 2006;135(2):323–4.

33. Carney AS, Timms MS, Marnane CN, et al. Radiofrequency coblation for the resection of head and neck malignancies. Otolaryngol Head Neck Surg 2008; 138(1):81–5.

34. Douglas R, Wormald PJ. Endoscopic surgery for juvenile nasopharyngeal angiofibroma: where are the limits? Curr Opin Otolaryngol Head Neck Surg 2006;14(1):1–5.

35. Glade RS, Pearson SE, Zalzal GH, et al. Coblation adenotonsillectomy: an improvement over electrocautery technique? Otolaryngol Head Neck Surg 2006;134(5):852–5.
36. Lee JY, Lee JD. Comparative study on the long-term effectiveness between coblation- and microdebrider-assisted partial turbinoplasty. Laryngoscope 2006; 116(5):729–34.
37. Eloy JA, Walker TJ, Casiano RR, et al. Effect of coblation polypectomy on estimated blood loss in endoscopic sinus surgery. Am J Rhinol Allergy 2009;23(5): 535–9.
38. Kostrzewa JP, Sunde J, Riley KO, et al. Radiofrequency coblation decreases blood loss during endoscopic sinonasal and skull base tumor removal. ORL J Otorhinolaryngol Relat Spec 2010;72(1):38–43.
39. Smith NJ, Riley KO, Woodworth BA. Endoscopic coblator-assisted management of encephaloceles: a prospective study. Otolaryngol Head Neck Surg, in press.
40. Ferguson BJ, Stolz DB. Demonstration of biofilm in human bacterial chronic rhinosinusitis. Am J Rhinol 2005;19(5):452–7.
41. Ramadan HH. Chronic rhinosinusitis and bacterial biofilms. Curr Opin Otolaryngol Head Neck Surg 2006;14(3):183–6.
42. Sanclement JA, Webster P, Thomas J, et al. Bacterial biofilms in surgical specimens of patients with chronic rhinosinusitis. Laryngoscope 2005;115(4): 578–82.
43. Sanderson AR, Leid JG, Hunsaker D. Bacterial biofilms on the sinus mucosa of human subjects with chronic rhinosinusitis. Laryngoscope 2006;116(7): 1121–6.
44. Le T, Psaltis A, Tan LW, et al. The efficacy of topical antibiofilm agents in a sheep model of rhinosinusitis. Am J Rhinol 2008;22(6):560–7.
45. Chiu AG, Palmer JN, Woodworth BA, et al. Baby shampoo nasal irrigations for the symptomatic post-functional endoscopic sinus surgery patient. Am J Rhinol 2008;22(1):34–7.
46. Meltzer EO, Hamilos DL, Hadley JA, et al. Rhinosinusitis: establishing definitions for clinical research and patient care. J Allergy Clin Immunol 2004;114(Suppl 6): 155–212.
47. Desrosiers M, Myntti M, James G. Methods for removing bacterial biofilms: in vitro study using clinical chronic rhinosinusitis specimens. Am J Rhinol 2007; 21(5):527–32.
48. Inoue T, Ikezaki K, Sato Y. Ultrasonic surgical system (SONOPET) for microsurgical removal of brain tumors. Neurol Res 2000;22(5):490–4.
49. Nagasawa S, Shimano H, Kuroiwa T. [Ultrasonic aspirator with controllable suction system–variable action suction adapter and clinical experience with it]. No Shinkei Geka 2000;28(12):1083–5 [in Japanese].
50. Yura S, Kato T, Ooi K, et al. Oral tumor resection and salivary duct relocation with an ultrasonic surgical aspirator. J Craniofac Surg 2009;20(4):1250–1.
51. Yura S, Kato T, Ooi K, et al. Tongue reduction techniques with an ultrasonic surgical aspirator. J Oral Maxillofac Surg 2009;67(7):1568–71.
52. Samy RN, Krishnamoorthy K, Pensak ML. Use of a novel ultrasonic surgical system for decompression of the facial nerve. Laryngoscope 2007;117(5): 872–5.
53. Sivak-Callcott JA, Linberg JV, Patel S. Ultrasonic bone removal with the Sonopet Omni: a new instrument for orbital and lacrimal surgery. Arch Ophthalmol 2005; 123(11):1595–7.

54. Yamasak T, Moritake K, Nagai H, et al. A new, miniature ultrasonic surgical aspirator with a handpiece designed for transsphenoidal surgery. Technical note. J Neurosurg 2003;99(1):177–9.

55. Gassner HG, Ponikau JU, Sherris DA, et al. CSF rhinorrhea: 95 consecutive surgical cases with long term follow-up at the Mayo Clinic. Am J Rhinol 1999; 13(6):439–47.

56. Mattox DE, Kennedy DW. Endoscopic management of cerebrospinal fluid leaks and cephaloceles. Laryngoscope 1990;100(8):857–62.

57. Schick B, Ibing R, Brors D, et al. Long-term study of endonasal duraplasty and review of the literature. Ann Otol Rhinol Laryngol 2001;110(2):142–7.

58. Woodworth BA, Schlosser RJ, Palmer JN. Endoscopic repair of frontal sinus cerebrospinal fluid leaks. J Laryngol Otol 2005;119(9):709–13.

59. Woodworth BA, Neal JG, Schlosser RJ. Sphenoid sinus cerebrospinal fluid leads. Op Tech Otolaryngol 2006;17:37–42.

60. Woodworth BA, Schlosser RJ. Repair of anterior skull base defects and CSF leaks. Op Tech Otolaryngol 2006;18:111–6.

61. Hubbard JL, McDonald TJ, Pearson BW, et al. Spontaneous cerebrospinal fluid rhinorrhea: evolving concepts in diagnosis and surgical management based on the Mayo Clinic experience from 1970 through 1981. Neurosurgery 1985;16(3): 314–21.

62. Schlosser RJ, Bolger WE. Spontaneous nasal cerebrospinal fluid leaks and empty sella syndrome: a clinical association. Am J Rhinol 2003;17(2):91–6.

63. Schlosser RJ, Bolger WE. Significance of empty sella in cerebrospinal fluid leaks. Otolaryngol Head Neck Surg 2003;128(1):32–8.

64. Schlosser RJ, Wilensky EM, Grady MS, et al. Cerebrospinal fluid pressure monitoring after repair of cerebrospinal fluid leaks. Otolaryngol Head Neck Surg 2004;130(4):443–8.

65. Banks C, Palmer JN, Chiu AG, et al. Endoscopic closure of CSF rhinorrhea: 193 cases over 21 years. Otolaryngol Head Neck Surg 2009;140(6):826–33.

66. Schlosser RJ, Woodworth BA, Wilensky EM, et al. Spontaneous cerebrospinal fluid leaks: a variant of benign intracranial hypertension. Ann Otol Rhinol Laryngol 2006;115(7):495–500.

67. Schlosser RJ, Wilensky EM, Grady MS, et al. Elevated intracranial pressures in spontaneous cerebrospinal fluid leaks. Am J Rhinol 2003;17(4):191–5.

68. Woodworth BA, Prince A, Chiu AG, et al. Spontaneous CSF leaks: a paradigm for definitive repair and management of intracranial hypertension. Otolaryngol Head Neck Surg 2008;138(6):715–20.

69. Zuckerman JD, DelGaudio JM. Utility of preoperative high-resolution CT and intraoperative image guidance in identification of cerebrospinal fluid leaks for endoscopic repair. Am J Rhinol 2008;22(2):151–4.

70. Gehrking E, Wisst F, Remmert S, et al. Intraoperative assessment of perilymphatic fistulas with intrathecal administration of fluorescein. Laryngoscope 2002;112(9):1614–8.

71. Keerl R, Weber RK, Draf W, et al. Use of sodium fluorescein solution for detection of cerebrospinal fluid fistulas: an analysis of 420 administrations and reported complications in Europe and the United States. Laryngoscope 2004; 114(2):266–72.

72. Locatelli D, Rampa F, Acchiardi I, et al. Endoscopic endonasal approaches for repair of cerebrospinal fluid leaks: nine-year experience. Neurosurgery 2006; 58(4 Suppl 2):ONS-246–256 [discussion: ONS-256–7].

73. Lue AJ, Manolidis S. Intrathecal fluorescein to localize cerebrospinal fluid leakage in bilateral mondini dysplasia. Otol Neurotol 2004;25(1):50–2.

74. Meco C, Oberascher G. Comprehensive algorithm for skull base dural lesion and cerebrospinal fluid fistula diagnosis. Laryngoscope 2004; 114(6):991–9.

75. Ricchetti A, Burkhard PR, Rodrigo N, et al. Skull base cerebrospinal fluid fistula: a novel detection method based on two-dimensional electrophoresis. Head Neck 2004;26(5):464–9.

76. Mahaley MS Jr, Odom GL. Complication following intrathecal injection of fluorescein. J Neurosurg 1966;25(3):298–9.

77. Moseley JI, Carton CA, Stern WE. Spectrum of complications in the use of intrathecal fluorescein. J Neurosurg 1978;48(5):765–7.

78. Tabaee A, Placantonakis DG, Schwartz TH, et al. Intrathecal fluorescein in endoscopic skull base surgery. Otolaryngol Head Neck Surg 2007;137(2):316–20.

79. Park KY, Kim YB. A case of myelopathy after intrathecal injection of fluorescein. J Korean Neurosurg Soc 2007;42(6):492–4.

80. Woodworth BA, Palmer JN. Spontaneous cerebrospinal fluid leaks. Curr Opin Otolaryngol Head Neck Surg 2009;17:59–65.

81. Bleier BS, Palmer JN, Gratton MA, et al. In vivo laser tissue welding in the rabbit maxillary sinus.
Am J Rhinol 2008;22(6):625–8.

82. Yahr WZ, Strully KJ. Blood vessel anastamosis by laser and other biomedical applications. J Assoc Adv Med Instrum 1966;1:28–31.

83. Gil Z, Shaham A, Vasilyev T, et al. Novel laser tissue-soldering technique for dural reconstruction. J Neurosurg 2005;103(1):87–91.

84. Kirsch AJ, Miller MI, Hensle TW, et al. Laser tissue soldering in urinary tract reconstruction: first human experience. Urology 1995;46(2):261–6.

85. Barrieras D, Reddy PP, McLorie GA, et al. Lessons learned from laser tissue soldering and fibrin glue pyeloplasty in an in vivo porcine model. J Urol 2000; 164(3 Pt 2):1106–10.

86. Foyt D, Johnson JP, Kirsch AJ, et al. Dural closure with laser tissue welding. Otolaryngol Head Neck Surg 1996;115(6):513–8.

87. Wright EJ, Poppas DP. Effect of laser wavelength and protein solder concentration on acute tissue repair using laser welding: initial results in a canine ureter model. Tech Urol 1997;3(3):176–81.

88. Carrau RL, Snyderman CH, Kassam AB. The management of cerebrospinal fluid leaks in patients at risk for high-pressure hydrocephalus. Laryngoscope 2005; 115(2):205–12.

89. Hegazy HM, Carrau RL, Snyderman CH, et al. Transnasal endoscopic repair of cerebrospinal fluid rhinorrhea: a meta-analysis. Laryngoscope 2000;110(7): 1166–72.

90. Zweig JL, Carrau RL, Celin SE, et al. Endoscopic repair of cerebrospinal fluid leaks to the sinonasal tract: predictors of success. Otolaryngol Head Neck Surg 2000;123(3):195–201.

91. Hadad G, Bassagasteguy L, Carrau RL, et al. A novel reconstructive technique after endoscopic expanded endonasal approaches: vascular pedicle nasoseptal flap. Laryngoscope 2006;116(10):1882–6.

92. El-Sayed IH, Roediger FC, Goldberg AN, et al. Endoscopic reconstruction of skull base defects with the nasal septal flap. Skull Base 2008;18(6):385–94.

93. Fortes FS, Carrau RL, Snyderman CH, et al. The posterior pedicle inferior turbinate flap: a new vascularized flap for skull base reconstruction. Laryngoscope 2007;117(8):1329–32.

94. Kassam AB, Thomas A, Carrau RL, et al. Endoscopic reconstruction of the cranial base using a pedicled nasoseptal flap. Neurosurgery 2008;63(1 Suppl 1):ONS44–52 [discussion: ONS52–3].

95. Shah RN, Surowitz JB, Patel MR, et al. Endoscopic pedicled nasoseptal flap reconstruction for pediatric skull base defects. Laryngoscope 2009;119(6): 1067–75.

96. Bolger WE, McLaughlin K. Cranial bone grafts in cerebrospinal fluid leak and encephalocele repair: a preliminary report. Am J Rhinol 2003;17(3): 153–8.

97. Perry JH, Rosenbaum AE, Lunsford LD, et al. Computed tomography/guided stereotactic surgery: conception and development of a new stereotactic methodology. Neurosurgery 1980;7(4):376–81.

98. Siewerdsen JH, Jaffray DA. Cone-beam computed tomography with a flat-panel imager: magnitude and effects of x-ray scatter. Med Phys 2001; 28(2):220–31.

99. Chennupati SK, Woodworth BA, Palmer JN, et al. Intraoperative IGS/CT updates for complex endoscopic frontal sinus surgery. ORL J Otorhinolaryngol Relat Spec 2008;70(4):268–70.

100. Woodworth BA, Chiu AG, Cohen NA, et al. Real-time computed tomography image update for endoscopic skull base surgery. J Laryngol Otol 2008; 122(4):361–5.

101. Donias HW, Karamanoukian HL, D'Ancona G, et al. Minimally invasive mitral valve surgery: from port access to fully robotic-assisted surgery. Angiology 2003;54(1):93–101.

102. O'Malley BW Jr, Weinstein GS, Snyder W, et al. Transoral robotic surgery (TORS) for base of tongue neoplasms. Laryngoscope 2006;116(8):1465–72.

103. Smith JA Jr, Herrell SD. Robotic-assisted laparoscopic prostatectomy: do minimally invasive approaches offer significant advantages? J Clin Oncol 2005; 23(32):8170–5.

104. Bandera CA, Magrina JF. Robotic surgery in gynecologic oncology. Curr Opin Obstet Gynecol 2009;21(1):25–30.

105. Hockstein NG, O'Malley BW Jr, Weinstein GS. Assessment of intraoperative safety in transoral robotic surgery. Laryngoscope 2006;116(2):165–8.

106. O'Malley BW Jr, Weinstein GS. Robotic skull base surgery: preclinical investigations to human clinical application. Arch Otolaryngol Head Neck Surg 2007; 133(12):1215–9.

107. O'Malley BW Jr, Weinstein GS. Robotic anterior and midline skull base surgery: preclinical investigations. Int J Radiat Oncol Biol Phys 2007;69(Suppl 2):S125–8.

108. Hanna EY, Holsinger C, DeMonte F, et al. Robotic endoscopic surgery of the skull base: a novel surgical approach. Arch Otolaryngol Head Neck Surg 2007;133(12):1209–14.

Rhinologic Surgical Training

Eng H. Ooi, MBBS, PhD, FRACS, Ian J. Witterick, MD, MSc, FRCSC*

KEYWORDS

- Rhinology fellowship • Endoscopic sinus surgery simulators
- Surgical education • Endoscopic sinus surgery training
- Surgical skills

The specialty of otolaryngology–head and neck surgery has expanded into multiple subspecialties due to advances in technology, surgical techniques, medical care, and research. Rhinology is a relatively new field compared with more established subspecialties, such as oncologic head and neck surgery and otology. Rhinology surgery, however, is arguably one of the more complex subspecialties in otolaryngology. Surgeons operate within a small bony anatomic space with vital structures, such as the brain and orbit, in close relation. Skills are required to maneuver the endoscope, manipulate instruments, and dissect within this space. The field of rhinology is rapidly growing due to advancements in instrumentation, technology, and research. Examples of the changes in rhinologic surgery in the past 2 decades include endoscopic sinus surgery (ESS) in the management of inflammatory sinus disease, endoscopic transphenoidal pituitary surgery, and, more recently, endoscopic skull base surgery.[1–3] This has implications for residency or specialist surgical training programs and post-training fellowships.

RESIDENCY TRAINING

Residency or specialist surgical training is the preparation of recently graduated medical students with knowledge, skills, ability, and judgment to practice as otolaryngologists. The period of training ranges between 4 and 6 years depending on individual programs and whether or not a period of research is undertaken as part of training. For the purposes of this article, the terms resident and trainee are used interchangeably.

The history of surgical training and different models have been previously reviewed.[4] In brief, the most common and well-established method of training is the

EHO is supported by the Royal Australasian College of Surgeons Margorie Hooper traveling scholarship and the South Australian Postgraduate Medical Education Association Mark Jolly traveling scholarship.

Department of Otolaryngology–Head and Neck Surgery, University of Toronto, Mount Sinai Hospital, 600 University Avenue, Room 413, Toronto, ON M5G 1X5, Canada

* Corresponding author.

E-mail address: iwitterick@mtsinai.on.ca

apprenticeship model, where a trainee observes and then practices surgical procedures under direct supervision of a consultant. It is the origin of the saying, "see one, do one, teach one," that has been passed on through the years.

The Halsted model of training is an apprenticeship style of training where surgical trainees are supervised and taught by skilled and experienced surgeons with trainees receiving increasing responsibility with each advancing year of training. The level of supervision and mentoring varies depending on a trainee's level of experience. The Osler model of training, adopted for clinical clerkships in medical school, is similar to the Halsted model, but with greater emphasis on the role of mentoring.[4] Both models are based on an apprenticeship style of training. Trainees learn preoperative preparation, performing incisions, tissue handling and dissection techniques, postoperative care, and managing complications, thus learning the art as well as the science of surgery. Today's training programs, based on the Halsted and Osler models, use a combination of various methods of teaching and assessment (**Table 1**).[5]

Today's training programs face new challenges, however, due to resident work hour restrictions. This issue arose due to a concern about possible fatigue, sleep deprivation, and potential for medical errors. It was thought that limiting work hours would address these concerns. The Accreditation Council for Graduate Medical Education (ACGME) in 2003 mandated an 80-hour resident workweek in the United States (**Table 2**).[6,7] In France, the resident workweek restriction is now 52.5 hours per week whereas Canada has adopted workweek hour restriction similar to the ACGME mandate.[8] In Australia, the Royal Australasian College of Surgeons released a position statement on safe working conditions for surgeons and trainees.[9] Unlike the ACGME, however, these are guidelines and recommendations rather than mandatory requirements.

Anonymous surveys were performed in 2005 and 2006 to assess the perceptions of otolaryngology residents and residency program directors to the ACGME changes in residency training.[6,7] Residents reported an average of 67.5 hours per week worked (range 40 to 120 hours) but less than half of the responders felt that the work hour restrictions had led to improved patient care or resident education.[6] Similarly, less than half reported no change in fatigue or errors. Most residents, however, reported an improvement in morale, a reduction in noneducational duties, and increased time

Table 1
Training and assessment methods

Skills Assessed in Training[5]	Methods of Teaching Surgical Skills	Assessment Tools Used
Cognitive	Didactic lectures, self-directed study, grand rounds, participation in continuing medical education, research and publications in peer-reviewed literature	Multiple choice questions, other written or computerized tests, case-based presentations, and patient management problems
Clinical	Bedside teaching, operating room cases	Objective structured clinical examination
Technical	Operating room cases, surgical simulators	OSATS, surgical simulators, surgical logbooks, morbidity and mortality audits

Table 2
List of key ACGME resident work hour regulations

1. Maximum of 80 duty hours per week, including in-house call, averaged over 4 weeks

2. 1 Day of 7 free from all clinical and educational responsibilities averaged over 4 weeks

3. Cannot be scheduled for in-house call more than once every 3 nights, averaged over 4 weeks

4. Duty periods cannot last for more than 24 hours, although residents may remain on duty for 6 additional hours to transfer patients, maintain continuity of care, or participate in educational activities

5. At least 10 hours for rest and personal activities between daily duty periods and after hours call

6. In-house moonlighting counts toward the weekly limit

for self-study. The majority of program directors reported making minor changes to comply with ACGME requirements but most disagreed that the duty hour restrictions led to improvements in residency training. Program directors' negative perceptions included decreased operative cases and continuity of care.

In general surgery research, the rate of bile duct injury was found reduced after the implementation of the ACGME requirements.[10] A recent retrospective study of one institution compared several parameters related to otolaryngology residency training before and after institution of the ACGME duty hour mandate.[11] It found no significant differences in the otolaryngology training examination results, number of operative cases, 30-day hospital readmission rates, length of stay, or hospital mortality rates. The conclusions from this study were that the ACGME requirements did not improve certain patient care measurements or adversely affect the number of operative cases in otolaryngology training.

Today's trainees may or may not have sufficient exposure to the number of cases to feel competent in ESS at the end of their training period. Due to workweek restrictions, trainees may see certain operations only a few times whereas previously they may have observed ESS procedures more frequently. Furthermore, if trainees have not acquired sufficient skills for basic ESS, they may not be able to progress to more advanced sinus surgery cases during their training. Therefore, they may not feel confident in managing certain major or revision cases after finishing their training. Lengthening the period of training is an alternative that is used in some European countries where supervision of junior consultants is required for an additional period of time by more experienced colleagues before they are allowed to practice autonomously.[12] This is unlikely to be embraced in North America or Australia where the current trend is to shorten training time.

Furthermore, the need to improve patient safety and reduce the threat of litigation has resulted in trainee surgeons having less opportunity to learn by operating on patients. There is also greater complexity of cases in teaching hospitals resulting in more cases performed by consultant staff rather than allowing a resident to be the primary surgeon. Research into surgical education has identified use of surgical simulators as a method of improving surgical training. Simulators allow trainees to practice and master skills to perform an operation before they lay hands on a patient.

The Fitts-Posner 3-stage theory of acquiring motor skills—cognition, integration, and automation—was discussed in a review article on surgical education.[13] The theory emphasizes practice of basic skills until they become automatic, resulting in the tasks gradually being completed smoothly without interruptions (**Table 3**). Mastery

Table 3			
Models for skill learning			
Stages	**Fitts-Postner Model**[13]	**Implicit Motor Learning Model**[14]	**Description of surgical performance at each Stage**
Cognitive	Trying to understand the task, explicit hypothesis testing, building declarative knowledge, requires explanation	Bypasses this stage to prevent declarative knowledge build up	Erratic, slow, procedure performed in distinct steps, hesitates
Integration	Understands the task, repeated practice, receives feedback from expert	Learn by expert demonstration, frees up "mental space" for decision making, skills thought more robust under stress	Movement more fluid, less thinking about the steps
Automatic	Automated movements, requires little cognitive input, can concentrate on other aspects of the procedure	Automated movements, requires little cognitive input, can concentrate on other aspects of the procedure	Continuous movements performed with ease and precision

of these basic skills allows trainees to focus on more complex issues in an operating room. A recent editorial discussed an alternate view where circumventing the cognitive stage of skill learning by directly observing without instructions promotes development of enhanced procedural skills.[14] This view of implicit motor learning is thought to be more stable over time and under conditions of psychological stress because learners are more likely to automatically perform a movement and less likely to think about previous instructions.

A large volume of cases used to be the hallmark of surgical training and a method of measuring technical skills of trainees was to use the logbook system. The number of cases performed, however, does not necessarily correlate with surgical competence.[15] The number of hours spent in deliberate practice, not just the number of hours spent in surgery, is critical to achieving a level of expertise. Therefore, it could be argued that learning to do a case well is better than doing many cases poorly.

Trainees acquire skills with manipulating an endoscope and instruments, maintaining a good surgical field, recognizing anatomic structures, and having the setup ergonomically positioned. Many basic skills must be acquired by trainees before they perform ESS. The 3-D nature of structures is also not easily appreciated when trainees begin ESS using a camera and monitor-type system. Trainees have to build a 3-D picture in their head of a patient's sinus anatomy from 2-D CT scan images. A major development with ESS is use of a monitor as a teaching tool, allowing trainees to observe surgery and, vice versa, consultants to observe and teach trainees, compared with performing sinus surgery with the use of a headlight or looking directly through an endoscope. An alternative teaching method is to use an endoscope with a beam splitter and observation arm. The traditional method for trainees acquiring these skills is performing as many procedures as possible on patients while they are supervised. This follows the time-honored tradition of the apprenticeship model for surgical training. Otolaryngology chief residents were surveyed recently regarding their rhinology experience in terms of teaching, research opportunities, and surgical experience using a 5-point Likert scale.[16] Although the response rate was poor, at 17.6%, the overall experience in rhinology was reported as positive (median 4 points) with no negative effects reported in programs with rhinology fellowships.

Research in surgical education has led to a change from the traditional methods of teaching.[13] The teaching of basic skills should take place outside the operating room, for example in surgical skill centers, and trainees would only be allowed to operate on patients once they had met predetermined criteria.[13,17] The focus on surgical training is changing to competency based rather than time or caseload based. Previous methods of training might not be applicable for teaching rhinology surgical skills in today's training programs. This has resulted in a need for newer methods of assessing surgical skills. Further research is required to develop and validate safer and more effective methods of teaching rhinologic surgical skills. In the future, program directors may need to restructure the rhinology component of their training program to implement newer methods of training.

RHINOLOGY FELLOWSHIPS

Otolaryngology fellowships refer to a period of focused, intensive, education experience in a recognized subspecialty area.[18] There has been a rapid growth in the number and type of otolaryngology fellowships in North America.[19] In 1994 there were only 8 rhinology fellowships listed in the fellowship directory of the American Academy of Otolaryngology–Head and Neck Surgery.[18] Currently, there are 23 rhinology fellowship positions listed on the San Francisco matching program (SF Match) Web site (http://www.sfmatch.org) at the end of June 2009.[20] The American Rhinologic Society sponsors the rhinology fellowship match through the SF Match program and provides a directory of fellowship programs available in the United States but does not certify or monitor any of these programs. There are also many rhinology fellowships available in countries other than United States. Rhinology fellowships are generally 1 year in duration and usually located at academic institutions.

There are various reasons why people might choose to do a fellowship after their training. A survey of postgraduate fellows, with a reasonable response rate (46.2%), found that inadequate operative caseload during residency training was the most common reason.[21] An article by Byron Bailey in 1994 stated, "there is not place in the fellowship world for remedial fellowships in which individuals pursue additional training because of deficiencies."[18] A survey found that most residents felt pursuing a fellowship was necessary due to inadequate residency training.[22] This implies that for some residents a fellowship is used to compensate for a perceived weakness in their training program. Other reasons for pursuing a fellowship include perception of inadequate didactic teaching in a subspecialty during residency, need to secure an academic position,[23] desire to enhance private practice, and an extra year for additional certification or board examination.[21,22] More than 70% of respondents thought, "there should be a centralized system of standards and accreditation of fellowships rather than the present system," and a majority preferred a certificate of added qualifications.

One of the concerns is the variability of the quality of these fellowships. Some fellowships have a significant quantity of hands-on surgical experience, research, didactic lectures, and one-on-one teaching whereas others might be deficient in 1 or more of these areas. Bailey in his article argued that fellowship training should go beyond simply providing surgical case numbers and provide education, training, and intellectual challenge.[18] He controversially argued against preceptorship-style fellowship training, stating, "preceptorship training was eliminated from residency training 50 years ago but we tolerate preceptorships in fellowship training today. That is illogical and I believe that it is no longer acceptable." He proposed that accreditation and regulation of fellowships are required to ensure they are of high quality. This was echoed in previous surveys of fellows and residents.[21,22]

More recently, a survey of rhinology fellows found that most were satisfied with the overall experience of their fellowship training.[24] Most respondents were more comfortable with advanced endoscopic procedures for the frontal sinus, anterior skull base, and orbit, and most were in academic practice, highlighting the value of fellowship training for future rhinologists. In contrast, lower comfort levels were associated with craniofacial procedures, frontal sinus obliteration, and dacryocystorhinostomy. Again, the survey highlighted issues with lack of a formalized process for fellowship accreditation, assessment of core competencies after training, and determining the minimum criteria for a fellowship program.

Therefore, more than 15 years later, the same issues of accreditation are present with today's rhinology fellowships. The question remains, Who needs to do a rhinology fellowship and is such a fellowship necessary? Many expert rhinologists today did not do a rhinology fellowship and trained themselves to become experts in their field. There are also competent otolaryngologists today who did not do a rhinology fellowship but are skilled in ESS due to the standards of their training program. It is essential that ESS remains part of training for general otolaryngologists whereas advanced procedures, which remain to be defined, should be part of fellowship training. Future research needs to define minimum requirements and curriculum for rhinology fellowship training and an accreditation body in order to provide training that advances the skills of fellowship trainees, not simply providing a substitute for inadequate residency training.

RHINOLOGY SURGICAL SIMULATORS

Simulators are widely used in the aviation and military fields whereas their use in surgical training is more recent.[25] Surgical simulators offer significant advantages over traditional didactic teaching and learning by operating on patients. They cause no harm to patients, can be used as teaching tools, shorten learning curves, allow learners to make mistakes, and enable standardized training and repeat assessment of technical skills. These simulators have to be validated before they can be widely and effectively implemented into the surgical training program. Validity can be defined in many ways (**Table 4**) and there are different methods of assessing validity.[25,26] Time to complete a task is often used as a measure of success but speed is not necessarily indicative of better outcomes. The definitions of novice and expert are variable as well. Some studies define novices as those with no surgical experience at all (eg, medical students) whereas others define novices as trainees who have not performed much of the study procedure.[25] Other studies define experts by an arbitrary number of cases performed per year and some studies do not even define what constitutes being an expert. There is no conclusive proof regarding the minimum cases a surgeon needs to perform to be classified as an expert. This is an important issue in validation studies as experts generally form the benchmark level of competency.

A recent review discussed the advances in surgical education with the use of different simulators as a way of preparing trainees before they begin to operate on patients.[13] A summary of the different simulators available with their respective advantages and disadvantages is presented in **Table 5**. The move toward

Table 4
The validation of tools for the assessment of surgical skills

Different Types of Validity in Testing Instruments	Definition[26]	Use of the Different Validity Tools
Face	Having experts review the contents of the test to see if it measures what it is supposed to measure	To initially design a test (subjective)
Content	An estimate of the validity of a testing instrument based on a detailed examination of the contents of the test item	Experts review whether or not the test contains the logical steps and skill used in a procedure (subjective)
Construct	A set of procedures for evaluating a testing instrument based on the degree to which the test items identify the quality, ability, or trait it was designed to measure	To differentiate between novices and experts (objective)
Concurrent	An evaluation in which the relationship between the test scores and the scores on another instrument purporting to measure the same construct are related	To compare the new test with the current gold standard test (objective)
Discriminate	An evaluation that reflects the extent to which the scores generated by the assessment tool actually correlate with factors they should correlate with	Does the test differentiate skill levels within a group of similar experience, such as all 3rd-year trainees (objective)
Predictive	The extent to which the scores on a test are predictive of actual performance	Test used to measure skill predicts who will actually perform the procedure well and who will not in the operating room. This provides the most clinically useful assessment (objective)

Reproduced from Reznick RK, MacRae H. Teaching surgical skills—changes in the wind. N Engl J Med 2006;355(25):2664–9; with permission.

competency-based training and pressures from threat of medical litigation and patient safety have made using surgical simulators an attractive option for teaching and training and as an assessment tool. Multiple studies have shown improvement in technical skills after training with simulators.[27] Transfer validity studies of laparoscopic simulators have shown positive results with specific in-theater operative skills (eg, knot tying) after training with simulators.[28] Studies have demonstrated that simulators differentiate between novices and experts. A review of the literature found surgical simulators useful for novices and the skills acquired in virtual reality (VR) simulation transfer to the operating room but simulators do not seem to benefit more experienced operators.[27,29]

Table 5
Types of surgical simulations available

Simulation	Advantages	Disadvantages	Best Use
Bench models	Cheap, portable, reusable, minimal risks	Acceptance by trainees, low fidelity, basic tasks, not operations	Basic skills for novice learners, discrete skills
Live animals	High fidelity, availability, can practice hemostasis and entire operations	Cost, special facilities and personnel required, ethical concerns, single use, anatomic differences	Advanced procedural knowledge, procedure in which blood flow is important, dissection skills
Cadavers	High fidelity, only "true" anatomic simulator, currently can practice entire operations	Cost, availability, single use, compliance of tissues, infection risk	Advanced procedural knowledge, dissection, continuing medical education
Human performance simulators	Reusable, high fidelity, data capture, interactivity	Cost, maintenance, and downtime, limited "technical" applications	Team training, crisis management
VR surgical simulators	Reusable, data capture, minimal setup time	Cost, maintenance, and downtime, acceptance by trainees, 3-D not well simulated	Basic laparoscopic skills, endoscopic and transcutaneous procedural skills

Data from Reznick RK, MacRae H. Teaching surgical skills—changes in the wind. N Engl J Med 2006;355(25):2664–9.

Cost remains a significant issue with VR simulators due to their higher fidelity (more lifelike). Cheaper low-fidelity simulators have been developed as an alternative (eg, box trainers). Studies of laparoscopic skills comparing time to task completion with number of errors showed no difference between a VR box trainer and a VR simulator.[30] Research from the field of general surgery has provided evidence that surgical simulators reduce operative errors and, therefore, shorten the learning curve for novices. A small group of residents was randomized to VR training until the residents reached a predefined expert level of performance or to the control group (no training). They subsequently performed laparoscopic cholecystectomies under supervision and their videotaped performance was independently assessed. Results showed that competency-based VR training significantly reduced the error rate in residents performing their first 10 laparoscopic cholecystectomies.[31] In summary, surgical simulators seem to have a role as part of a surgical curriculum and training program but their role continues to evolve.[32] Simulators can shorten the learning curve for novice trainees, allow testing of trainees to establish a predefined competency before trainees operate on patients, and allow trainees to focus attention on subtleties in the operating room after having mastered the basic skills (cognitive stage).[33]

In otolaryngology, temporal bone simulators have been developed to teach and train temporal bone drilling skills.[34,35] The authors' department recently demonstrated construct validity with a VR temporal bone simulator (developed in Hamburg, Germany) to assess the surgical drilling skills of trainees using motion tracking analysis and blinded expert reviewers.[35] ESS is another area suitable for surgical simulators. A survey of European otolaryngologists to assess the training needs for ESS found that tasks related to spatial orientation, such as recognizing and learning to make a 3-D mental representation of anatomy, were considered hardest whereas manual skills, such as manipulating an endoscope, were judged easier.[36] Therefore, models simulating the realistic endoscopic anatomy might be more important in the development of future ESS simulators whereas training manual tasks may be performed on a simple low-cost simulator.

The authors' department recently developed a low-fidelity, low-cost ESS simulator to develop basic skills in ESS.[37] The models were constructed to emphasize atraumatic scope navigation (**Fig. 1**), depth perception, manipulation of instrumentation, and performing a maxillary antrostomy. Hand motion analysis, expert evaluation, and comparison with performance on a cadaver were used to assess novice trainees (years 1 and 2) versus experienced trainees (years 3 to 5). Unfortunately, the model did not demonstrate construct validity, probably due to the choice of tasks and participants used in the study.

The ESS simulator (ES3, Lockheed Martin, Bethesda, MA, USA) is a VR device developed and extensively validated.[38–41] A Silicon Graphics workstation runs the simulation and a rubber head mannequin serves as the physical patient model (**Fig. 2**). The position of the endoscope is tracked through an electromechanical component outside and inside the mannequin head. A second personal computer provides haptic control with a replica of an endoscope and a surgical tool handle. Haptic feedback replicates resistance and vibration on the surgical instrument's handle by applying force in 3 axes but it does not apply force to the endoscope replica. The ES3 also simulates bleeding and image degradation similar to the dirty endoscope during surgery. It has 3 modes: novice, intermediate, and advanced. In the novice mode, a subject must complete 3 tasks, navigation, injection, and dissection, thereby testing basic hand-eye coordination and bimanual tasks. In the intermediate mode, ESS is performed with a simulated patient and labels on the sinus anatomy. The difference with the advanced mode is that the patient has middle meatal polyps and there are no labels or teaching aids. Haptics and simulated bleeding are introduced in the advanced mode. The simulator has been tested with several studies demonstrating

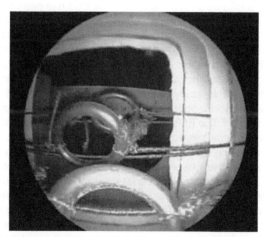

Fig. 1. Low- fidelity model involving manipulation of an endoscope through a series of suspended rings in different orientations. The aim of this simple task is to simulate atraumatic endoscope navigation. (*Courtesy of* Randy Leung, MD, Toronto, ON.)

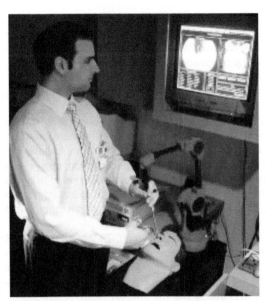

Fig. 2. The ESS simulator (ES3, Lockheed Martin, Bethesda, MA, USA). (*Reproduced from* Fried MP, Sadoughi B, Weghorst SJ, et al. Construct validity of the endoscopic sinus surgery simulator: II. Assessment of discriminant validity and expert benchmarking. Arch Otolaryngol Head Neck Surg 2007;133[4]:350–7. Copyright [2007] American Medical Association. All rights reserved; with permission.)

face and construct validity.[41–44] The ES3 can train novices (medical students) to perform simulated ESS to a level within 80% of experienced surgeons (performed more than 300 endoscopic sinus procedures).[45] Those with a prior history of frequent video gaming initially performed better in the novice mode for the ES3, but this advantage was short lived, and those with no history of gaming eventually reached the same level with repeated testing on the ES3.[43] Medical students were generally positive toward the use of the ES3 as a teaching tool.[46] The ES3 has been shown more effective for teaching surgical anatomy to medical students compared with textbooks.[47] The control group in this study spent on average 78 minutes studying paranasal sinus anatomy from textbooks and it is debatable if this was sufficient preparation for the comparative test. The ES3 has also been used to assess the performance of residents in the novice mode before and after a 24-hour call period finding no change in scores.[48] A limitation of this study is the small numbers tested. The ES3 has also been used as a training tool for ophthalmology residents in preparation for endoscopic dacryocystorhinostomy.[49] The ES3 so far has not demonstrated predictive validity.

The Dextroscope (Volume Interactions, Bracco AMT, Bracco Group, Singapore) VR simulator is another training tool for ESS.[50] Residents trained on it and then performed a real operation under the observation of a consultant surgeon. The simulator improved the residents understanding of anatomy but failed to translate into improved real-time operative performance. Other VR simulators have been developed using CT paranasal sinus images.[51] The Stanford group recently published work on constructing 3-D anatomic models of patient's anatomy in a virtual surgical environment from preoperative CT scans.[52] This system uses a commercially available haptic interface device modified by attaching it to a shaft of an endoscope providing force feedback as the user manipulates the endoscope in a virtual environment. The cost of this system was estimated at under $10,000 whereas the ES3 has been estimated to cost more than $200,000.[53] Furthermore, this system can be used to practice patient-specific operations before the real operation, mistakes can be made, and experimentation can occur without any harm to the patient. The investigators acknowledge several issues, including the lack of realistic tissue manipulation effects (eg, users cannot medialize the middle turbinate, there is no bleeding, and the sinus instruments used are not realistic).

Anatomic models simulating the paranasal sinus anatomy have been developed from polymers to closely resemble human tissue and represent an alternative to cadaveric dissection. They allow operations to be performed using real endoscopic sinus instruments. The main limitation with the model developed by the University of Zurich is the higher rigidity of the soft tissues, which made work in the frontal recess more difficult than in a human specimen.[54] The tissues were easily removed with cutting instruments but more difficult with noncutting forceps. A realistic model composed of an external and internal parts, the Sinus Model Otorhino-Neuro Trainer, has been developed in Brazil.[55] The external part is composed of a proprietary material called Neoderma (Pro Delphus, Recife, Brazil) to form the human face that is reusable as many times as required. The internal part is not reusable and consists of 7 separate structures (nasal septum, turbinates, uncinate process, sinuses, ethmoidal bulla, orbit, intersinus sphenoid septum, and the sella with a pituitary tumor) realistically similar to a live human patient. A newer model is being developed with additional anatomic detail and with bleeding capacity to provide an even more realistic experience. More recently, an anatomic model generated from 3-D CT data and silicone was developed and presented at the recent North American Skull Base Society meeting.[56] These anatomic models are promising and seem realistic but are yet to be validated.

In summary, the use of surgical simulators seems positive and eventually will be part of surgical training. Their effectiveness has been demonstrated for novice learners. There are several endoscopic sinus surgical models currently available. Some of them are not validated and cost remains a significant issue. Questions remain about whether or not they are required to practice whole operations or to practice different parts of an operation on a simulator and how to transfer these skills to ESS in the operating room. Results have not been validated in large-scale studies and additional research is needed to demonstrate their applicability to different institutions. Further research is needed to address the use of rhinology surgical simulation for trainees and current surgeons in practice.

ASSESSMENT OF RHINOLOGIC SURGICAL SKILLS

The assessment of training and surgical skills is increasingly recognized as an important issue. In the future it may be used to select prospective trainees, assess the ability of trainees to progress successfully with their training, and even assess current surgeons continuing to practice surgery on the basis of these tests. The move toward competency-based surgical training has resulted in the need to develop alternative methods of assessing surgical skills besides surgical logbooks. One method is to have supervising surgeons assess the surgical skills of trainees in the form of periodic training evaluation forms but these are subjective, lack validity, and have poor inter-rater reliability.[15] They are often based on 1 or more supervising surgeon's reports and can be subjected to bias, with well-liked trainees receiving better reports than other trainees.

Measuring technical performance in surgery is difficult. One method is to use a standardized assessment process where a candidate performs a series of standardized objective tasks under the direct observation of an expert. This objective structured assessment of objective skills (OSATS) includes a task-specific checklist consisting of essential surgical procedures for that task and a global rating scale that assesses the surgical performance.[57] Other methods include the McGill Inanimate System for Training and Evaluation of Laparoscopic Skills that uses a box to simulate skills required for laparoscopic surgery.[58] The Imperial College Surgical Assessment Device uses hand motion sensors to track movement of trainees' hands during a specific procedure and time taken to complete a specific task.[59] This study showed that more experienced operators took less time and movements to complete small bowel anastomosis. This is consistent with the frequent observation that the expert surgeons seem slower in their movements but are actually more efficient and deliberate in their actions and avoid doing the same thing twice.

Recently, a competency assessment tool specific for ESS was developed and tested for face, content, and construct validity.[60] It was based on the OSATS and consists of a task-specific checklist of 22 items and an ESS global rating assessment. A member of staff assessed residents performing cadaveric ESS using a 5-point Likert rating scale for each item. The tool was easy to use and took a median of 7 minutes to complete. A score of 3 was considered the minimum level for achieving competence. Another competency-based tool for ESS was developed in the United Kingdom.[61] The ESS competence assessment tool (ESSCAT) was developed as a pilot study for in-theater assessment of higher surgical trainees. The ESSCAT contains 8 tasks assessed with a 5-point Likert scale showing good inter-rater reliability. These tests show promise as a tool for assessing the competency of trainees performing ESS. The limitation with these tools is the definition of who is an expert and what is a minimum benchmark for competency. Future research is needed, directed toward ongoing development and validation of specific assessment tools for rhinologic surgical training.

THE EXPERT RHINOLOGIST AND HEURISTICS

It is estimated that an expert in music or sport typically takes at least 10 years or 10,000 hours of deliberate practice to achieve a level of expertise and the same probably applies for expertise in surgery.[62] Research on expertise has described perceptual, cognitive, and motor skills that differentiate experts from the nonexperts (**Table 6**). In surgery, an expert is generally defined as an experienced surgeon with consistently better outcomes than nonexperts.[62]

Heuristics are rules of thumb that experts learn through trial and error.[63] Often these maneuvers are performed unconsciously and may seem simple to an expert but without them a procedure becomes more difficult, takes longer, or is not possible to do safely. Three main types of heuristics are used in surgical dissection: motor, perceptual, and cognitive. These heuristics have not previously been validated. A discussion of rhinology heuristics has identified several important principles when performing ESS.[64] One of the most important principles is achieving a good surgical field by maintaining hemostasis as a small amount of bleeding can deteriorate the quality of the surgical field. Trauma to the septum or middle turbinate with an endoscope causes bleeding, degrading the surgical field, and may lead to postoperative adhesions. Trainees need to understand these simple principles to maintain a good surgical field thus allowing surgery to progress.

Cognitive heuristics, where a surgeon thinks 1 or 2 steps ahead, are important in rhinology, especially with the choice of instruments. There are many instruments available for ESS with a dual purpose (eg, suction Freer) or different angles and lengths (eg, frontal sinus curettes) to choose from. An important principle with sinus surgery is to create dependent areas initially with the dissection by starting low as blood flows

Table 6
Differentiating the expert from the nonexpert surgeon—an expertise-based approach to training

	Expert	Nonexpert
Perceptual	Superior visual spatial perceptual ability, ability to recognize and recall domain-specific patterns and anticipate potential events from past experiences	Poor depth perception has to pass sinus surgery instruments under direct vision, poor recognition of safe versus unsafe structures
Cognition	Superior declarative and procedural knowledge and spends considerable time analyzing the situation before arriving at a solution to the problem. Forward directed reasoning	Lacks procedural knowledge (how to do it). Approaches problems by using backward reasoning
Motor	Movements more consistent, makes more effective use of external forces, seems slower but make fewer mistakes or less need to repeat movement	Apply forces unnecessarily or inefficiently, frequently repeats steps in performing a procedure, hesitates
Attention	Increased automatic movements and ability to multitask	Thinks more about the steps in the procedure
Feedback monitoring	Superior ability at self-monitoring cognitive and motor tasks. More aware of when mistakes are made	Relies on feedback from external sources to detect and correct errors

Data from Abernethy B, Poolton JM, Masters RS, et al. Implications of an expertise model for surgical skills training. ANZ J Surg 2008;78(12):1092–5.

to dependent areas, thus aiding the surgical field. Trainees also must understand that sometimes performing a limited endoscopic septoplasty improves access for ESS.

Perceptually, trainee surgeons have to recognize important buried structures in the walls of the operated sinus, such as the lamina papyracea in the ethmoid sinus or the internal carotid artery in the sphenoid sinus, so as to avoid injury to them. Visually and mentally, experts appreciate depth of field on a monitor by moving the endoscope in and out short distances relative to recognizable anatomic landmarks. Haptic heuristics in rhinology involves recognizing the feedback from the feel of anatomic structures. This includes the softer feel of lamina papyracea bone versus the generally firmer bone of the skull base (excluding the lateral lamella of the fovea ethmoidalis). Motor heuristics in rhinology emphasize the importance of surgeon ergonomics. These include placing a monitor in a favorable position for the surgeon or holding an endoscope steady by a surgeon sitting down with the elbow resting on an arm board support.[64]

SUMMARY
Implications for Research

Traditional methods of assessing and teaching surgical skills need to change due to advancements in rhinologic surgical techniques. Use of simulators in surgical training has potential benefits but their value remains unclear. Further research is required to develop and validate newer methods of assessing rhinologic surgical skills and the use of surgical simulators. Economic analysis studies are also required to demonstrate a cost-benefit analysis before incorporating changes for training programs.

Implications for Clinical Practice

Rhinology fellowships should involve an educational experience as well as training in advanced endoscopic rhinologic surgical techniques. The formation of an organizational body to oversee the accreditation of rhinology fellowships is required to ensure that future trainees receive appropriate rhinology training. Surgical simulators have the potential to revolutionize operations in the future by allowing clinicians to practice a real operation, using patient CT and MRI data, in a VR or anatomic model.

REFERENCES

1. Uren B, Vrodos N, Wormald PJ. Fully endoscopic transsphenoidal resection of pituitary tumors: technique and results. Am J Rhinol 2007;21(4):510–4.
2. Snyderman CH, Carrau RL, Kassam AB, et al. Endoscopic skull base surgery: principles of endonasal oncological surgery. J Surg Oncol 2008;97(8):658–64.
3. Wormald PJ. Salvage frontal sinus surgery: the endoscopic modified Lothrop procedure. Laryngoscope 2003;113(2):276–83.
4. Franzese CB, Stringer SP. The evolution of surgical training: perspectives on educational models from the past to the future. Otolaryngol Clin North Am 2007;40(6):1227–35, vii.
5. Satava RM, Gallagher AG, Pellegrini CA. Surgical competence and surgical proficiency: definitions, taxonomy, and metrics. J Am Coll Surg 2003;196(6):933–7.
6. Reiter ER, Wong DR. Impact of duty hour limits on resident training in otolaryngology. Laryngoscope 2005;115(5):773–9.
7. Brunworth JD, Sindwani R. Impact of duty hour restrictions on otolaryngology training: divergent resident and faculty perspectives. Laryngoscope 2006; 116(7):1127–30.
8. Woodrow SI, Segouin C, Armbruster J, et al. Duty hours reforms in the United States, France, and Canada: is it time to refocus our attention on education? Acad Med 2006;81(12):1045–51.
9. RACS. Standard for safe working hours and conditions for fellows, surgical trainees, and international medical graduates: position statement. 1st edition. Royal Australasian College of Surgeons; 2007. Available at: http://www.surgeons. org/publications. Accessed February 26, 2010.
10. Yaghoubian A, Saltmarsh G, Rosing DK, et al. Decreased bile duct injury rate during laparoscopic cholecystectomy in the era of the 80-hour resident workweek. Arch Surg 2008;143(9):847–51 [discussion: 851].
11. Shonka DC Jr, Ghanem TA, Hubbard MA, et al. Four years of accreditation council of graduate medical education duty hour regulations: have they made a difference? Laryngoscope 2009;119(4):635–9.
12. Sakorafas GH, Tsiotos GG. New legislative regulations, problems, and future perspectives, with a particular emphasis on surgical education. J Postgrad Med 2004;50(4):274–7.
13. Reznick RK, MacRae H. Teaching surgical skills—changes in the wind. N Engl J Med 2006;355(25):2664–9.
14. Masters RS, Poolton JM, Abernethy B, et al. Implicit learning of movement skills for surgery. ANZ J Surg 2008;78(12):1062–4.

15. Fried GM, Feldman LS. Objective assessment of technical performance. World J Surg 2008;32(2):156–60.

16. Tabaee A, Anand VK, Stewart MG, et al. The rhinology experience in otolaryngology residency: a survey of chief residents. Laryngoscope 2008;118(6): 1072–5.

17. MacRae HM, Satterthwaite L, Reznick RK. Setting up a surgical skills center. World J Surg 2008;32(2):189–95.

18. Bailey BJ. Fellowship proliferation. Impact and long-range implications. Arch Otolaryngol Head Neck Surg 1994;120(10):1065–70.

19. Ryan MW, Johnson F. Fellowship training in otolaryngology-head and neck surgery. Otolaryngol Clin North Am 2007;40(6):1311–22, viii–ix.

20. Rhinology SF. Match 2009; report of the June 2009 match. Available at: http://www.sfmatch.org/vacancies/f_rhinology.htm#2011. Accessed October 20, 2009.

21. Crumley RL. Survey of postgraduate fellows in otolaryngology-head and neck surgery. Arch Otolaryngol Head Neck Surg 1994;120(10):1074–9.

22. Miller RH. Otolaryngology residency and fellowship training. The resident's perspective. Arch Otolaryngol Head Neck Surg 1994;120(10):1057–61.

23. Nadol JB Jr. Training the physician-scholar in otolaryngology-head and neck surgery. Otolaryngol Head Neck Surg 1999;121(3):214–9.

24. Tabaee A, Luong A, Fried MP. Fellowship training in rhinology: a survey of fellows from the past 6 years. Arch Otolaryngol Head Neck Surg 2009;135(6):571–4.

25. Schout BM, Hendrikx AJ, Scheele F, et al. Validation and implementation of surgical simulators: a critical review of present, past, and future. Surg Endosc 2010;24(3):536–46.

26. Gallagher AG, Ritter EM, Satava RM. Fundamental principles of validation, and reliability: rigorous science for the assessment of surgical education and training. Surg Endosc 2003;17(10):1525–9.

27. Fitzgerald TN, Duffy AJ, Bell RL, et al. Computer-based endoscopy simulation: emerging roles in teaching and professional skills assessment. J Surg Educ 2008;65(3):229–35.

28. Verdaasdonk EG, Dankelman J, Lange JF, et al. Transfer validity of laparoscopic knot-tying training on a VR simulator to a realistic environment: a randomized controlled trial. Surg Endosc 2008;22(7):1636–42.

29. Seymour NE. VR to OR: a review of the evidence that virtual reality simulation improves operating room performance. World J Surg 2008;32(2):182–8.

30. Newmark J, Dandolu V, Milner R, et al. Correlating virtual reality and box trainer tasks in the assessment of laparoscopic surgical skills. Am J Obstet Gynecol 2007;197(5):e541–4, 546.

31. Ahlberg G, Enochsson L, Gallagher AG, et al. Proficiency-based virtual reality training significantly reduces the error rate for residents during their first 10 laparoscopic cholecystectomies. Am J Surg 2007;193(6):797–804.

32. Dankelman J. Surgical simulator design and development. World J Surg 2008; 32(2):149–55.

33. Gurusamy K, Aggarwal R, Palanivelu L, et al. Systematic review of randomized controlled trials on the effectiveness of virtual reality training for laparoscopic surgery. Br J Surg 2008;95(9):1088–97.

34. O'Leary SJ, Hutchins MA, Stevenson DR, et al. Validation of a networked virtual reality simulation of temporal bone surgery. Laryngoscope 2008; 118(6):1040–6.

35. Zirkle M, Roberson DW, Leuwer R, et al. Using a virtual reality temporal bone simulator to assess otolaryngology trainees. Laryngoscope 2007;117(2):258–63.

36. Bakker NH, Fokkens WJ, Grimbergen CA. Investigation of training needs for functional endoscopic sinus surgery (FESS). Rhinology 2005;43(2):104–8.
37. Leung RM, Leung J, Vescan A, et al. Construct validation of a low-fidelity endoscopic sinus surgery simulator. Am J Rhinol 2008;22(6):642–8.
38. Edmond CV Jr, Heskamp D, Sluis D, et al. ENT endoscopic surgical training simulator. Stud Health Technol Inform 1997;39:518–28.
39. Edmond CV Jr. Impact of the endoscopic sinus surgical simulator on operating room performance. Laryngoscope 2002;112(7 Pt 1):1148–58.
40. Fried MP, Uribe JI, Sadoughi B. The role of virtual reality in surgical training in otorhinolaryngology. Curr Opin Otolaryngol Head Neck Surg 2007;15(3): 163–9.
41. Weghorst S, Airola C, Oppenheimer P, et al. Validation of the Madigan ESS simulator. Stud Health Technol Inform 1998;50:399–405.
42. Arora H, Uribe J, Ralph W, et al. Assessment of construct validity of the endoscopic sinus surgery simulator. Arch Otolaryngol Head Neck Surg 2005;131(3): 217–21.
43. Glaser AY, Hall CB, Uribe SJ, et al. The effects of previously acquired skills on sinus surgery simulator performance. Otolaryngol Head Neck Surg 2005; 133(4):525–30.
44. Fried MP, Sadoughi B, Weghorst SJ, et al. Construct validity of the endoscopic sinus surgery simulator: II. Assessment of discriminant validity and expert benchmarking. Arch Otolaryngol Head Neck Surg 2007;133(4):350–7.
45. Uribe JI, Ralph WM Jr, Glaser AY, et al. Learning curves, acquisition, and retention of skills trained with the endoscopic sinus surgery simulator. Am J Rhinol 2004;18(2):87–92.
46. Glaser AY, Hall CB, Uribe SJ, et al. Medical students' attitudes toward the use of an endoscopic sinus surgery simulator as a training tool. Am J Rhinol 2006;20(2): 177–9.
47. Solyar A, Cuellar H, Sadoughi B, et al. Endoscopic sinus surgery simulator as a teaching tool for anatomy education. Am J Surg 2008;196(1):120–4.
48. Jakubowicz DM, Price EM, Glassman HJ, et al. Effects of a twenty-four hour call period on resident performance during simulated endoscopic sinus surgery in an accreditation council for graduate medical education-compliant training program. Laryngoscope 2005;115(1):143–6.
49. Weiss M, Lauer SA, Fried MP, et al. Endoscopic endonasal surgery simulator as a training tool for ophthalmology residents. Ophthal Plast Reconstr Surg 2008; 24(6):460–4.
50. Caversaccio M, Eichenberger A, Hausler R. Virtual simulator as a training tool for endonasal surgery. Am J Rhinol 2003;17(5):283–90.
51. Bockholt U, Muller W, Voss G, et al. Real-time simulation of tissue deformation for the nasal endoscopy simulator (NES). Comput Aided Surg 1999;4(5):281–5.
52. Parikh SS, Chan S, Agrawal SK, et al. Integration of patient-specific paranasal sinus computed tomographic data into a virtual surgical environment. Am J Rhinol Allergy 2009;23(4):442–7.
53. Rudman DT, Stredney D, Sessanna D, et al. Functional endoscopic sinus surgery training simulator. Laryngoscope 1998;108(11 Pt 1):1643–7.
54. Briner HR, Simmen D, Jones N, et al. Evaluation of an anatomic model of the paranasal sinuses for endonasal surgical training. Rhinology 2007;45(1): 20–3.
55. Nogueira JF, Stamm AC, Lyra M, et al. Building a real endoscopic sinus and skull-base surgery simulator. Otolaryngol Head Neck Surg 2008;139(5):727–8.

56. Snyderman C, Grunert R, Moeckel H, et al. A surgical training model for endoscopic skull base surgery. Skull Base 2009;19(Suppl 3):14–5.
57. Anastakis DJ, Regehr G, Reznick RK, et al. Assessment of technical skills transfer from the bench training model to the human model. Am J Surg 1999;177(2): 167–70.
58. Fried GM, Feldman LS, Vassiliou MC, et al. Proving the value of simulation in laparoscopic surgery. Ann Surg 2004;240(3):518–25 [discussion: 525–8].
59. Datta V, Mackay S, Mandalia M, et al. The use of electromagnetic motion tracking analysis to objectively measure open surgical skill in the laboratory-based model. J Am Coll Surg 2001;193(5):479–85.
60. Lin SY, Laeeq K, Ishii M, et al. Development and pilot-testing of a feasible, reliable, and valid operative competency assessment tool for endoscopic sinus surgery. Am J Rhinol Allergy 2009;23(3):354–9.
61. Syme-Grant J, White PS, McAleer JP. Measuring competence in endoscopic sinus surgery. Surgeon 2008;6(1):37–44.
62. Abernethy B, Poolton JM, Masters RS, et al. Implications of an expertise model for surgical skills training. ANZ J Surg 2008;78(12):1092–5.
63. Patkin M. Surgical heuristics. ANZ J Surg 2008;78(12):1065–9.
64. Weitzel EK, Floreani S, Wormald PJ. Otolaryngologic heuristics: a rhinologic perspective. ANZ J Surg 2008;78(12):1096–9.

Erratum to Anosmia: Loss of Smell in the Elderly from Otolaryngologic Clinics February 2009, page 126

Fig. 2 in the article, Anosmia: Loss of Smell in the Elderly, published in the issue: Palliative Therapy in Otolaryngology - Head and Neck Surgery in February 2009 should be credited as "Modified from Morphology of the human olfactory epithelium by Morris EE and Costonzo RM in J Comp Neurol 1990;297:1–13, Fig. 4A; Wiley InterScience."

Otolaryngol Clin N Am 43 (2010) 691
doi:10.1016/j.otc.2010.04.023
0030-6665/10/$ – see front matter © 2010 Elsevier Inc. All rights reserved.

oto.theclinics.com

Index

Note: Page numbers of article titles are in **boldface** type.

Otolaryngol Clin N Am 43 (2010) 693–699
doi:10.1016/S0030-6665(10)00108-8
0030-6665/10/$ – see front matter © 2010 Elsevier Inc. All rights reserved.

oto.theclinics.com

Moving?

Make sure your subscription moves with you!

To notify us of your new address, find your **Clinics Account Number** (located on your mailing label above your name), and contact customer service at:

Email: journalscustomerservice-usa@elsevier.com

800-654-2452 (subscribers in the U.S. & Canada)
314-447-8871 (subscribers outside of the U.S. & Canada)

Fax number: 314-447-8029

Elsevier Health Sciences Division
Subscription Customer Service
3251 Riverport Lane
Maryland Heights, MO 63043

*To ensure uninterrupted delivery of your subscription, please notify us at least 4 weeks in advance of move.

Printed and bound by CPI Group (UK) Ltd, Croydon, CR0 4YY

03/10/2024

01040461-0008